6/30/93

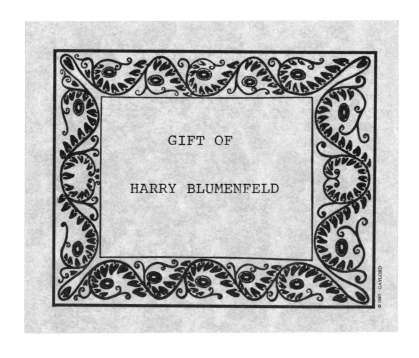

GIFT OF

HARRY BLUMENFELD

MODERN PERSPECTIVES IN PSYCHIATRY
Edited by John G. Howells

10

MODERN PERSPECTIVES IN CLINICAL PSYCHIATRY

MODERN PERSPECTIVES IN PSYCHIATRY

Edited by John G. Howells

1. Modern Perspectives in Child Psychiatry (2nd ed., 1967)

2. Modern Perspectives in World Psychiatry (1968). Introduction by Lord Adrian, O.M. and Gene Usdin, M.D.

3. Modern Perspectives in International Child Psychiatry (1969). Introduced by Leo Kanner, M.D.

4. Modern Perspectives in Adolescent Psychiatry (1971)

5. Modern Perspectives in Psycho-Obstetrics (1972)

6. Modern Perspectives in the Psychiatry of Old Age (1975)

7. Modern Perspectives in the Psychiatric Aspects of Surgery (1976)

8. Modern Perspectives in the Psychiatry of Infancy (1979)

9. Modern Perspectives in the Psychiatry of Middle Age (1981)

10. Modern Perspectives in Clinical Psychiatry (1988)

Modern Perspectives in Clinical Psychiatry

Edited by

JOHN G. HOWELLS
M.D., F.R.C.Psych., D.P.M.

BRUNNER/MAZEL, *Publishers* • New York

Library of Congress Cataloging-in-Publication Data

Modern perspectives in clinical psychiatry / edited by John G.
  Howells.
        p.   cm. — (Modern perspectives in psychiatry; 10)
      Includes bibliographies and indexes.
      ISBN 0-87630-499-4
      1. Psychiatry.   2. Psychotherapy.   I. Howells, John G.
      II. Series.
      [DNLM: 1. Mental Disorders.   2. Psychiatry — trends.   W1 M0167P v.
      10   WM 100 M691]
      RC480.M62   1988   616.89 — dc19   87-36742
      DNLM/DLC   CIP
      for Library of Congress

Copyright © 1988 by John G. Howells

Published by
BRUNNER/MAZEL, INC.
19 Union Square
New York, New York 10003

MANUFACTURED IN THE UNITED STATES OF AMERICA

10   9   8   7   6   5   4   3   2   1

EDITOR'S PREFACE

The Modern Perspectives Series can be regarded as an international encyclopedia of psychiatry. The nine volumes already published deal with the psychiatry of all age periods — infancy, childhood, adolescence, adulthood, middle age, and old age — together with explorations into world psychiatry, into the special fields of psychoobstetrics, and into the psychiatric aspects of surgery.

The Series will now continue with a volume on psychosocial pathology, followed by three volumes devoted to the main nosological entities — the neuroses, the affective disorders, and schizophrenia. But before doing so, the opportunity is taken to prepare this special volume on general clinical psychiatry, which stands, as it were, on the shoulders of the last nine volumes.

The aim of each volume in the Series has remained as stated in the first volume of the Series. *Modern Perspectives in Clinical Psychiatry* is thus planned to bring the facts from the growing points of psychiatry, and pertinent related fields, to the attention of the clinician at as early a stage as possible. A complete coverage of the field is not attempted. A single volume is not a textbook. To give an international flavor to the Series, the Editor feels free to wander over the world inviting acknowledged experts to present a topic to the readership. Each contributor has the task of selecting, appraising, and explaining the available knowledge on his subject for the benefit of colleagues who may be less well acquainted with that field. Special consideration is given to the requirements of psychiatrists in training.

The Editor eschews any interests or biases of his own. Thus, ranging over the possible topics, it becomes apparent that those to be covered select themselves. Together, they speak of eclecticism. Although they lean toward the clinical, applied and basic sciences, clinical and biobehavioral sciences, dynamic and biological psychiatry stand comfortably together.

v

This volume on Clinical Psychiatry starts with chapters on a number of general issues of topical interest before moving on to subjects in symptomatology and diagnosis, ending with aspects of management and treatment.

In this volume, as in all previous volumes in the Series, the Editor has profited by the zeal and flair of his assistant editor, Mrs. Livia Osborn. This he gratefully acknowledges.

CONTENTS

MODERN PERSPECTIVES IN PSYCHIATRY
Edited by John G. Howells

10

MODERN PERSPECTIVES IN CLINICAL PSYCHIATRY

1

EPIDEMIOLOGY IN PSYCHIATRY

MYRNA M. WEISSMAN, PH.D.

Professor of Epidemiology in Psychiatry,
College of Physicians and Surgeons
of Columbia University and New York State Psychiatric Institute,
New York, New York

INTRODUCTION

Epidemiology is the study of the distribution of diseases, disorders, or health-related phenomena in populations. It relates the distribution of disease (incidence and prevalence) to factors (e.g., time, place, person) existing in or affecting that population. These factors are called risks. The unit of study in epidemiology is an aggregate population or group, rather than the individual. Whereas the clinician deals with individual cases, the epidemiologist deals with aggregates of cases in a population. The epidemiologist may start with a population and seek out cases in it or may start with cases and refer back to a population. However, whatever the starting point, the epidemiologist ends up with some estimate of cases per population (i.e., numerator and denominator). Unlike the clinician, the epidemiologist is interested in calculating the rates of occurrence or, equally important, the nonoccurrence of a phenomenon. Epidemiology has been called the "basic science of preventive medicine" (6). By understanding the risks for occurrence of a disorder, clues are sought as to interventions that might lead to its control or prevention. Ultimately, the purpose of epidemiology is to provide knowledge leading to abolishing the clinical condition (16).

This chapter presents an overview of key concepts and definitions of epidemiology, a brief historical perspective to current research in psychiatric epidemiology, and a guide to future directions. The theme underlying this chapter is the new dialogue between psychiatric epidemiology and clinical psychiatry. This dialogue was first described by Shepherd in the late 1970s in London (29). This dialogue is possible because in the last decade there has been an increase of information on the epidemiology of major psychiatric disorders in adults and families, including information on the rates of psychiatric disorders and who is at increased risk for these disorders.

The availability of new information is due to the major achievements in clinical psychiatry, including more precise and reliable diagnoses and the development of methods for collecting information on signs and symptoms to make diagnoses. These achievements have enabled the conduct of large psychiatric epidemiological studies. Between 1975 and 1980 the methodological work for the conduct of these studies was undertaken in the United States. The majority of substantive studies were only begun within this decade, so that the major information is still forthcoming. This information has direct value for clinical practice and treatment, and for the prevention of psychiatric disorders in adults and in their offspring.

CONCEPTS, DEFINITIONS, AND SCOPE

Good discussions of epidemiological methods can be found in the literature (9,13,27,33). The fundamental quantitative unit in epidemiology is a *rate*, which may be defined as the number of persons affected with a disease, disorder, or characteristic, per unit of population, per unit of time. The numerator reflects the number of persons affected, or "cases." A person can qualify as a case as defined by the investigator, who may observe presence of a disease, disorder, abnormal laboratory finding, or symptoms in that person. The denominator indicates the reference population among whom the affected persons are observed. This reference group is often defined as the *population at risk* and quantifies the number of people in a population capable of manifesting the specific disorder under study. The population at risk may be any defined group of people, such as a demographically defined community, a family, or a group of patients. The epidemiologist may begin with a population at risk and seek out cases or may start with cases and refer back to a population.

The epidemiologist is concerned not only with rates, but also with identification of factors associated with variations in these rates. A *risk factor* is a specific characteristic or condition that seemingly increases the probability of present or future occurrence of a specific disorder. This implies a statistically significant association between presence of a disorder in one group with the risk factor when compared to a comparable group without the risk factor. The risk factor associated with the disorder may be causative; innocuous but correlated with another risk factor; or a sequela of the disorder. Risk factors can be defined by time, place, or person. Personal characteristics include sociodemographic factors (e.g., age, sex, race, occupation, level of education, marital status); biological and genetic factors (physiological functioning of specific organ systems, biochemical levels, hormonal status); or personal habits (alcohol and drug use, diet, exercise). An investigator may isolate a population with the appropriate risk factor and compare the differential rate of occurrence of a disorder to that of a comparable population without the factor. Conversely, one may identify cases with the disorder, select a comparable sample of noncases or "controls," and compare the differential rates of occurrence of the risk factor in question. Statistical significance would suggest association.

Epidemiological analysis utilizes a variety of rates in measuring the frequency of disorders. It must be emphasized that in the rates defined below, the numerator and denominator must be similarly restricted as to sex, age, race, and so forth.

Incidence is the number of new cases of a disorder with onset during a defined period of time among individuals referred to a population at risk. Most incidence rates reflect onset of disorder over a one-year period. In the recurrent affective disorders, these rates may reflect onset of previously remitted cases.

Prevalence is the number of both old and new cases in a population for a defined period of time. *Point prevalence* is the proportion of a population manifesting the disorder being studied at a given point in time. *Period prevalence* is the proportion of a population with the disorder for a given period of time (e.g., one year, six months). *Lifetime prevalence* is the proportion of a population alive on a given day of ascertainment that has ever had the disorder under study. In essence, it reflects the proportions of survivors affected with the disorder at some point during their lifetime.

Lifetime risk differs from lifetime prevalence in that it attempts to include the entire lifetime of a birth cohort, past and future, and includes those deceased at the time of survey. It is the proportion of a birth cohort that would be expected to have the disorder develop before a specified age, if all unaffected persons survived to that age.

Morbid risk is an individual's lifetime risk of having a first episode of illness. For major depression, the period of risk is greater than it is for bipolar disorder, where incidence rates fall dramatically by the fifth and sixth decades of life. Thus, morbid risk has some meaningful applications in bipolar disorder.

Two commonly used measures of the degree of association between hypothesized risk factors and disorders are relative risk and attributable risk.

Relative risk is the ratio of the incidence of disorder among the exposed and nonexposed groups. It is also termed the "risk ratio." *Attributable risk* is the incidence of the disorder in exposed individuals that can be attributed to their exposure to a hypothesized risk factor. It is derived by subtracting the rate of the disorder among persons without the risk factor from the corresponding rate among individuals with the risk factor. Its determination provides an assessment of the causal association between risk factor and disorder.

Psychiatric epidemiology includes: (1) descriptive studies, in which the extent and type of psychiatric disorder in a defined population are determined; (2) analytical studies, which attempt to determine why rates differ among particular groups by identifying the risk factors that influence origin and clinical course of a disorder; and (3) experimental studies, in which the investigator has control over the population and the risk factors under study and can manipulate these factors to determine the effects on the disorder or its component. (See References 1, 9, 33, for a comprehensive discussion of these strategies.)

Descriptive and analytical study designs are the most common, and three basic approaches can be identified. Descriptive data provide the first step in elucidating the causes of a disorder by identifying groups with high or low rates of a specific disease. Once such identification has been made, the next step is to question why the rates are high or low in a particular group, place, or time. These observations lead to hypotheses which can then be tested through more focused analytical or experimental studies. The analytical or etiological studies are conducted when enough is known about a disorder to test specific hypotheses.

In the experimental approach the study factor is manipulated by experiments of nature (e.g., floods, fires, hurricanes, closing of a factory, nuclear accidents) or by the investigator (as in clinical trials or laboratory experiments, etc.).

Although there are numerous variations, the basic study design under these three approaches can be broadly classified as cross-sectional, cohort, case control. (See Reference 9 for a detailed discussion of design.)

Cross-sectional studies, also called survey and prevalence studies, employ a naturalistic sampling frame that selects samples from a larger population and then determines the frequency of the disorder and the variation in distribution by person, time, place, and so forth. Measurements of the disorder and its variation are done at the same time. Although basic descriptive associations can be made, it is not possible to determine the temporal sequence between the factor and the disorder or, more important, whether the factor(s) associated with the disorder was present before the onset and, thus, is related etiologically to the disorder. The cross-sectional design can answer questions about the frequency of the disorder; the ages, groups, and segments of a community affected; the proportion of known cases under medical care; the range of the clinical phenomena; and the similarity between patients seen in treatment and those who never seek care. The NIMH Epidemiologic Catchment Area (ECA) study (21) (to be described), which estimated rates of psychiatric disorders in adults selected by probability sampling from five urban communities, is an example of a cross-sectional study. The major obstacle to such large-scale descriptive studies in psychiatry has been the unreliability of psychiatric diagnosis. The ability to carry out the ECA is directly related to improvements in diagnostic reliability.

Cohort studies, also called follow-up, incidence, or prospective studies, follow a population at risk of developing the disease for a given period of time during which new cases are identified. A cohort can also be defined as a group of patients, and information on the clinical course and natural history of the disease can be obtained. A cohort study is expensive and inefficient for rare diseases. The follow-up can be prospective or retrospective. In a prospective study the investigator follows a health cohort over a period of time (e.g., Vaillant's [32] study of a Harvard University class to determine their health and social functioning over a 40-year period).

In a retrospective cohort study the investigator selects a study group and then goes back in time and traces the factor of interest in these groups over time. Robins' follow-up study (23) of over 500 persons 30 years after they were first identified as attending a child guidance clinic is an example of a cohort study in retrospect. In the Vaillant study (32) the investigators followed the cohort over the 40-year study period.

Case-control studies, also known as retrospective studies, follow a paradigm that proceeds from effect to cause (27). This strategy involves the study of a predetermined number of individuals with the disorder of interest (the cases) who are compared to individuals who are similar to the cases in as many ways as possible, but for whom the disorder of interest is absent (the controls). Cases and controls are compared with respect to attributes considered relevant to the disorder under study. The controls provide an estimate of the frequency of exposure expected in persons free of disease. The ratio of the rates in exposed persons and unexposed persons is the relative risk or odds ratio. The Weissman et al. (37) study, which examined differential risk of psychiatric illness in families of psychiatrically ill patients compared with families of nonpsychiatrically ill normal controls, is an example of a case-control study.

There is some controversy over the range of experimental studies to be included under the rubric of epidemiology. Kleinbaum et al. (9), in their outstanding textbook of epidemiology, include: laboratory experiments, which estimate the effect of some biological or behavioral responses believed to be risk factors for disease; and clinical trials, which include random assignment of an intervention or treatment for a disorder (e.g., the study of Prien et al. [20] of maintenance pharmacological treatment for prevention of relapse of a recurrent depression). The purpose is to test the efficacy of an intervention either as therapy or as prophylaxis. The treatment can be at the individual or at the community level.

HISTORICAL TRENDS

There have been approximately three generations of increasingly sophisticated techniques aimed at establishing true prevalence of mental disorder in communities. (See References 3, 24, 33, 35, 36, for review of studies cited.)

The first community study of psychiatric disorder, defined as "insanity" and "idiocy," in the United States was conducted in 1855 by Dr. Edward Jarvis in Massachusetts. Information was collected indirectly from reports of key informants (general practitioners, clergymen) as well as from hospital and other records.

Subsequent studies in the United States were similarly characterized by use of indirect methods of ascertainment and comprise the "first generation" of epidemiological studies. Comparison of findings with future research would be restricted by the presence of incomplete "case" assessments, diagnosed unreliably at face value by clinicians. However, these studies were not without contributions for future conceptualizations. For example, Faris and Dunham in 1967 (4) demonstrated the significance of social variables in their classic examination of mental hospital admission rates in Chicago during the 1930s.

The experience of World War II had an important impact on the evolution of epidemiological investigations. These would rely on direct interviews of community residents, a distinction of "second-generation" studies.

During World War II, military psychiatrists and social scientists investigated such phenomena as combat fatigue, transient functional psychoses, dissociative states, and stress reactions. Studies were conducted with rigorous precision, reflected in advanced sampling and survey techniques yielding data exposed to statistical analysis. The employment of screening questionnaires and scales of impairment disclosed an apparent correlation between symptomatology and the environmental stresses of combat or captivity in concentration camps. Thus, the identification of "stress" as an important precipitating factor of mental illness was established, and subsequent studies in civilian settings proposed analogous "stress" factors such as poverty, social class, rapid social change, and urbanization.

The unanticipated finding that psychiatric reactions had also occurred among those men previously screened as mentally fit for selective service focused even more attention on precipitating stresses rather than predisposing vulnerabilities. In addition, the publicized prevalence of psychiatric disorder implied in the high rejection rates for selective service created heightened awareness of mental health problems and the need for information, prompting federal support for epidemiological studies in the general population at the close of the war.

The consequent community surveys of the 1950s and 1960s adopted not only the methodology developed during the military experience, but also the unifying concept of stress consistent with defining mental health and mental illness along one continuum, an orientation based on the theories of Adolf Meyer. Thus, rejecting the Kraepelinian models of discrete psychiatric disorders, these studies chose to measure overall impairment, independent of specific diagnosis, and to attribute etiology to social factors. Representative community surveys included the Stirling County Study by Leighton et al. (12) and the Baltimore Morbidity Survey (31). Overall, these studies reported high rates of impairment (e.g., 81% in the Midtown Manhattan Study [31]). Other studies, such as that of Hollingshead and Redlich (8), established social class in association with treated mental illness, especially schizophrenia.

The development of methodology and attention to psychosocial variables engendered significant contributions to the understanding of psychiatric disorders and the use of mental health services. However, the intentional lack of rates for specific psychiatric disorders severely limited application of previous findings to the issues of public policy and to the research in psychopharmacology, genetics, and neuropsychiatry that would emerge in the 1970s.

In response to this recognition as well as to the research gaps identified by Carter's Presidential Commission on Mental Health (PCMH) in 1977, a "third generation" of epidemiological studies was to evolve in the 1980s. Its recent convergence with the allied fields of clinical psychiatry and basic research is readily observed in the development of reliable and systematic techniques of assessment by direct interview or family history. This refined methodology is actually the legacy of the psychopharmacological revolution, initiated almost three decades earlier.

The psychopharmacological revolution, begun in the 1950s, initiated a resurgence of interest in descriptive psychopathology as the basis for diagnostic assessment. Early clinical trials delineated differential responses to pharmacotherapy in patients with differing mental disorders. The development of subsequent pharmacotherapies and their clinical trials was motivated by the desire to find the most appropriate medication for the individual patient. For example, in the treatment of affective disorders, the discovery of antidepressants and lithium disclosed the need for establishing more refined and reliable differential diagnoses. Furthermore, clinical trials required the selection of homogeneous groups of patients in order to reliably test the efficacy and safety of the drugs, to propose and verify etiological hypotheses, to allow comparisons between studies, and finally, to foster communication with the practicing clinician.

The Washington University Department of Psychiatry in St. Louis strove to meet these needs and recommended use of operational criteria in establishing diagnosis of a number of psychiatric illnesses. These diagnostic criteria were subsequently incorporated into the Research Diagnostic Criteria (RDC) published in 1978 by Spitzer, Endicott, and Robins (30). The RDC were developed to enable research investigators to apply a consistent set of criteria for the description or selection of samples of subjects with functional psychiatric illness. The RDC were thus constructed with the deliberate purpose of obtaining relatively homogeneous groups of subjects, ensuring as few "false positives" as possible despite a certain number of false negatives. The DSM-III, published in 1980, was based on this approach.

A logical extension of the operational criteria set forth by the RDC was the development of other standardized instruments used to obtain quantitative assessment of the duration and overall intensity of the requisite symptom patterns experienced by the research subject. A structured interview, the Schedule for Affective Disorders and Schizophrenia (SADS), was designed to supplement the RDC. Its purpose was to obtain information on a patient's functioning and symptoms. It elicited details on the current episode as well as historical information.

Application of the standardized instruments in epidemiological research proved feasible in a pilot study of 511 community residents by Weissman and Myers in 1975–1976 (40). At that time, limitations in broader applications for the intended multisite surveys prompted by the PCMH of 1977 were recognized. Namely, administration required clinically trained interviewers in order to achieve reliability, RDC and not DSM-III diagnoses were generated, and computerized scoring of the instrument had not been developed.

In response, the NIMH developed the Diagnostic Interview Schedule (DIS) by Robins et al. (25). The DIS is a highly structured interview designed for use by lay interviewers in epidemiological surveys. It is designed to elicit the elements of diagnosis (symptom severity, frequency, and distribution) and is capable of generating computer diagnosis in terms of DSM-III, Feighner, or RDC criteria. It has been used primarily in the NIMH–ECA program. Recent investigators in family-study research have similarly created standardized instruments for eliciting pedigree information and family psychiatric history. These are amenable to use by lay interviewers and in programming for computer-assisted analysis.

Finally, it should be noted that a parallel development of a refined methodology has occurred in the United Kingdom in the form of the Present State Examination (PSE) by Wing et al. (42). Diagnoses, set by the hierarchical rules of the International Classification of Diseases, (ICD-9, the British analog of DSM-III), are generated by computer. An Index of Definition (ID) establishes threshold levels for the various symptoms reported on the PSE.

THE EPIDEMIOLOGICAL CATCHMENT AREA PROGRAM

With the development of the structured diagnostic assessments, the demonstration of their feasibility in community surveys, and the need for accurate information on rates of specific psychiatric disorders, in 1980 the NIMH organized a five-site Epidemiologic Catchment Area (ECA) Program (21). Each site had a large degree of autonomy in collecting specific data for its area, but there was a collaborative design in which all centers collected the same core information and used the DIS.

The objectives of the multisite longitudinal study were to provide information on the following:

- The prevalence and incidence of specific mental disorders in the community by means of appropriate surveys in single-family households, multiple dwelling units, group quarters, and in institutional settings such as nursing homes, homes for the aged, prisons, schools, and mental institutions.

- Estimation of the relationship between having a diagnosis and receiving treatment and when treatment was first initiated, and if not in treatment, the reasons for not seeking and/or receiving treatment.
- For newly developed mental disorders (incidence), the concomitant risk factors associated with or causative of the disorder.

Each of the five catchment areas has at least 200,000 inhabitants and boundaries that coincide with one or more contiguous comprehensive community mental health center (CMHC) catchment areas. Yale University in New Haven, Connecticut, received the first such grant, followed by Johns Hopkins University in Baltimore, Washington University in St. Louis, and subsequently Duke University in Durham, North Carolina, and the University of California at Los Angeles. Each site assessed at least 3,000 subjects (in addition, some sites have oversamples of specific subgroups, such as the elderly, Hispanics, and blacks). Data are available on at least 18,000 subjects at two or more points in time, based on probability samples from the community in each of the five U.S. sites. Data on the epidemiology of psychiatric disorders, who is at risk, and who is receiving treatment are beginning to emerge (see References 18, 26, 28, 34).

The first achievement of the ECA study has been to demonstrate the magnitude of psychiatric disorders in the community, as well as the consistency in findings between sites for most disorders.

Overall, approximately 14/100 men and 12/100 women experience a DSM-III Axis I disorder in a six-month period. The rates are comparable between the sexes. Young people are at greatest risk for a current psychiatric disorder. The age of highest risk is 18–44 years, particularly 18–24 years. The rates are highest for anxiety disorders (primarily phobias); affective disorders (primarily major depression); and substance abuse (primarily alcohol abuse). The rates are comparable in all sites for most disorders with the exception of phobias, which are highest in Baltimore. For the young men (aged 18–24) alcohol abuse, drug abuse, and phobias are the most common disorders. Phobias, drug abuse, and major depression are the most common disorders for the young women. The affective disorders (major depression) are most prevalent in ages 18–44 for both men and women.

How does the magnitude of these disorders compare with who comes for treatment? Only a small proportion (about 20%) of persons with a recent DIS/DSM-III disorder receive any treatment for this problem in any section of the health care system. This finding not only demonstrates the unmet need for treatment of a large portion of affected persons, but also demonstrates the importance of community samples to obtain rates of psychiatric disorders. If we surveyed only those who are in treatment, we would have a limited view of affected persons.

Other intriguing findings have to do with possible secular changes in rates of major depression. There is some evidence that for major depression, the age of onset is decreasing and that there is a birth cohort effect. Observations regarding a birth cohort effect were first made clinically by Klerman in 1976 (10) and were later confirmed in his family study (11) and in several other studies (7,22,38). The age of onset of major depression is younger and the rates are higher in the cohort that came to maturity after World War II — the cohort born after 1935. Preliminary ECA results suggest that this finding is consistent across all five sites.

For the clinician, this means that there are a greater number of younger persons affected with major depression and that their age of first episode is younger. The mean age of first onset is in the twenties. We do not know the rates of psychiatric disorders among children in the community in the United States.

GENETIC EPIDEMIOLOGY

Because of the promising results about familial factors in some of the psychiatric disorders, a familial-genetic approach is being integrated into epidemiological studies. This is accomplished by studies of large pedigrees of biologically related relatives; studies of adoptees separated at birth from a biological parent who is ill with a psychiatric disorder; studies of individuals at high risk for a disorder because of family history; and studies of twins. There is increasing realization that genetics and epidemiology have much in common. Both disciplines are interested in familial resemblance, and there is an overlap in methodology (14,17). Both depend on collection of data dealing with disease frequency, and both draw heavily on the application of mathematics to understand the patterns of disease distribution. Since few diseases are determined solely by either genes or environment, and since it frequently cannot be determined a priori whether a disease should best be studied by an epidemiologist or by a geneticist, there is emerging an exciting new hybrid discipline termed "genetic epidemiology." This approach is being applied in the Framingham study (5) of cardiovascular disease and, with increasing frequency, in studies of psychiatric disorders.

In psychiatry, there is emerging a technology of family studies (39) including: systematic approaches to obtaining pedigrees, and methods of obtaining family history when direct interviews with relatives are not possible. Such techniques have improved the quality of these studies and are quite applicable to ordinary clinical practice.

The family genetic techniques have been applied to studies of several psychiatric disorders, and the largest studies have included the families of affectively ill patients. The results from these family studies consistently show that major depression is familial. There is a two- to threefold increase in major depression in the first-degree adult relatives of probands with major depression, as compared to the relatives of nonill controls.

Moreover, the earlier the onset of the major depression, especially onset before age 20, the higher the familial loading. Clinicians treating patients with an onset of major depression in childhood or adolescence can expect that other members of the patient's family are likely to be ill. Also, the relatives themselves are more likely to have major depression with an early onset (41).

Assortative mating in these families is high — a depressed patient is frequently married to a depressed spouse. Where there is assortative mating, the risk of marital problems in the couples and psychiatric problems in the children is increased (15).

Recently, as methods for assessing psychopathology in children have been developed, attention has turned to studying the children of depressed patients. The results of these studies show high rates of depression in children aged 6–17 of depressed parents. Similar to the adults, there is a two- to threefold increase of depression in these children (19).

The children report more depression when asked directly themselves than do their parents when asked about their children. The parents don't always seem to know the extent of their children's illness. Similar findings concerning discrepancies between child and mother reports of children's behaviors have been presented now in a number of studies.

Anxiety and alcohol/substance abuse are also increased in these children — again, the parents are unaware of the extent. The children's problems are apparent in all aspects of their lives with friends and siblings and in school. We don't yet know the long-term significance of these clinical states in children. Longitudinal studies of these children will yield this information.

GAPS IN UNDERSTANDING AND FUTURE DIRECTIONS

As mentioned previously, the early 1980s was a period of new energy in psychiatric epidemiology. The application of new techniques in psychiatric research has produced opportunities for new studies, particularly those in community surveys. However, there are also those efforts in familial studies using twins and large pedigrees, as well as case-control methods and follow-up studies of high-risk samples. These studies embody new conceptual approaches and a redirection from previous concern exclusively with social factors. There has been a broadening of the domains of relevant risk factors, including familial-genetic, nutrition, and environmental toxins; new advances in virology; as well as better understanding of social class, cross-cultural differences, and the important roles of social processes, such as urbanization, changes in the composition of the labor force, economic developments, and industrialization.

Despite the progress that has been made there are many problems. Some of these problems are common to understanding the epidemiology of any chronic noninfectious disorder, and some are unique to psychiatric disorders.

In most chronic disorders, etiology is multifactorial, and many domains of risk factors (e.g., biological, behavioral) must be studied. The onset of the disorder is usually difficult to determine, making incidence data difficult to obtain. There is often a long latency period between the first symptoms and the full-blown episode, making it more difficult to sort out risk factors related to cause from those factors that are a consequence of the early stages of the disorder. In psychiatric disorders the lack of established biological indices and the lack of clear differentiation between the normal and the pathological pose additional difficulties.

In addition to these general problems, there are specific problems in psychiatric disorders. There are no large-scale epidemiological studies of children and adolescents similar to the ECA study. Efforts to develop an epidemiological assessment for this population are underway under the aegis of the NIMH Center for Epidemiological Studies. When these methods are ready, epidemiological studies comparable to the ECA for adults and the elderly should be possible for children. Findings from the recent ECA and other sources suggest an increased prevalence of certain psychiatric disorders in young persons. Therefore, this is an important population for future study.

Longitudinal studies of community samples to determine risk factors associated with development of new disorders are limited. The ECA will provide a follow-up of only one year. The risk factors included in the ECA study are limited, and no biological or familial assessments have been included. Case-control studies (i.e., studies of defined patient groups compared with a matched control group to determine how the groups differ on the defined risk factors under study) are probably the most profitable for generating hypotheses about risk factors for specific disorders. Promising ones should be included in epidemiological studies either prospectively in the full sample or in case-control groups drawn from the community samples.

Historically, the great success of epidemiology has been in understanding the basis for infectious and nutritional disorders and in providing the scientific foundation for public-health efforts at control and prevention. With the conquest of infectious disorders and the gradual conquest of nutritional deficiency, attention focused, particularly in modern urbanized societies, on issues of chronic disease. The application of epidemiological methods to cardiovascular and cancer disorders has led to considerable knowledge of important risk factors, such as cigarette smoking for cardiovascular disorder and for cancer of the lung, the role of diet in arteriosclerosis, and the role of industrial toxins as carcinogens, and allows for the development of preventive efforts, even though the exact etiology and pathogenesis of these disorders remain unknown. For example, the death rate from cardiovascular disease, hypertension, and stroke has been reduced from 10% to 15% in the United States, probably owing to changes in salt ingestion, reduced fat content of diet, increased exercise, control of cigarette smoking, and early detection and treatment of hypertension. Nevertheless, the etiology of arteriosclerosis and hypertension remains unknown.

It is hoped that a similar application of epidemiological knowledge will lead to public health approaches to psychiatric disorders. In this respect, it is important to recognize that many psychiatric disorders that were of high prevalence and, in some cases, high mortality in the late 19th and early 20th centuries are no longer problems. Included in this category are pellagra, bromide psychosis, general paresis due to syphilis of the brain, and involutional melancholia. As knowledge of the risk factors associated with these disorders became available, it led to various types of preventive efforts and to public-health, legal, and health care innovations. Similarly, knowledge of the role of stress and group support has led the military to alter its practices, resulting in decreased incidents of combat-related neurotic reaction in the Korean and Vietnam wars. Similar opportunities for secondary prevention may exist in the emerging data on children of depressed parents and studies of the recently divorced and separated, or the unemployed.

In the long run, primary prevention is the goal. The public-health approach to primary prevention has been through identification of risk factors that are modifiable before the individual becomes ill, through either individual behavior change, health care interventions, or societal, public-health, or legal interventions. Recent development of the first genetic tests for detecting Huntington's disease prenatally and in as-yet-unaffected individuals provides a potential model for the future collaboration between psychiatric epidemiologists and geneticists for primary prevention. Using the new molecular genetic techniques of gene-splicing and searching for genetic markers in large and informative families with Huntington's disease, a potential for case identification is now possible. Although it is likely that most of the psychiatric disorders are more heterogeneous and multifactorial in etiology than Huntington's disease, these new techniques may be useful for subgroups of some psychiatric disorders.

ACKNOWLEDGMENTS

Portions of this chapter have appeared in:

Weissman, M. M., & Klerman, G. L. (1978). The epidemiology of mental disorders: Emerging trends. *Archives of General Psychiatry,* *35*, 705–712. (Copyright 1978, American Medical Association.)

Weissman, M. M., & Klerman, G. L. (1985). Epidemiology: Purpose and historical overview. In R. Michels (Chair, Ed. Bd.) & J. O. Cavenar, Jr. (Ed.), *Psychiatry, Vol. 3.* Philadelphia: Lippincott.

Weissman, M. M. (1987). Epidemiology overview. In R. E. Hales and A. J. Frances (Eds.), *American Psychiatric Association annual review, Vol. 6* (pp. 574–588). Washington, DC: American Psychiatric Press, Inc. (Copyright 1987. Used with permission.)

Weissman, M. M. (1985). Psychiatric epidemiology and clinical psychiatry: The new dialogue. Presented in acceptance of the 1985 Rema Lapouse Mental Health Epidemiology Award, at the American Public Health Association Annual Meeting, Washington, D.C. (Nov. 18).

This research was supported in part by the Yale Mental Health Clinical Research Center, National Institute of Mental Health grant MH30929; by the John D. and Catherine T. MacArthur Foundation Mental Health Research Network on Risk and Protective Factors in the Major Mental Disorders; and by the Yale ECA–NIMH grant MH40603-01A1. The Epidemiologic Catchment Area Program was established as a series of five epidemiologic research studies performed by independent research teams in collaboration with staff of the Division of Biometry and Epidemiology of the National Institute of Mental Health. The five sites are Yale University, U01 MH34224; Johns Hopkins University, U01 MH33870; Washington University, U01 MH33883; Duke University, U01 MH35386; University of California, Los Angeles, U01 MH35865.

REFERENCES

1. CHARNEY, E. A., & WEISSMAN, M. M. (in press). Epidemiology of depressive and manic syndromes. In A. Georgotas & R. Cancro (Eds.), *Depression and mania: A comprehensive textbook*. New York: Elsevier.
2. *Diagnostic and Statistical Manual of Mental Disorders* (Third edition) (DSM-III). (1980). Washington, DC: American Psychiatric Association.
3. DOHRENWEND, B. P., & DOHRENWEND, B. S. (1982). Perspectives on the past and future of psychiatric epidemiology. *American Journal of Public Health, 72*, 1271.
4. FARIS, R. E. L., & DUNHAM, H. W. (1967). *Mental disorders in urban areas: An ecological study of schizophrenia and other psychoses*. Chicago: The University of Chicago Press.
5. FEINLEIB, M., KANNEL, W. B., GARRISON, R. J., McNAMARA, P. M., & CASTELLI, W. P. (1975). The Framingham offspring study: Design and preliminary data. *Preventive Medicine, 4*, 518–525.
6. GRUENBERG, E. M., & TURNS, D. M. (1975). Epidemiology. In A. M. Freedman, H. I. Kaplan & B. J. Sadock (Eds.), *Comprehensive textbook of psychiatry – II*. Baltimore: Williams & Wilkins.
7. HAGNELL, O., LANKE, J., RORSMAN, B., & OJESJO, L. (1982). Are we entering an age of melancholy? Depressive illness in a prospective epidemiological study over 25 years: The Lundby Study, Sweden. *Psychological Medicine, 12*, 279.
8. HOLLINGSHEAD, A. B., & REDLICH, F. D. (1958). *Social class and mental illness*. New York: John Wiley & Sons.
9. KLEINBAUM, D. G., KUPPER, L. L., & MORGENSTERN, H. (1982). *Epidemiologic research: Principles and quantitative methods*. Belmont, CA: Wadsworth.
10. KLERMAN, G. L. (1976). Age and clinical depression: Today's youth in the twenty-first century. *Journal of Gerontology, 31*, 318.
11. KLERMAN, G. L., LAVORI, P. W., RICE, J., REICH, T., ENDICOTT, J., ANDREASEN, N. C., KELLER, M. B., & HIRSCHFELD, R. M. A. (1985). Birth cohort trends in rates of major depressive disorder among relatives of patients with affective disorders. *Archives of General Psychiatry, 42*, 689.
12. LEIGHTON, D. C., HARDING, J. S., MACKLIN, D. B., et al. (1963). *The character of danger: Stirling County study #3*. New York: Basic Books.
13. LILIENFELD, A. M. (1976). *Foundations of epidemiology*. New York: Oxford University Press.
14. MACMAHON, B., & PUGH, T. (1970). *Epidemiology: Principles and methods*. Boston: Little, Brown.
15. MERIKANGAS, K. R. (1984). Divorce and assortative mating for depression. *American Journal of Psychiatry, 141*, 74.
16. MORRIS, J. N. (1975). *Uses of epidemiology* (3rd ed.). Edinburgh: Churchill Livingstone.
17. MORTON, N. E., & CHUNG, C. S. (Eds.) (1978). *Genetic epidemiology*. New York: Academic Press.
18. MYERS, J. K., WEISSMAN, M. M., TISCHLER, G. L., HOLZER, C. E., LEAF, P. J., ORVASCHEL, H., ANTHONY, J., BOYD, J. H., BURKE, J. D., KRAMER, M., & STOLTZMAN, R.

(1984). Six-month prevalence of psychiatric disorders in three communities. *Archives of General Psychiatry, 41,* 959.

19. ORVASCHEL, H., WEISSMAN, M. M., & KIDD, K. K. (1980). Children and depression: The children of depressed parents; the childhood of depressed patients; depression in children. *Journal of Affective Disorders, 2,* 1.

20. PRIEN, R. F., KUPFER, D. J., MANSKY, P. A., SMALL, J. G., TUASON, V. B., VOSS, C. B., & JOHNSON, W. E. (1984). Drug therapy in the prevention of recurrences in unipolar and bipolar affective disorders. *Archives of General Psychiatry, 41,* 1096.

21. REGIER, D. A., MYERS, J. K., KRAMER, M., ROBINS, L. N., BLAZER, D. G., HOUGH, R. L., EATON, W. W., & LOCKE, B. Z. (1984). The NIMH Epidemiologic Catchment Area Program: Historical context, major objectives, and study population characteristics. *Archives of General Psychiatry, 41,* 934.

22. RICE, J., REICH, T., ANDREASEN, N. C., LAVORI, P. W., ENDICOTT, J., CLAYTON, P. J., KELLER, M. S., HIRSCHFELD, R. M. A., & KLERMAN, G. L. (1984). Sex related differences in depression: Familial evidence. *Journal of Affective Disorders, 7,* 199.

23. ROBINS, L. N. (1966). *Deviant children grown up: A sociological and psychiatric study of sociopathic personality.* Baltimore: Williams & Wilkins.

24. ROBINS, L. N. (1978). Psychiatric epidemiology. *Archives of General Psychiatry, 35,* 697.

25. ROBINS, L. N., HELZER, J., CROUGHAN, J., & RATDIFF, K. S. (1981). The NIMH diagnostic interview schedule: Its history, characteristics, and validity. *Archives of General Psychiatry, 38,* 381–389.

26. ROBINS, L. N., HELZER, J. E., WEISSMAN, M. M., ORVASCHEL, H., GRUENBERG, E., BURKE, J. D., & REGIER, D. (1984). Lifetime prevalence of specific psychiatric disorders in three sites. *Archives of General Psychiatry, 41,* 949.

27. SCHLESSELMAN, J. J. (1982). *Case-control studies: Design and conduct of analysis.* New York: Oxford University Press.

28. SHAPIRO, S., SKINNER, E. A., KESSLER, L. G., VONKORFF, M., GERMAN, P. S., TISCHLER, G. L., LEAF, P. J., BENHAM, L., COTTER, L., & REGIER, D. A. (1984). Utilization of health and mental health services. *Archives of General Psychiatry, 41,* 971.

29. SHEPHERD, M. (1978). Epidemiology and clinical psychiatry. *British Journal of Psychiatry, 133,* 289.

30. SPITZER, R. L., ENDICOTT, J., & ROBINS, E. (1978). Research diagnostic criteria: Rationale and reliability. *Archives of General Psychiatry, 35,* 773–779.

31. SROLE, L., LANGNER, T. S., MICHAEL, S. T., et al. (1962). *Mental health in the metropolis: The midtown Manhattan study, Vol. 1.* New York: McGraw-Hill.

32. VAILLANT, G. E. (1983). *The natural history of alcoholism.* Cambridge, MA: Harvard University Press.

33. WEISSMAN, M. M. (1987). Epidemiology overview. In R. E. Hales & A. J. Frances (Eds.), *American Psychiatric Association annual review, Vol. 6* (pp. 574–588). Washington, DC: American Psychiatric Press.

34. WEISSMAN, M. M. (1985). Psychiatric epidemiology and clinical psychiatry: The new dialogue. Presented at the American Public Health Association Annual Meeting, Washington, DC (Nov. 18).

35. WEISSMAN, M. M., & KLERMAN, G. L. (1985). Epidemiology: Purpose and historical overview. In R. Michels (Chair, Ed. Bd.) & J. O. Cavenar, Jr. (Ed.), *Psychiatry, Vol. 3.* Philadelphia: Lippincott.

36. WEISSMAN, M. M., & KLERMAN, G. L. (1978). The epidemiology of mental disorders: Emerging trends. *Archives of General Psychiatry, 35,* 705.

37. WEISSMAN, M. M., GERSHON, E. S., KIDD, K. K., PRUSOFF, B. A., LECKMAN, J. F., DIBBLE, E., HAMOVIT, J., THOMPSON, W. D., PAULS, D. L., & GUROFF, J. J. (1984). Psychiatric disorders in the relatives of probands with affective disorders: The Yale-NIMH collaborative family study. *Archives of General Psychiatry, 41,* 13.

38. WEISSMAN, M. M., LEAF, P. J., HOLZER, C. E., MYERS, J. K., & TISCHLER, G. L. (1984).

The epidemiology of depression: An update on sex differences in rates. *Journal of Affective Disorders, 7*, 179.

39. WEISSMAN, M. M., MERIKANGAS, K. R., JOHN, K., WICKRAMARATNE, P., PRUSOFF, B. A., & KIDD, K. K. (1986). Family-genetic studies of psychiatric disorders: Developing technologies. *Archives of General Psychiatry, 43*, 1104–1116.

40. WEISSMAN, M. M., & MYERS, J. K. (1978). Affective disorders in a U.S. urban community. *Archives of General Psychiatry, 35*, 1304–1311.

41. WEISSMAN, M. M., WICKRAMARATNE, P., MERIKANGAS, K. R., LECKMAN, J. F., PRUSOFF, B. A., CARUSO, K. A., KIDD, K. K., & GAMMON, G. D. (1984). Onset of major depression in early adulthood: Increased familial loading and specificity. *Archives of General Psychiatry, 41*, 1136.

42. WING, J. K., COOPER, J. E., & SARTORIUS, N. (1974). *The measurement and classification of psychiatric symptoms*. London: Cambridge University Press.

2

DSM-III: AN EVALUATION

MURRAY A. MORPHY, M.D.

Chief, Psychiatry Service,
Buffalo VA Medical Center;
Associate Professor,
SUNY at Buffalo, Department of Psychiatry,
Buffalo, New York

INTRODUCTION

The American Psychiatric Association (APA) adopted the third edition of the *Diagnostic and Statistical Manual of Mental Disorders* (DSM-III) (6) as its official classification system in 1980. This concluded six years of concerted and often controversial effort to develop a major new psychiatric nosology for use in the United States. This task was entrusted by the APA to the Task Force on Nomenclature and Statistics appointed in May 1974 under the chairmanship of Robert Spitzer, M.D. Debate over the goals, direction, and product of this ambitious enterprise has often been heated, has spread well beyond American shores, and shows little sign of abating even though several years have passed since the publication of DSM-III.

Unlike its native-born predecessors, DSM-III has aroused the intense interest and engagement of American psychiatry and attracted considerable attention and reaction around the world as well. Its stormy six-year gestational period has now been followed by several years of widespread clinical application. Extensive efforts have been made to examine its reliability, validity, acceptability to clinicians, and a host of other factors directly relevant to an official classificatory scheme. In this chapter an attempt will be made to review and account for this impressive degree of concern and to offer an evaluation of DSM-III's overall impact. While the emphasis will be on the effects felt in the clinical arena, DSM-III's influence on administrative, teaching, and research concerns of the specialty will also be considered.

19

An extensive literature exists regarding DSM-III to aid in such an evaluation. The sheer volume of this material in fact attests to the level of interest generated by this document throughout the mental health professions. This literature ranges from heated attacks and equally impassioned defenses to scientific efforts to test the diagnostic hypotheses encompassed in DSM-III. This chapter reviews a representative, but still reasonably substantial portion of these publications. It is hoped that this will be sufficient to accurately reflect the major viewpoints that currently exist regarding DSM-III, and to assess its contribution to the advancement of psychiatric nosology.

HISTORICAL DEVELOPMENT

Psychiatric diagnosis has been widely acknowledged as problematic in recent decades (15,16,60,63,76,77,134). This state of affairs is not confined to our own historical area, however. Hippocrates and his followers who compiled a classification of mental disorders in the 5th century B.C. undoubtedly had their detractors. In the intervening centuries the critiques of psychiatric diagnosis have been at least as numerous as the various categories and systems proposed (2).

Lack of knowledge regarding the etiology and pathophysiology of most mental disorders remains the central, though not sole, source of this difficulty. In the absence of such information all approaches to psychiatric classification have been and continue to be arbitrary and thus subject to debate. Even when some consensus has been achieved on the disease categories to be used, variation in gathering and interpreting clinical information has generally led to poor diagnostic reliability (16,76). Diagnostic categories were often seen as offering little in the way of guidance for treatment or prognosis (48). For psychoanalysts and the majority of psychotherapists the primary goal of assessment has been formulation of an individual's unique intrapsychic and occasionally interpersonal difficulties. Descriptive classifications that attempted to group patients based on shared behaviors were thus often seen as irrelevant.

Critics such as Eysenck et al. (32,33) have felt that all such diagnostic efforts were doomed to fail in that behavioral phenomena were simply not amenable to a categorical approach. Menninger (89) was among those arguing a continuum model for behavioral disturbance, while Szasz (130) raised some of the most strenuous objections to the application of the "medical model" in psychiatry.

In the face of these widely recognized problems and quite salient criticisms, attempts to improve categorical approaches to psychiatric diagnosis nonetheless continued. The U.S.-U.K. Cross National Diagnostic Project (75) was quite important in this regard. Together with other transcultural efforts (109), this study demonstrated the sources for much of the diagnostic difficulty in psychiatry and ways in which this might be reduced. In the United States dissatisfaction with the first two editions of the *Diagnostic and Statistical Manual of Mental Disorders*, DSM-I (4) and DSM-II (5), introduced in 1952 and 1968, respectively, fueled several productive research undertakings. Most notable were the accomplishments of the St. Louis group that culminated in the production of the "Feighner criteria" in 1972 (35). Named after the senior author of the paper and generated primarily for research purposes, these criteria were described for 15 diagnostic conditions for which it was believed the most evidence for validity existed. Building on these developments, Spitzer et al. (121) then went on to formulate and publish the Research Diagnostic Criteria (RDC). Such criteria were felt to be of critical importance to psychiatric research where clearly defined homogeneous categories were essential for comparative purposes. The value of such criteria for clinical work was also increasingly evident, and their development thus became a priority for the architects of DSM-III (120).

Diagnostic efforts on the international scene at this time culminated in the ninth revision of the International Classification of Diseases (ICD-9) published in 1977 (145). While a clinical modification of this system was created for use in the United States, work on DSM-III continued to accelerate. The original Task Force appointed 14 advisory committees, each charged with development of a major diagnostic section of the document. The Task Force, whose membership continued to increase over the next five years, served as a steering committee and retained responsibility for the key choices made in DSM-III's overall design.

From the outset, the Task Force on Nomenclature and Development intended to redesign the DSM to reflect current empirical knowledge. Unlike its predecessors, DSM-III would be developed after careful scrutiny of all the available scientific literature. Etiological theories would be avoided, and individuals and associations representing all the mental health professions were to be consulted as much as possible. Early in its existence the Task Force also made its critical commitments to the use of diagnostic criteria, a multiaxial format, and extensive field testing.

Progress reports on DSM-III's development were made regularly, beginning at the American Psychiatric Association's Annual Meeting in May 1975. A conference entitled, "DSM-III in Midstream" was held in St. Louis in June 1976. One important outcome of this meeting was the adoption of DSM-III's multiaxial format. A first draft of the manual appeared in 1977, and that fall the NIMH-sponsored field trials began. Over 800 clinicians in more than 200 private and public settings evaluated over 12,000 patients (54,122,123) with this draft, and this experience led to a number of modifications incorporated in the final version. The Task Force then submitted this document to the Council on Research and Development at the American Psychiatric Association's Annual Meeting in May 1979. This body approved and forwarded it to the organization's Board of Trustees where, not without additional controversy, it was ultimately endorsed for adoption and publication in 1980.

The goals set for DSM-III were thus ambitious ones. Questions remain over the choice and desirability of these goals, and how successfully they were met. The remainder of this chapter is devoted to an evaluation of the available answers to these questions.

CRITICAL REVIEW

Examination of the responses to DSM-III will be done in three stages, beginning with reviews of the document as a whole. This will be followed by critiques of the multiaxial format and each of the major diagnostic sections. The final portion of this chapter will deal with DSM-III's acceptance in the United States, additional international opinion, and the conclusions that are now possible regarding DSM-III's success as a diagnostic instrument.

OVERALL REACTIONS TO DSM-III

This section reviews the efforts that have been made to examine DSM-III in its entirety. They primarily include book reviews, editorials, "insider" opinion, and debate. More "scientific" evaluations examining questions of reliability and validity have generally been focused on particular diagnostic categories. These will be included when the appropriate subsections of DSM-III are being considered.

Critical overviews of DSM-III to date have been mixed. While each commentary might be categorized as either primarily positive or negative, it is the rare reviewer who is either entirely pleased or displeased with the document. The size and complexity of DSM-III, one frequently cited source of concern, and the improbability of meeting all possible expectations that can be brought to bear on a diagnostic system help ensure such an outcome.

Book Reviews

Consecutive issues of the *American Journal of Psychiatry* in late 1980 and early 1981 contained in their book review sections first a British (65) and then an American (22) overview of the manual. These two critiques aptly summarize many of the concerns raised both before and after DSM-III's publication and thus provide an appropriate starting point for this discussion.

Author of the British perspective was R. E. Kendell, who has made many thoughtful contributions to the literature on psychiatric classification (62–64,66,67). While suggesting that the overall design of the diagnostic system was admirable and well informed, he did point to several problems. Among these was the additional burden placed on international communication caused by the differences in DSM-III's content from the World Health Organization's ICD-9.

While Kendell generally supported the incorporation of diagnostic criteria and praised the corresponding gain in nosologic reliability, doubts were raised about the validity of some specific items. Among these were the age (under 45) and duration (over six months) requirements for the diagnosis of schizophrenia. The absence of criteria for schizoaffective disorder was seen as a serious shortcoming, and the increased complexity of the multiaxial approach was viewed as a potential liability. More logical distinctions between Axes I and II were recommended, including moving mental retardation to Axis II with the personality and developmental disorders. This axis would then include all lifelong but stable handicaps, while Axis I would be reserved for disorders that were either progressive or potentially reversible. Sadness over the departure of such familiar terms as hysteria, neurosis, and manic depressive illness was predicted, as was a lack of enthusiasm for the harsher new vocabulary that included such items as substance use disorder, paraphilia, and somatoform disorder. Finally, it was pointed out that if clinically accepted, DSM-III had the potential to advance psychiatry in the direction of a more rational and scientific specialty. If most clinicians ignored, rejected, or failed to master DSM-III, however, the entire enterprise would be a failure, "a psychiatric Concorde" (65).

Cooper and Michels, who wrote the American review (22), must also be counted among those who have made significant contributions to the literature on psychiatric nosology (41) and, somewhat literally, the debate on DSM-III (73). After wisely predicting best-seller status for the volume (over 425,000 copies were sold in the subsequent five-year period), they went on to raise many of the more important questions that are still being asked about DSM-III. Are more precise diagnostic criteria really helpful for the practitioner, or are they primarily of value to the clinical investigator? Was the desirability of excluding all theoretical models of mental functioning, including the popular psychodynamic viewpoint, from DSM-III worth the price of a nomenclature that would seem so much less familiar to so many? Are questions of etiology really being avoided when, for example, dysthymic disorder is assigned to the affective disorders as opposed to being seen as a "conflictual disorder" or as a form of personality disorder?

Concern regarding the difficulty of teaching and learning DSM-III in the absence of broad organizing principles was also expressed. One potential hazard predicted was the "laundry list" approach to psychiatric assessment, which might be particularly prevalent in students new to the field.

Despite the reservations outlined above and several others addressed in their review, the authors concluded by pronouncing DSM-III "a major achievement in psychiatry" that will benefit the field for many years into the future. They also suggested, however, that DSM-III can only be judged positively in the long run if it helps to generate new knowledge about many of the present conceptual and diagnostic problems in psychiatry. If successful in this regard, DSM-III would "lead to a DSM-IV that will be different in important ways, and the profession will be further enriched by the process of its evolution" (22).

Views from Within

In addition to these early assessments, the literature of the past decade contains several overall descriptions of DSM-III from those who were directly involved in its creation. Robert Spitzer, the acknowledged chief architect of DSM-III and thus a figure of considerable controversy himself, coauthored a summary (125) that appeared just as the manual was beginning to roll off the presses. Not every issue raised in the creation and content of DSM-III was obviously addressed nor was the author claiming an absence of bias. The review did, however, provide a valuable early introduction for a large number of clinicians struggling to come to terms with this complex document.

Other "insider" reports have followed. Bayer and Spitzer (13) reviewed the prolonged and highly politicized struggle over use of the term neurosis and a variety of other psychodynamic issues that were of particular concern to the psychoanalytic community. Another major contributor to DSM-III, Theodore Millon, has provided interesting commentary (91,92) on the document's development. Historians, should they deem DSM-III worthy of study in the future, will be abundantly supplied with source material.

Editorials

Many of the papers published on DSM-III might well be described as editorials though they are not labeled as such. Where this has been made explicit, the reviews of DSM-III have again been largely positive, though with a variety of reservations expressed.

Feighner (34) supported the notion of a more systematic data-oriented approach to nosology and repeated Guze's request (49) for resolution of diagnostic issues by data, not debate. Wolberg, writing in the *Journal of the American Academy of Psychoanalysis* (144), cautioned against excessive expectations for any diagnostic system. He defended the medical model as "a viable paradigm for the structuring of diagnosis" and suggested that the apparent "superfluity of categories" in DSM-III actually reflected an effort to provide more precise designations.

McKegney suggested that we should not expect psychiatric diagnoses to completely describe an individual and his treatment any more than we would elsewhere in medicine. He lamented the absence of a distinct category for the suicidal individual, but felt on balance that DSM-III would be particularly useful for psychiatrists working in a general hospital setting (83).

Writing in *Psychological Medicine* (94), Morphy offered a capsule summary of some of the main controversies concerning DSM-III, including the apparent disappearance of the neuroses and the narrowing of the concept of schizophrenia. He went on to contend that DSM-III reflected a hopeful degree of scientific maturation for the specialty and stood as a landmark in psychiatry's increasing medical identity.

Wortis (146) suggested that "you either try to bring system and science into psychiatric research by defining your terms, or you continue the confusions and wasted efforts of the past." He noted that nosological efforts become increasingly questionable the farther one moves from "the major psychoses and gross pathology into the realm of character development and the common anxieties." He cautioned against regarding the descriptive categories of DSM-III as diseases or fixed entities and supported their value in guiding better future research.

Other reviews to which editorial characteristics might be ascribed have not been so charitable. While Robin Murray wrote that "the incorporation of operational definitions into the diagnostic manual gives the U.S.A. an everyday classificatory system potentially superior to those in use elsewhere in the world" (95), an anonymous review published in *Psychological Medicine* (17) described the manual as a "hodgepodge" that would be confusing to non-Americans more familiar with ICD-9. Allen (3) suggested that DSM-III had left "the darkness unobscured," and that the architects of the system had made a serious error in not actively involving the insurance companies in their deliberations. Zubin, a major figure in the U.S.-U.K. Cross National Diagnostic Project (75) and a frequent contributor to the nosological literature (149), raised the question of DSM-III's value to science (150). Concern was expressed that political, economic, and other guild issues may have overwhelmed scientific values. Responding to an earlier draft of DSM-III that suggested mental disorders were a subset of medical disorders (71,119), he argued against the "gratuitous predominance of the medical model." Further, he warned of the risk of prematurely accepting the validity of the diagnostic categories as currently constituted.

Zubin's concern with politics versus science as applied to DSM-III is a common refrain in the literature. One of the more thorough discussions of this issue is provided in papers by Schacht (110) and Spitzer (117). From different vantage points they speak of the need to openly acknowledge the inevitable mix of practical or political considerations and scientific data in any classification system.

Sex Bias

Discriminatory diagnostic practices based on sex have been researched in the area of mental health in recent years (18,20,46,61). DSM-III has been examined in this regard by Kaplan (56) and found wanting. Her paper argues that masculine-based assumptions about which behaviors are healthy and which are not are somehow codified in DSM-III's diagnostic criteria. Companion articles by Williams and Spitzer (141) and Kass et al. (59) dispute this claim. There is little elsewhere in the literature to suggest this concern is widespread. However, as DSM-III is modified to possibly include such entities as premenstrual dysphoric disorder, these issues will again be raised, and quite likely with more passion.

Guild Concerns

Suspicions about possible ulterior motives on psychiatry's part in creating DSM-III have been prevalent among other mental health professionals. Such feelings were more commonly expressed prior to DSM-III's official arrival than subsequently (111). Organized psychiatry was seen as being primarily interested in establishing medical hegemony over all mental disorders. Particularly since the range and number of these disorders was dramatically increased in DSM-III, the economic consequences were viewed as alarming. Fueling such feeling was the inclusion in an early draft of DSM-III of the aforementioned claim that mental disorders were in fact a subset of medical disorders. When this claim was abandoned in later editions, the sense of alarm diminished.

Concern about the "medicalization" of such a large number of psychological ills and behavior patterns persists, however (86). Other diagnostic approaches have certainly been proposed as a result (85). Despite the possible desire for alternatives (116), none have as yet been formally adopted by any of the other mental health professional groups such as the American Psychological Association.

Formal Debate

A popular institution at recent meetings of the American Psychiatric Association has been the formal debate. Many issues important to the field have been engaged in this way. An entertaining and informative debate was held at the Toronto meeting in 1982. Arguing the affirmative of the question "Do the advantages of DSM-III outweigh the disadvantages?" were two major contributors to the nosological literature, Robert Spitzer (125) and Gerald Klerman (72). Equally articulate points on the negative side of the question were provided by Robert Michels and George Vaillant. With the loss of some of the humor, the substance of the debate was subsequently published in the *American Journal of Psychiatry* (73). Included are statements rapidly approaching "classic" status, such as Michel's admonition that "Dr. Spitzer and his group have led us from the brainless psychiatry of the 1950's to the threat of a mindless psychiatry for the 1980's." Winners are not anointed, but the exchange is valuable in that many of the more important issues regarding psychiatric diagnoses in general and DSM-III in particular are raised.

MULTIAXIAL FORMAT AND SECTION REVIEW

As a supplement to the evaluation of DSM-III as a whole, a brief review of the multiaxial format and of each major diagnostic section will now be undertaken. Following the discussion of the axes, the order selected for the diagnostic categories matches that in which they appear in DSM-III.

Multiaxial System

Along with inclusion of diagnostic criteria, the decision to utilize a multiaxial format is generally viewed as one of DSM-III's major contributions to nosological advancement in psychiatry. Credit in this regard has nothing to do with originating the concept of multiaxial diagnosis. As long ago as 1947, Essen-Moller and Wohlfahrt (31) proposed that the official Swedish psychiatric classification adopt a distinction between syndromes and causes of those syndromes. Although Sweden did not do so, the Danish Psychiatric Association did adopt a biaxial system in 1952 (129). In the 1970s a number of additional articles appeared on multiaxial systems (30,98,143), and these and others were well reviewed in 1979 by Mezzich (90). What DSM-III can take credit for is being the first official classification by such a large and influential body as the American Psychiatric Association to incorporate a multiaxial approach.

The history of how DSM-III's particular multiaxial format evolved and the subsequent critiques, reliability and validity studies, and suggestions for change are well summarized by Williams (139,140). Only a few of the major findings from that review will be highlighted here.

Axes I and II

The separation of mental disorders into the clinical syndromes of Axis I and the personality and developmental disorders of Axis II has added substantially to the reliability with which both are diagnosed (123). Future versions of the DSM-III are likely to retain this distinction, though Kendell's aforementioned criticism (65) of logical inconsistency here probably will result in the movement of mental retardation to Axis II.

Axis III

Some sympathy exists for broadening the physical disorders listed on Axis III beyond those "potentially relevant to the understanding or management of the individual" (6). Kendell (65) has suggested that any etiological factor, proven or suspected, be included here. Although some coding procedures may be introduced in the future to help address the issue of etiology, other changes in Axis III are unlikely. The one major exception to this conclusion would occur if the suggestion to incorporate Axis III in Axis I were followed (139).

Axes IV and V

These axes, which deal with psychosocial stressors and level of functioning, have been the subject of the most criticism despite their "optional" status. On Axis IV, is it most useful to note an average person's reaction to the stress or to give a more individualized description? Are stressors to be left nonspecific, and how can acute versus chronic stressors best be distinguished? Would any change here be worth the burden of further complicating the system? On Axis V should functioning currently or perhaps over several years be included, rather than just the highest level during the past year? Despite these and other questions, the field trials have demonstrated that the reliability of Axes IV and V ($k = .6$ and $.7$, respectively) compares favorably with that of Axes I and II ($k = .7$ and $.6$) (123), and some support for their validity also exists in the literature (148).

Other Axes

Axes other than the five selected for inclusion in DSM-III have been proposed. Treece (132) suggested a separate axis for substance-related disorders, while Fleck (36) and Frances et al. (40) have commented on DSM-III's multiaxial shortcomings for family therapy purposes. Karasu and Skodol (57) recommended a sixth axis for psychodynamic evaluation, and others (73) have suggested using this axis for at least a description of a patient's coping styles or defense mechanisms. An axis for coding response to treatment was suggested by Schacht and Nathan (111), while Schover et al. (112) proposed an alternative multiaxial system for describing psychosexual dysfunctions.

While all the above suggestions have merit, an overriding consideration may be the limits of complexity necessary for such a widely utilized system. Williams (140) provides some compelling reasons for caution in this regard, and it seems likely that the architects of future DSM's will take a conservative approach to any changes in DSM-III's multiaxial format.

Infancy, Childhood, and Adolescence

The section on disorders usually arising in these early years has been the subject of some of DSM-III's most heated criticism. Garmezy (42), responding to the first widely circulated draft of DSM-III, suggested that the entire taxonomy was endangered by "an overreaching effort by the creators of the children's section to bring under psychiatry's wing deficits and disabilities that are not mental disorders." He spoke of a "children's crusade" to battle the notion that millions of American children might suddenly be implicated as mentally ill (45). Few data have subsequently accumulated to support this fear, and later reviews have been more encouraging. Cantwell et al. (19), in the final of a series of four papers, concluded that the childhood section of DSM-III compared to DSM-II was more reliable and easier to use. Rutter and Shaffer (108) also commented on improvements introduced, such as the multiaxial format, though they did criticize the particular multiaxial structure chosen. Earls (27) supported the appropriateness of DSM-III categories for very young children, and Russell et al. (107) predicted wide acceptance among child psychiatrists. Excellent interrator reliability has been found in both children (137) and adolescents (128). Overall, despite early reservations and continuing dissatisfaction with certain specific categories (e.g., does attention deficit disorder without hyperactivity exist?), this section of DSM-III has been seen as a distinct improvement over its predecessors.

Organic Mental Disorders

While questions of reliability and validity have generally been less pressing with diagnoses in this area in the past, DSM-III nonetheless incorporates several significant changes. Basic concepts such as "dementia" are more explicitly defined. Lipowski (80) supports the broadened range of organic mental disorders included, the dismissal of such inappropriate dichotomies as psychotic/nonpsychotic, and the recognition that the traditional boundary between the organic and functional mental disorders is largely an artificial one.

Barnes and Raskind (10) have reported that DSM-III criteria for dementia are useful for more accurate assessment of nursing-home patients. Ellison (28) has suggested that the DSM-III organic mental disorder categories are of value in emergency-room work. The availability of specific diagnostic criteria is applauded by Fox (38), who, like Lipowski, suggests that this will help remedy the neglect of these disorders by psychiatry.

Substance Abuse

The substance-induced subsection of the organic mental disorders is considerably expanded to reflect the increases in knowledge and experience in this area. As further data accumulate, new categories, such as cocaine withdrawal, will appear and existing ones will be modified.

For the substance use section of the manual, proposed changes have already been suggested by Rounsaville et al. (106). While diagnostic reliability and in some cases validity are already rather high in this portion of DSM-III, it's thus clear that further modifications are inevitable as knowledge in this area continues to expand.

Schizophrenic Disorders

Few sections in DSM-III have generated more concern than the one dealing with the schizophrenic disorders. The term "Kraepelinian" has been used by critics in a pejorative sense to describe this category as arbitrarily narrow, with an overemphasis on poor outcome (44). The requirements for age of onset (prior to 45) and duration (greater than six months) have been questioned (65). The DSM-III concept of schizophrenia is indeed more restrictive than that offered by DSM-II, and the incidence of the disorder should thus decline (114). Whether in fact this will happen in at least some settings remains uncertain (79).

The U.S.-U.K. Cross National Diagnostic Project (75) was among the pre-DSM-III studies that demonstrated the generosity with which American psychiatrists conferred the diagnosis of schizophrenia (102,109). Attempts to better define and reduce the heterogeneity in this patent group had already led to the "Feighner" (35) and Research Diagnostic Criteria (121). While alternatives are available (43,69), it was on these models that the DSM-III category was built.

DSM-III does provide explicit criteria for making the diagnosis of schizophrenia, and greater reliability of diagnosis has already been demonstrated in the field trials (122,123). This reliability has been shown to rise with the increasing clinical experience of the rater (100). Validity remains far more elusive, particularly in the absence of any symptom criteria pathognomonic for schizophrenia (21). The long-standing problem of determining the boundary with affective disorders (68,70) also persists. Subsequent studies have shown the DSM-III definition of schizophrenia to have predictive validity (29,51), though the six-month duration requirement was not crucial in this regard (52). When examined, the schizophreniform disorder category that DSM-III offers to define illnesses of briefer duration (two weeks to six months) has generated less certain data. Coryell and Tsuang found outcomes in this group that were intermediate between schizophrenic and affective disorder and suggested shortening the duration criteria (24). Fogelson et al. (37), however, found the group to more closely represent a subset of affective disorder. Pope et al. (103) reported similar findings for patients diagnosed as schizoaffective. The absence of diagnostic criteria for this latter group in DSM-III has been widely lamented (65), as has the absence of implications for treatment for schizophrenia and the "schizophreniclike" illnesses in DSM-III (131). Despite failing to solve these and other schizophrenia-related problems, DSM-III has at least made a contribution to the quality and quantity of research in this important area.

Affective Disorders

Concepts of affective disorders have a long evolutionary history (7), with important contributions from many of the major figures in psychiatry (105). The frequency of affective disorders in the general population and psychiatric practice makes accurate assessment all the more compelling.

Most classification efforts have utilized dichotomies, with the primary-secondary distinction being popular (1,136). DSM-III explicitly incorporates a unipolar-bipolar dichotomy and implies a major-minor distinction (major depression versus dysthymic disorder, bipolar versus cyclothymic disorder). Van Praag (133) suggests that this at least has helped bring order out of chaos, and certainly much research has been stimulated as a result. Validation efforts have been numerous (9,14,23,96,127,147) and generally supportive of the DSM-III approach. While refinement and some restructuring of the categories are likely in the future, this section of the manual has held up well.

Anxiety and Somatoform Disorders

The "dismantling" of the neuroses carried out in DSM-III and the emergence of the anxiety and somatoform disorder sections are directly related phenomena. Most of the neuroses of DSM-II are included here.

The reliability for the new anxiety disorder categories has been supported (25). More important, the separation of panic from generalized anxiety disorder, long argued on the basis of different treatment indications, appears valid (104). Another generally lauded feature of this section of the manual is the "rediscovery" of trauma-related psychopathology now described as post-traumatic stress disorder (47). Experience with Vietnam veterans was obviously important in this regard, and in turn the recognition of this entity has been helpful, especially to the Veterans Administration, in assessing and treating this challenging patient group.

Hyler and Sussman (53), in their 1984 review of somatoform disorders before and after DSM-III, provide a thorough evaluation of the literature in this area. Although less "hard" research is available on these disorders compared to other common psychiatric conditions, they suggest that evidence for the validity of at least somatization disorder is quite solid. A more recent report is similarly supportive of the validity of DSM-III criteria for hypochondriasis (11). Further research on the other conditions in this group is clearly necessary. As is the case with the anxiety disorders, satisfaction with the current scheme is by no means universal, and future modifications are likely.

Personality Disorders

One of the principal reasons that a multiaxial format was adopted in DSM-III was to highlight the importance of the personality disorders. Placing them on a separate axis was designed to ensure that they not be overlooked when attending to the often more florid Axis I disorders. In this regard, DSM-III has generally been judged a success.

Nonetheless, many long-standing conceptual and procedural problems related to the personality disorders persist in DSM-III. These problems, which include the lack of clear boundaries demarcating the personality disorders from normal behavior and from one another, are well reviewed by Frances (39). Contradictions introduced by competing categorical and dimensional paradigms remain (138). Not surprisingly, reliability has been lower with this group of diagnoses (88). Some support for the validity of the DSM-III definitions has been forthcoming, however (26), and little interest has been expressed in abandoning the search for better criteria (74).

Again, the quantity of research stimulated at least in part by DSM-III has been impressive. Much of this has focused on the more recently incorporated categories of borderline and schizotypal personality disorder. Although reviews of the definitions chosen for these diagnoses by DSM-III have been mixed (45,50,82,97,99,101,113), inclusion of these somewhat controversial categories has generally been regarded as helpful for both clinical and research purposes. Meanwhile, other lines of inquiry may well lead to the emergence of additional entities, such as masochistic or self-defeating personality disorder (58), in future versions of the DSM. The state of flux in diagnostic convention is likely to remain very much in evidence in this still troublesome group of disorders.

Other Specific Features

Many other features and categories included in DSM-III are deserving of review. Among these are the implications for consultation-liaison psychiatry and psychosomatic medicine contained particularly in the Axis III concept (78,84,87), and the more thorough approach taken to psychosexual dysfunction. Adjustment disorders have also been seen as more adequately described in DSM-III (8), and the volume of literature on ego-dystonic homosexuality is impressive (12,118). Nonetheless, in the interests of eventually bringing this chapter to a close, these additional issues will be left to other reviews. The final section of the present evaluation will instead be confined to a brief review of DSM-III's acceptance in America and abroad and some conclusions about its overall successes and shortcomings.

ACCEPTANCE IN THE UNITED STATES

DSM-III's best-seller status, mentioned earlier in this chapter, is one measure of its acceptance in the United States. Another is its virtually universal utilization in public psychiatric institutions despite problems caused by a design so different from that of its predecessor (81).

Teaching and learning DSM-III has been easier than expected (115), assisted by a variety of specially developed teaching aids (124,135). The impact on residency training has been considerable and generally positive (142). Residents and their teachers appreciate the common language that DSM-III provides and feel that it contributes to learning basic psychopathology. On the negative side, a mechanistic "cookbook" approach to assessment can be fostered. The comprehensiveness of DSM-III can also help sustain the illusion that far more is known about the mental disorders than is actually the case (142). Overall, however, teaching difficulties predicted by Cooper and Michels (22) in their early review of DSM-III have for the most part not materialized.

Clinicians have responded to DSM-III with varying degrees of enthusiasm, as would be expected. The difference between psychiatrists and other mental health professionals in this regard has not been striking (93). In a recent survey, 35 % of practicing psychiatrists and 20 % of residents did say they would stop using it if it were not required (55). These individuals were among the most skeptical about the validity of DSM-III criteria. They were also most concerned about losing a deeper understanding of patient problems in the quest for detailing more superficial phenomena. On the other hand, DSM-III's acceptance by a majority of practitioners and by an even larger percentage of residents suggests that it will not in fact become "a psychiatric Concorde" (65).

INTERNATIONAL PERSPECTIVES

Transcultural issues in psychiatric diagnosis have been raised earlier in this chapter, and some comments from abroad specifically on DSM-III have already been included (65,95). What seems most impressive here is the magnitude of interest in DSM-III expressed by the international community.

Much of this response has been gathered in an interesting volume entitled, appropriately enough, *International Perspectives on DSM-III* (126). This book is quite thorough in its coverage of world opinion, and reviewing this extensive collection would well reward any student of psychiatric nosology. General as well as regional perspectives are offered, as well as a summary of empirical studies that had been completed by the early 1980s on a variety of reliability and validity issues.

The overall tone of these assessments is positive despite the elaboration of a long list of criticisms. DSM-III's descriptive approach is often found valuable, though its departures from traditional nosological concepts such as neurosis are frequently regretted. Some critics feel that DSM-III is contaminated by etiological assumptions beyond the awareness of its architects, while others argue that current knowledge regarding etiology is insufficiently incorporated in the manual. The adoption of a multiaxial approach is generally praised, though the actual structure of the axes selected is widely criticized. The inclusion of diagnostic criteria is also seen as a major advance, but the validity of the criteria selected is questioned in many cases. Some categories, such as the affective disorders, are now seen as too broad, while others, such as schizophrenia, are felt to be overly restrictive. The absence of some conditions that have a high degree of cultural determination is noted, as are the difficulties of applying such a complex system in Third World countries. The consensus that emerges, however, is that DSM-III has helped more than hindered progress toward a more legitimate and useful psychiatric nomenclature. Ultimately future revisions of the International Classification of Diseases may reflect this worldwide response, despite the ICD's inherent conservatism.

CONCLUSION

Much of the international commentary outlined here is, of course, in line with the domestic criticism that has been the subject of much of this chapter. Opinion remains varied as to how well DSM-III has met the goals set for it by its own architects, let alone those that have been suggested by a variety of other constituencies within the specialty. Although in general the adoption of diagnostic criteria and a multiaxial format has certainly been widely applauded, many particulars of the criteria and axes actually selected have received equally widespread criticism. The ambitious scope of the document and its resulting complexity certainly provide many opportunities for disagreement. This is true even for those who welcome the major changes it incorporates. For those less sympathetic to a descriptive approach that eschews etiological theories and features instead adynamic symptom lists and a complicated multiaxial format, DSM-III is an even greater assault on diagnostic sensibilities.

Some, but certainly not all, of the current conflict and controversy over DSM-III can be resolved by further research. The structure of the document lends itself readily to change, and a work group to supervise such a process has been in place virtually since the ink on DSM-III began drying. In looking ahead to DSM-IV and beyond, it seems safe to predict both the retention of DSM-III's major features and the revision of many of its details. From the outset DSM-III was designed to be a state-of-the-art expression of psychiatric diagnostic knowledge. Its successors, in turn, will reflect whatever advancements are possible in that knowledge. Data and not debate may indeed become the basis for most diagnostic decision making. Certainly this was attempted in DSM-III, and the revisions that follow may eventually be even more successful in this regard. Perhaps this will prove DSM-III's most valuable legacy.

REFERENCES

1. AKISKAL, H. S., ROSENTHAL, R. H., ROSENTHAL, T. L., et al. (1979). Differentiation of primary affective illness from situational, symptomatic, and secondary depressions. *Archives of General Psychiatry, 36,* 635.

2. ALEXANDER, F. G., & SELESNICK, S. T. (1966). *The history of psychiatry*. New York: Harper & Row.
3. ALLEN, J. R. (1980). DSM-III: Leaving the darkness unobscured. *Oklahoma State Medical Association, 73*, 343.
4. American Psychiatric Association (1952). *Diagnostic and statistical manual of mental disorders* (1st ed.). Washington, DC: American Psychiatric Association.
5. American Psychiatric Association (1968). *Diagnostic and statistical manual of mental disorders* (2nd ed.). Washington, DC: American Psychiatric Association.
6. American Psychiatric Association (1980). *Diagnostic and statistical manual of mental disorders* (3rd ed.). Washington, DC: American Psychiatric Association.
7. ANDREASEN, N. C. (1982). Concepts, diagnosis and classification. In E. S. Paykel (Ed.), *Handbook of affective disorders*. New York: Guilford Press.
8. ANDREASEN, N.C., & HOENK, P. R. (1982). The predictive value of adjustment disorders: A follow-up study. *American Journal of Psychiatry, 139*, 584.
9. ANDREASEN, N. C., SCHEFTNER, W., REICH, T., et al. (1986). The validation of the concept of endogenous depression. A family study approach. *Archives of General Psychiatry, 43*, 246.
10. BARNES, R. F., & RASKIND, M. A. (1980). DSM-III criteria and the clinical diagnosis of dementia: A nursing home study. *Journal of Gerontology, 36*, 20.
11. BARSKY, A. J., WYSHAK, G., & KLERMAN, G. L. (1986). Hypochondriasis. An evaluation of the DSM-III criteria in medical outpatients. *Archives of General Psychiatry, 43*, 493.
12. BAYER, R., & SPITZER, R. L. (1982). Edited correspondence on the status of homosexuality in DSM-III. *Journal of the History of Behavioral Science, 18*, 32.
13. BAYER, R., & SPITZER, R. L. (1985). Neurosis, psychodynamics, and DSM-III. A history of the controversy. *Archives of General Psychiatry, 42*, 187.
14. BEARDSLEE, W. R., KLERMAN, G. L., KELLER, M. B., et al. (1985). But are they cases? Validity of DSM-III major depression in children identified in a family study. *American Journal of Psychiatry, 142*, 687.
15. BECK, A. T. (1962). Reliability of psychiatric diagnoses: 1. A critique of systematic studies. *American Journal of Psychiatry, 119*, 210.
16. BECK, A. T., WARD, C. H., MENDELSON, M., et al. (1962). Reliability of psychiatric diagnoses: 2. A study of consistency of clinical judgments and ratings. *American Journal of Psychiatry, 119*, 351.
17. Book Review (1981). Diagnostic and statistical manual of mental disorders. DSM-III. *Psychological Medicine, 11*, 215.
18. BROVERMAN, I. D., BROVERMAN, D. M., CLARKSON, F. E., et al. (1970). Sex-role stereotypes and clinical judgments of mental health. *Journal of Consulting and Clinical Psychology, 34*, 1.
19. CANTWELL, D. P., MATTISON, R., RUSSELL, A. T., & WILL, L. (1979). A comparison of DSM-II and DSM-III in the diagnosis of childhood psychiatric disorders. IV. Difficulties in use, global comparison, and conclusions. *Archives of General Psychiatry, 36*, 1217.
20. CARMEN, E. H., RUSSO, N. F., & MILLER, J. B. (1981). Inequality in women's mental health: An overview. *American Journal of Psychiatry, 138*, 1319.
21. CARPENTER, W. T., STRAUSS, J. S., & MULLEH, S. (1973). Are there pathognomonic symptoms in schizophrenia? An empiric investigation of Schneider's first-rank symptoms. *Archives of General Psychiatry, 28*, 847.
22. COOPER, A. M., & MICHELS, R. (1981). DSM-III: An American view (Book Forum). *American Journal of Psychiatry, 138*, 128.
23. CORYELL, W., GAFFNEY, G., & BURKHARDT, P. E. (1982). DSM-III melancholia and the primary-secondary distinction: A comparison of concurrent validity by means of the dexamethasone suppression test. *American Journal of Psychiatry, 139*, 120.
24. CORYELL, W., & TSUANG, M. T. (1982). DSM-III schizophreniform disorder. Compari-

sons with schizophrenia and affective disorder. *Archives of General Psychiatry, 38,* 66.

25. Di Nardo, P. A., O'Brien, G. T., Barlow, D. H., et al. (1983). Reliability of DSM-III anxiety disorder categories using a new structured interview. *Archives of General Psychiatry, 40,* 1070.

26. Drake, R. E., & Vaillant, G. E. (1985). A validity study of axis II of DSM-III. *American Journal of Psychiatry, 142,* 553.

27. Earls, F. (1982). Application of DSM-III in an epidemiological study of preschool children. *American Journal of Psychiatry, 139,* 242.

28. Ellison, J. M. (1984). DSM-III and the diagnosis of organic mental disorders. *Annals of Emergency Medicine, 13,* 521.

29. Endicott, J., Nee, J., Cohen, J., et al. (1986). Diagnosis of schizophrenia. Prediction of short-term outcome. *Archives of General Psychiatry, 43,* 13.

30. Essen-Moller, E. (1971). Suggestions for further improvement of the international classification of mental disorders. *Psychological Medicine, 1,* 308.

31. Essen-Moller, E., & Wolhfahrt, S. (1947). Suggestions for the amendment for the official Swedish classification of mental disorders. *Acta Psychiatrica Scandinavica, 47* (Suppl), 551.

32. Eysenck, H. J. (1970). A dimensional system of psychodiagnostics. In A. R. Mahrer (Ed.), *New approaches to personality classification.* London: Columbia University Press.

33. Eysenck, H. J., Wakefield, J. A., & Friedman, A. F. (1983). Diagnosis and clinical assessment: The DSM-III. *Annual Review of Psychology, 34,* 167.

34. Feighner, J. P. (1979). Nosology: A voice for a systematic data-oriented approach. *American Journal of Psychiatry, 136,* 1173.

35. Feighner, J. P., Robins, E., & Guze, S. B. (1972). Diagnostic criteria for use in psychiatric research. *Archives of General Psychiatry, 26,* 57.

36. Fleck, S. (1983). A holistic approach to family typology and the axes of DSM-III. *Archives of General Psychiatry, 40,* 901.

37. Fogelson, D. L., Cohen, B. M., & Pope, H. G. (1982). A study of DSM-III's schizophreniform disorder. *American Journal of Psychiatry, 139,* 1281.

38. Fox, H. A. (1983). The DSM-III concept of organic brain syndrome. *British Journal of Psychiatry, 142,* 419.

39. Frances, A. (1980). The DSM-III personality disorders section: A commentary. *American Journal of Psychiatry, 137,* 1050.

40. Frances, A., Clarkin, J. F., & Perry, S. (1984). DSM-III and family therapy. *American Journal of Psychiatry, 141,* 406.

41. Frances, A., & Cooper, A. M. (1981). Descriptive and dynamic psychiatry: A perspective on DSM-III. *American Journal of Psychiatry, 138,* 1198.

42. Garmezy, N. (1978). DSM-III: Never mind the psychologists: Is it good for the children? *Clinical Psychology, 32,* 4.

43. Gift, T. E., Strauss, J. S., Ritzler, B. A., et al. (1980). How diagnostic concepts of schizophrenia differ. *Journal of Nervous and Mental Disease, 168,* 3.

44. Goldstein, W. N. (1983). DSM-III and the diagnosis of schizophrenia. *American Journal of Psychotherapy, 37,* 168.

45. Goldstein, W. N. (1983). DSM-III and the diagnosis of borderline. *American Journal of Psychotherapy, 37,* 312.

46. Gove, W. R., & Tudor, J. (1973). Adult sex roles and mental illness. *American Journal of Sociology, 73,* 812.

47. Green, B. L., Lindy, J. D., & Grace, M. C. (1985). Post traumatic stress disorder. Toward DSM-IV. *Journal of Nervous and Mental Disease, 173,* 406.

48. Grinker, R. R. (1977). The inadequacies of contemporary psychiatric diagnosis. In V. M. Rakoff, H. C. Stancer, & H. B. Kedward (Eds.), *Psychiatric diagnosis.* New York: Brunner/Mazel.

49. Guze, S. (1970). The need for tough mindedness in psychiatric thinking. *Southern Medical Journal, 63*, 662.

50. Hamilton, N. G., Green, H. J., Mech, A. W., et al. (1984). Borderline personality: DSM-III versus a previous usage. *Bulletin of the Menninger Clinic, 48*, 540.

51. Helzer, J. E., Brockington, I. F., & Kendell, R. E. (1981). Predictive validity of DSM-III and Feighner definitions of schizophrenia. A comparison with Research Diagnostic Criteria and CATEGO. *Archives of General Psychiatry, 38*, 791.

52. Helzer, J. E., Kendell, R. E., & Brockington, I. F. (1983). Contribution of the six-month criterion to the predictive validity of the DSM-III definition of schizophrenia. *Archives of General Psychiatry, 40*, 1277.

53. Hyler, S. E., & Sussman, N. (1984). Somatoform disorders: Before and after DSM-III. *Hospital and Community Psychiatry, 35*, 469.

54. Hyler, S. E., Williams, J. B. W., & Spitzer, R. L. (1982). Reliability in the DSM-III field trials. Interview versus case summary. *Archives of General Psychiatry, 39*, 1275.

55. Jampala, V. C., Sierles, F. S., & Taylor, M. A. (1986). Consumers' views of DSM-III: Attitudes and practices of U.S. psychiatrists and 1984 graduating psychiatric residents. *American Journal of Psychiatry, 143*, 148.

56. Kaplan, M. (1983). A woman's view of DSM-III. *American Psychology, 38*, 786.

57. Karasu, T. B., & Skodol, A. E. (1980). VIth axis for DSM-III: Psychodynamic evaluation. *American Journal of Psychiatry, 137*, 607.

58. Kass, F., MacKinnon, R. A., & Spitzer, R. L. (1986). Masochistic personality: An empirical study. *American Journal of Psychiatry, 143*, 216.

59. Kass, F., Spitzer, R. L., & Williams, J. B. W. (1983). An empirical study of the issues of sex bias in the diagnostic criteria of DSM-III axis II personality disorders. *American Psychology, 38*, 799.

60. Katz, M. M., Cole, J. O., & Lowery, H. A. (1969). Studies of the diagnostic process: The influence of symptom perception, past experience, and ethnic background on diagnostic decisions. *American Journal of Psychiatry, 125*, 109.

61. Kelly, J. A. (1983). Sex role stereotypes and mental health: Conceptual models in the 1970's and issues for the 1980's. In V. Franks & E. D. Rothblum (Eds.), *The stereotyping of women: Its effects on mental health.* New York: Springer.

62. Kendell, R. E. (1973). Psychiatric diagnoses: A study of how they are made. *British Journal of Psychiatry, 122*, 437.

63. Kendell, R. E. (1975). *The role of diagnosis in psychiatry.* Oxford: Blackwell Scientific Publications.

64. Kendell, R. E. (1975). Defining diagnostic criteria for research purposes. In P. Sainsbury & N. Kreitman (Eds.), *Methods in psychiatric research* (2nd ed.) Oxford: Oxford University Press.

65. Kendell, R. E. (1980). DSM-III: A British perspective (Book Forum). *American Journal of Psychiatry, 137*, 1630.

66. Kendell, R. E. (1981). The International Classification and the diagnoses of English psychiatrists 1968–1980. *British Journal of Psychiatry, 139*, 177.

67. Kendell, R. E. (1982). The choice of diagnostic criteria for biological research. *Archives of General Psychiatry, 39*, 1334.

68. Kendell, R. E., & Brockington, I. F. (1980). The identification of disease entities and the relationship between schizophrenic and affective psychoses. *British Journal of Psychiatry, 137*, 324.

69. Kendell, R. E., Brockington, I. F., & Leff, J. P. (1979). Prognostic implications of six alternative definitions of schizophrenia. *Archives of General Psychiatry, 36*, 25.

70. Kendell, R. E., & Gourlay, J. (1970). The clinical distinction between the affective psychoses and schizophrenia. *British Journal of Psychiatry, 117*, 261.

71. Klein, D. F. (1978). A proposed definition of mental illness. In R. L. Spitzer & D. F. Klein (Eds.), *Critical issues in psychiatric diagnosis.* New York: Raven Press.

72. KLERMAN, G. L. (1978). Evolution of a scientific nosology. In J. Shershow (Ed.), *Schizophrenia*. Cambridge: Harvard University Press.
73. KLERMAN, G. L., VAILLANT, G. E., SPITZER. R. L., & MICHELS, R. (1984). A debate on DSM-III. *American Journal of Psychiatry, 141*, 539.
74. KOENIGSBERG, H. W., KAPLAN, R. D., GILMORE, M. M., & COOPER, A. M. (1985). The relationship between syndrome and personality disorder in DSM-III: Experience with 2,462 patients. *American Journal of Psychiatry 142*, 207.
75. KRAMER, M., ZUBIN, J., COOPER, J. E., et al. (1969). Cross-national study of diagnosis of the mental disorders. *American Journal of Psychiatry, 125* (suppl.), 1.
76. KREITMAN, N. (1961). The reliability of psychiatric diagnosis. *Journal of Mental Science, 107*, 876.
77. KREITMAN, N., SAINSBURY, P., MORRISSEY, J., et al. (1961). The reliability of psychiatric assessment: An analysis. *Journal of Mental Science, 107*, 887.
78. LINN, L., & SPITZER, R. L. (1982). DSM-III: Implications for liaison psychiatry and psychosomatic medicine. *Journal of the American Medical Association, 247*, 3207.
79. LIPKOWITZ, M. H., & IDUPUGANTI, S. (1985). Diagnosing schizophrenia in 1982: The effect of DSM-III. *American Journal of Psychiatry, 142*, 634.
80. LIPOWSKI, S. J. (1980). A new look at organic brain syndromes. *American Journal of Psychiatry, 137*, 674.
81. LIPTON, A. A., & WEINSTEIN, A. S. (1981). Implementing DSM-III in New York State mental health facilities. *Hospital and Community Psychiatry, 32*, 616.
82. MCGLASHIN, T. H. (1983). The borderline syndrome. I. Testing three diagnostic systems. *Archives of General Psychiatry, 40*, 1311.
83. MCKEGNEY, F. P. (1982). DSM-III: A definite advance, but the struggle continues. *General Hospital Psychiatry, 4*, 281.
84. MCKEGNEY, F. P., MCMAHON, T., & KING, J. (1983). The use of DSM-III in a general hospital consultation-liaison service. *General Hospital Psychiatry, 5*, 115.
85. MCLEMORE, C. W., & BENJAMIN, L. S. (1979). Whatever happened to interpersonal diagnosis? A psychosocial alternative to DSM-III. *American Psychologist, 34*, 17.
86. MCREYNOLDS, W. T. (1979). DSM-III and the future of applied social science. *Professional Psychology, 10*, 123.
87. MACKENZIE, T. B., POPKIN, M. K., & CALLIES, A. L. (1983). Clinical applications of DSM-III in consultation-liaison psychiatry. *Hospital and Community Psychiatry, 34*, 628.
88. MELLSOP, G., VARGHESE, F., JOSHUA, S., & HICKS, A. (1982). The reliability of Axis II of DSM-III. *American Journal of Psychiatry, 139*, 1360.
89. MENNINGER, K. (1963). *The vital balance: The life processes in mental health and illness*. New York: Viking.
90. MEZZICH, J. E. (1979). Patterns and issues in multiaxial psychiatric diagnosis. *Psychological Medicine, 9*, 125.
91. MILLON, T. (1983). The DSM-III: Some historical and substantive reflections. In N. Endler & J. McV. Hunt (Eds.), *Personality and the behavioral disorders* (2nd ed.). New York: Wiley.
92. MILLON, T. (1983). The DSM-III: An insider's perspective. *American Psychology, 38*, 304.
93. MOREY, L. C. (1980). Differences between psychologists and psychiatrists in the use of DSM-III. *American Journal of Psychiatry, 137*, 1123.
94. MORPHY, M. A. (1982). DSM-III and the future orientation of American psychiatry. *Psychological Medicine, 12*, 241.
95. MURRAY, R. M. (1979). A reappraisal of American psychiatry. *Lancet, 1*, 255.
96. NELSON, J. C., CHARNEY, D. S., & QUINLAN, D. M. (1981). Evaluation of the DSM-III criteria for melancholia. *Archives of General Psychiatry, 38*, 555.

97. NUETZEL, E. J. (1985). DSM-III and the use of the term borderline. *Bulletin of the Menninger Clinic, 49*, 124.
98. OTTOSSON, J. O., & PERRIS, C. (1973). Multidimensional classification of mental disorders. *Psychological Medicine, 3*, 238.
99. PERRY, J. C., O'CONNELL, M. E., & DRAKE, R. (1984). An assessment of the Schedule for Schizotypal personalities and the DSM-III criteria for diagnosing schizotypal personality disorder. *Journal of Nervous and Mental Disease, 172*, 674.
100. PFOHL, B. (1980). Effects of clinical experience on rating DSM-III symptoms of schizophrenia. *Comprehensive Psychiatry, 21*, 233.
101. POPE, H. G., JONAS, J. M., HUDSON, J. I., et al. (1983). The validity of DSM-III borderline personality disorder. A phenomenologic, family history, treatment response, and long-term follow-up study. *Archives of General Psychiatry, 40*, 23.
102. POPE, H. G., & LIPINSKI, J. F. (1978). Diagnosis in schizophrenia and manic depressive illness. A reassessment of the specificity of "schizophrenic" symptoms in the light of current research. *Archives of General Psychiatry, 35*, 811.
103. POPE, H. G., LIPINSKI, J. F., COHEN, B. M., & AXELROD, D. T. (1980). "Schizoaffective disorder": An invalid diagnosis? A comparison of schizoaffective disorder, schizophrenia and affective disorder. *American Journal of Psychiatry, 137*, 921.
104. RASKIN, M., PEEKE, H. V. S., DICKMAN, W., & PINSKER, H. (1982). Panic and generalized anxiety disorders. Developmental antecedents and precipitants. *Archives of General Psychiatry, 39*, 687.
105. ROTH, M. (1960). Depressive states and their borderlands: Classification, diagnosis and treatment. *Comprehensive Psychiatry, 1*, 135.
106. ROUNSAVILLE, B. J., SPITZER, R. L., & WILLIAMS, J. B. W. (1986). Proposed changes in DSM-III's substance use disorders: Description and rationale. *American Journal of Psychiatry, 143*, 463.
107. RUSSELL, A. T., MATTISON, R., & CANTWELL, D. P. (1983). DSM-III and the clinical practice of child psychiatry. *Journal of Clinical Psychiatry, 44*, 86.
108. RUTTER, M., & SHAFFER, D. (1980). DSM-III. A step forward or back in terms of the classification of child psychiatric disorders? *Journal of the American Academy of Child Psychiatry, 19*, 371.
109. SANDIFER, M. G., HORDERN, A., TIMBURY, G. C. & GREEN, L. M. (1968). Psychiatric diagnosis: A comparative study in North Carolina, London and Glasgow. *British Journal of Psychiatry, 114*, 1.
110. SCHACHT, T. E. (1985). DSM-III and the politics of truth. *American Psychologist, 40*, 513.
111. SCHACHT, T. E., & NATHAN, P. E. (1977). But is it good for the psychologists? Appraisal and status of DSM-III. *American Psychologist, 32*, 1017.
112. SCHOVER, L. R., FRIEDMAN, J. M., WEILER, S. J., et al. (1982). Multiaxial problem-oriented system for sexual dysfunctions. An alternative to DSM-III. *Archives of General Psychiatry, 39*, 614.
113. SIEVER, L. J., & GUNDERSON, J. G. (1983). The search for a schizotypal personality: Historical origins and current status. *Comprehensive Psychiatry, 24*, 199.
114. SILVERSTEIN, M. L., WARREN, R. A., HARROW, M., et al. (1982). Changes in diagnosis from DSM-II to the Research Diagnostic Criteria and DSM-III. *American Journal of Psychiatry, 139*, 366.
115. SKODOL, A. E., SPITZER, R. L., & WILLIAMS, J. B. W. (1981). Teaching and learning DSM-III. *American Journal of Psychiatry, 138*, 1581.
116. SMITH, D., & KRAFT, W. A. (1983). DSM-III: Do psychologists really want an alternative? *American Psychologist, 38*, 777.
117. SPITZER, R. L. (1985). DSM-III and the politics-science dichotomy syndrome. *American Psychologist, 40*, 522.
118. SPITZER, R. L. (1981). The diagnostic status of homosexuality in DSM-III: A reformulation of the issues. *American Journal of Psychiatry, 138*, 210.

119. SPITZER, R. L., & ENDICOTT, J. (1978). Medical and mental disorder: Proposed definition and criteria. In R. L. Spitzer & D. F. Klein (Eds.), *Critical issues in psychiatric diagnosis.* New York: Raven Press.
120. SPITZER, R. L., ENDICOTT, J., & ROBINS, E. (1975). Clinical criteria for psychiatric diagnosis and DSM-III. *American Journal of Psychiatry, 132,* 1187.
121. SPITZER, R. L., ENDICOTT, J., & ROBINS, E. (1978). Research Diagnostic Criteria: Rationale and reliability. *Archives of General Psychiatry, 35,* 773.
122. SPITZER, R. L., & FORMAN, J. B. W. (1979). DSM-III field trials: II. Initial experience with the multiaxial system. *American Journal of Psychiatry, 136,* 818.
123. SPITZER, R. L., FORMAN, J. B. W., & NEE, J. (1979). DSM-III field trials: I. Initial interrator diagnostic reliability. *American Journal of Psychiatry, 136,* 815.
124. SPITZER, R. L., SKODOL, A. E., GIBB, M., et al. (1981). *DSM-III case book.* Washington, DC: American Psychiatric Association.
125. SPITZER, R. L., WILLIAMS, J. B. W., & SKODOL, A. E. (1980). DSM-III: The major achievements and an overview. *American Journal of Psychiatry, 137,* 151.
126. SPITZER, R. L., WILLIAMS, J. B. W. & SKODOL, A. E. (1983). *International perspectives on DSM-III.* Washington, DC: American Psychiatric Press.
127. STEWART, J. W., MCGRATH, P. J., LIEBOWITZ, M. R., et al. (1985). Treatment outcome validation of DSM-III depressive subtypes. Clinical usefulness in outpatients with mild to moderate depression. *Archives of General Psychiatry, 42,* 1148.
128. STROBER, M., GREEN, J., & CARLSON, G. (1981). Reliability of psychiatric diagnosis and hospitalized adolescents. Interrator agreement using DSM-III. *Archives of General Psychiatry, 38,* 141.
129. STROMGREN, E. (1983). The strengths and weaknesses of DSM-III. In R. L. Spitzer, J. B. W. Williams, & A. E. Skodol (Eds.), *International perspectives on DSM-III.* Washington, DC: American Psychiatric Press.
130. SZASZ, T. S. (1974). *The myth of mental illness: Foundation of a theory of personal conduct* (rev. ed.). New York: Harper & Row.
131. TAMMINGA, C. A., & CARPENTER, W. T. (1982). The DSM-III diagnosis of schizophrenic-like illness and the clinical pharmacology of psychosis. *Journal of Nervous and Mental Disease, 170,* 744.
132. TREECE, C. (1982). DSM-III as a research tool. *American Journal of Psychiatry, 139,* 577.
133. VAN PRAAG, H. M. (1982). A transatlantic view of the diagnosis of depressions according to the DSM-III. II. Did the DSM-III solve the problem of depression diagnosis? *Comprehensive Psychiatry, 23,* 330.
134. WARD, C. H., BECK, A. T., MENDELSON, M., et al. (1962). The psychiatric nomenclature. Reasons for diagnostic disagreement. *Archives of General Psychiatry, 7,* 198.
135. WEBB, L. J., DiCLEMENTE, C. C., JOHNSTONE, E. E., et al. (Eds.). (1981). *DSM-III training guide.* New York: Brunner/Mazel.
136. WEISSMAN, M. M., POTTENGER, M., KLEBER, H., et al. (1977). Symptom patterns in primary and secondary depression. *Archives of General Psychiatry, 34,* 854.
137. WERRY, J. S., METHVEN, R. J., FITZPATRICK, J. & DICKSON, H. (1983). The interrater reliability of DSM-III in children. *Journal of Abnormal Child Psychology, 11,* 341.
138. WIDIGER, T. A., & FRANCES, A. (1985). The DSM-III personality disorders. Perspectives from psychology. *Archives of General Psychiatry, 42,* 615.
139. WILLIAMS, J. B. W. (1985). The multiaxial system of DSM-III: Where did it come from and where should it go? I. Its origins and critiques. *Archives of General Psychiatry, 42,* 175.
140. WILLIAMS, J. B. W. (1985). The multiaxial system of DSM-III: Where did it come from and where should it go? II. Empirical studies, innovations, and recommendations. *Archives of General Psychiatry, 42,* 181.
141. WILLIAMS, J. B. W., & SPITZER, R. L. (1983). The issue of sex bias in DSM-III. *American Psychologist, 38,* 793.

142. WILLIAMS, J. B. W., SPITZER, R. L., & SKODOL, A. E. (1985). DSM-III and residency training: Results of a national survey. *American Journal of Psychiatry, 142,* 755.
143. WING, L. (1970). Observations on the psychiatric section of the International Classification of Diseases and the British Glossary of Mental Disorders. *Psychological Medicine, 1,* 79.
144. WOLBERG, L. R. (1979). DSM-III and the taxonomic stew. *Journal of the American Academy of Psychoanalysis, 7,* 143.
145. World Health Organization (1977). *International classification of diseases* (9th rev.). Geneva: WHO.
146. WORTIS, J. (1982). DSM-III: The big debate. *Biological Psychiatry, 17,* 1363.
147. ZIMMERMAN, M., CORYELL, W., PFOHL, B., & STANGL, D. (1986). The validity of four definitions of endogenous depression. II. Clinical, demographic, familial and psychosocial correlates. *Archives of General Psychiatry, 43,* 234.
148. ZIMMERMAN, M., PFOHL, B., STANGL, D., & CORYELL, W. (1985). The validity of DSM-III axis IV (Severity of psychosocial stressors). *American Journal of Psychiatry, 142,* 1437.
149. ZUBIN, J. (1967). Classification of the behavior disorders. *Annual Review of Psychology, 18,* 373.
150. ZUBIN, J. (1977). But is it good for science? *Clinical Psychology, 31,* 5.

3

SYSTEMS THEORY IN PSYCHIATRY

WILLIAM GRAY, M.D., L.F.A.P.A.

Private Practice of Psychiatry,
Newton Center, Massachusetts

INTRODUCTION

Problems of Compatibility

Systems theory and psychiatry have not proven to be as compatible as was expected and hoped for in their initial formal introduction to each other in the 1960s when those of us who are both psychiatrists and systems theorists were invited to present programs at the annual meetings of the American Psychiatric Association in 1966, 1967, and 1968. The papers presented at these meetings were brought together in a 1969 publication, *General Systems Theory and Psychiatry* (14). The reasons for this incompatibility are interesting, instructive, and, to those who have been active in both areas, rather discouraging. In their own right both psychiatry and systems theory are and will remain active fields of human endeavor, and since a more compatible relationship between the two may yet develop, a careful examination of what has gone wrong in the relationship will constitute the major focus of this chapter. This is the third time I have been asked to prepare a chapter on systems theory, with the result that examining the two previous contributions (11,13) allows me the advantage of hindsight in preparing the present chapter.

Medlars search. That the state of incompatibility between systems theory and psychiatry still exists is confirmed by a Medlars search recently undertaken, utilizing all the key terms that would indicate linkage between the two fields. Over the past three years there have been only 125

44

references, the majority of which deal with physiology, neurobiology, animal research, and the use of computer-linked systems. A considerable number of studies deal with the effectiveness of DSM-III classifications; others describe the use of microcomputer systems to study drugs' effectiveness. Some 20 articles refer to the use of systems theory in the fields of family and occupational therapy. The most clear-cut evidence of congruence between the fields can be found in some 10 articles reporting on the use of personal construct theory and its relation to systems theory, particularly that of system-precursor/system-forming type. Three or four papers deal with the attempt to develop expert systems for use in medicine and psychiatry, and these stress the barriers against their development and clinical utilization, the authors ascribing this partly to the difficulty of their design.

But nowhere can one find an article reporting positively on the value of cross-fertilization between the two fields. One must add that the Medlars database did not include a number of journals in which more enthusiastic articles can be found, such as the *American Journal of Social Psychiatry*, a number of the family process journals, the *Journal of Strategic-Systemic Therapies*, and such systems theory publications as *General Systems* and *Systems Research*. But since the database deals with the usual journals read and utilized by psychiatrists, the negativity of the Medlars search is a valid indication that clinical psychiatry has not found systems theory to be of much value.

In system-precursor/system-forming language (18) the system precursor configurations of the two fields were too disparate for effective system forming to take place. In addition, the societal, political, economic, and governmental environments in which they exist have tended to promote a confrontational rather than a cooperative attitude between them. To gain an understanding of this we turn to a comparative evaluation of each of the two fields.

HISTORICAL EVOLUTION OF PSYCHIATRY AND SYSTEMS THEORY

Psychiatry

Early history. Psychiatry became recognized as a distinct and necessary profession in the 1800s, devoted initially to the diagnosis, protection, and treatment of citizens whose bizarre behavior was alien to the expected customs and mores of a society — thus the initial identity of psychiatrists as "alienists." Since there are also many people who are only partially alien in their behavior, and since many of these come from wealthy and influential families, the utilization of psychiatry rapidly expanded beyond the walls of mental institutions, and in the latter half of the 19th century its identity changed to a predominantly psychoneurological form. It became the aspect of medicine devoted to disorders of the brain and mind.

In the early 20th century its identity again shifted, primarily as a result of the introduction of Freudian theory and therapy. Psychiatry became a distinctive field separated from neurology and dealing only with the mind or psyche. Individuality was emphasized, and the norm of psychiatric treatment swung strongly to the side of an intense dyadic and confidential relationship. The psychoanalytic identity of psychiatry reached its apogee in the two decades following World War II, stimulated considerably by its adoption as the standard mode of treatment for the large number of psychiatrically disturbed veterans of that war, and so receiving governmental funding. But this period of integrated identity in psychiatry began to fade in the late 1950s and early 1960s as the limitations of its effectiveness were recognized and as governmental financial requirements for less extensive forms of therapy began to predominate.

The 20th century, particularly the latter half, has been featured by intense intellectual activity, primarily evident in, but not limited to, the areas of science and technology. There is much evidence that the human brain is best characterized as being an intensely system-forming organ (6,18). One has seen virtual blossoming of new theories of how best to model the human psyche and new schools of practice of how best to treat disorders in its functioning.

The Pavlovian concepts of stimulus-response and conditioned reflex have, through the work of B. F. Skinner, rapidly mushroomed into behavioral theory and practice. Here the Freudian view of the importance of the individual ego was reversed and the existence of the individual almost totally denied.

Recent developments. Suddenly the family was recognized as the matrix in which the individual grows and in which combinations of productive and pathological developments occur, with the result that family therapy has blossomed into a method of psychotherapy. "Psychotherapy" must now be used in a generic sense, for family therapy does not focus directly on the individual psyche, but on the patternings of familial interactions and their pathological or productive influence on the psyche of each individual member. It is in the fields of family process and family therapy that one finds the strongest evidence of a productive marriage between general systems theory and the mental health disciplines. The most striking shift from the psychoanalytic model is the abandonment of the strictly dyadic model — a shift from the dominant intrapsychic model to an interpersonal one.

A similar shift to a dominant focus on interpersonal relationships led to the new fields of group process and group therapy. Although occurring in the same time period as family therapy, they were developed by a different set of theorists and practitioners; the distinction between family therapists and group therapists remains active. Here again a productive marriage between general systems theory and group therapy developed, but not in as clear and useful a way as was the case in family therapy. This is related to the fact that family therapists deal with an already formed system, whereas group therapists must deal with system-forming processes. Systems theory for many years dealt exclusively with already formed systems, and it is only recently that attention has been paid to the origin of systems, that is, to system precursors and system-forming processes.

Psychosomatic medicine is another new development that has shattered the integrated model of psychiatry that existed in the period of psychoanalytic dominance. More recently sociosomatic medicine has developed — another differentiation and a related one.

Attempts to integrate. A new and important attempt to bring about some degree of integration in the fragmented identity of psychiatry as a science and profession centers around the concept of social psychiatry and has been institutionalized in the World Association for Social Psychiatry and its member societies, such as the American Association for Social Psychiatry. It is here that a productive marriage between psychiatry and its associated disciplines and systems theory, including its general form, is most likely, as evidenced by the decision by the American Association for Social Psychiatry to organize its 1985 Annual Meeting on the theme of "The Rapidly Escalating System-Forming/Systemic Factors Dominant in Today's World in Medical and Psychiatric Practice."

Connecting mind and brain. The redefinitions of the proper model and concern of psychiatry noted above have taken place in the area of the mind and have neglected recognition that properties of mind result from the functioning of a biological entity, the human brain. If one accepts that the human brain-mind is intensely system-forming in character, and if one accepts that the system-forming capacity is not patented or restricted to a few special individuals, but is a possession of all who have human brains, then it can be expected that system-forming activity will be applied to all areas of human life. This will inspire intellectual ferment and research leading to new and often startling models of how the universe and we, its human inhabitants, work.

Study of the human brain in the twin fields of biological psychiatry and psychopharmacology has resulted in leaps ahead in development; many consider this the primary locus of identity for the field of psychiatry. Starting with the neuroleptics and their profound, although complicated, usefulness in the treatment of psychotic states, and moving on to the discovery of effective psychopharmaceuticals for the treatment of depressive conditions and manic-depressive disorders, psychopharmacological skill has become an essential component of clinical psychiatry.

Introduction of system-precursor/system-forming concepts. Of all the areas that comprise the "new" in psychiatry, the utilization of system-precursor/system-forming concepts is most evident in the research, study, and reports of those who investigate neurotransmitter/receptor functioning. The same is true of those who are unraveling the functioning of the immune system, of viral infection, of genetic functioning and misfunctioning, of gene splicing and its potential for the correction of genetic errors, and of organ and tissue transplantation, including the brain—but in all these cases the utilization of system-precursor/system-forming terminology appears to have been an independent development without formal connection to those who identify themselves as systems theorists or practitioners.

Increasing division. The rift between biological and psychological psychiatrists has become increasingly wide and has presented a considerable dilemma to the medical schools, which must adequately prepare each student to assume the tasks of being a doctor and of specializing and, most important to our discussion, must train a doctor to be an effective psychiatrist. The attempt to establish a biopsychosocial model in teaching as a way to heal the rift between biological and psychic or relational models is meeting with success. It uses system-theoretical concepts but has developed independently of formal system-theoretical institutions and practitioners.

Systems theory makes it clear that systemic relationships always form between any series of relatively independent systems and that there is a danger of infinite expansion of the number of systems that could be considered as needing inclusion in a systems approach. This is avoided by subjective decisions as to which sets of systems are relevant and which may be disregarded. The same problem faces modern psychiatry, for the list of new models and approaches continues to expand at a rapid rate. We will mention only those we consider most relevant.

Shift to a financing ecology. In the United States, a dramatic change took place in the mid-1960s when federal financing was shifted to originating and funding interpersonally, ecologically, and multidisciplinary oriented community mental-health centers. There was a concomitant drive to shift from inpatient mental hospital care to outpatient community-oriented treatment. The community mental-health-center model was strongly linked to system-theoretical concepts developed in business and management organization theory and practice. Its commercial origins were obvious: patients were now consumers, mental-health professionals were now producers, and each center was allotted a "catchment area." Management control systems were quickly introduced to maximize cost effectiveness, and a new profession of hospital or mental-health administrators was developed.

The financial backing of such centers was provided for by the rapid development of health insurance programs, and payment of fees was now replaced by the concept and practice of "third-party payment." This was all part of Lyndon Johnson's "Great Society." Medicare was developed as a federally financed third-party payer for the elderly and disabled, and Medicaid health insurance was enacted for the care of the unemployed, the poor, and the indigent members of society.

Increasing hostility to systems concepts. This trend in health care met with considerable resistance on the part of psychiatrists and other physicians. The ideological argument was that it was destroying the doctor-patient relationship, and that the authority of the doctor in medical decision-making had been taken over by nonmedically trained managers, with profit or cost effectiveness the primary determinant. Since various systems concepts were frequently used to justify the changes that had been made, a great deal of animosity toward systems theory developed in the medical and psychiatric professions and is a major factor leading to an antagonistic rather than a productive relationship between the psychiatric and systems sciences.

The struggle over the economics of health care goes on at an increasing pace: cost control and computer systems enable third-party payers, including government, to become immediately aware of the costs of health care. The result has been the development, in the United States, of Diagnostic

Related Groups (DRGs), which limit the amount of hospital time a patient may have, and capitation schemes to cut down on the cost of care. Studies have proven that DRGs do not work out in the psychiatric area, and the result has been the expansion of for-profit chains of psychiatric hospitals. There has been much public debate over these issues, and the future of psychiatry may well be dependent on decisions about how much of the federal budget will go to psychiatric care. New diagnostic groups, such as eating disorders, have come to the fore, as have drug- and alcohol-related problems, for which special funding has developed.

The illusion of problem solving. So all this means that the complexity of the problems that face psychiatry and the medical profession continues to increase with each problem that we have solved. Here we will stop the discussion of the historical evolution of psychiatry because it ties in so very well with one of the important recent developments in the evolution of systems theory, in which system-forming and systemic concepts have been utilized by Jerzy Wojciechowski to elucidate two fundamental characteristics of the continued evolution and goals of the human knowledge process itself (24). The first is that knowledge quickly develops a life of its own, no longer under the control of the human brain-mind from which it was born. The second is that the notion of problem solution as ordinarily conceived is an illusion. It is abundantly clear that any problem solution becomes a system precursor for the system forming of more complex problems. Advancement in the human knowledge process makes it easier for our muscles, but never for our brains. And in a sense that is fair enough, for here, too, our brains, with the intensity of their system-forming characteristics, have to have new problems to work on or they will die of starvation.

Systems Theory

Early history. Systems theory had its origin in the 1930s and 1940s. Prior to that time its usage was restricted to the adjectival form "systematic," which meant that one was careful not to leave things out and careful to arrange things in an orderly fashion. Systematic approaches have developed into the field of systematics. Edward O. Wilson has stated,

> The magnitude and cause of biological diversity is not just the central problem of systematics; it is one of the key problems of science as a whole. It does matter a great deal whether there are 1 million or 30

million forms. It also matters why a certain subset exists in each region of the earth, and what is happening to each one year by year. Unless we go for the whole package, we will fall far short of understanding life, and due to the accelerating extinction of species, much of our opportunity will slip away forever. (23, p. 1057)

But systematics so described is a modern version of taxonomics and has little to do with the evolution of the modern concept of systems. The term "system" in the 1930s and 1940s came to be applied to dynamic processes in which parts somehow came together to function as a unified whole. The term "system" has its origin in the Greek language, meaning things that stand together or fall together. For the Greeks the term "stand" has the general connotation that we now apply to "understand," and so the term "system" meant situations in which a series of parts understood each other and so functioned in an integrated way; should their understanding disappear, they would fall together or become a collection of parts that no longer function.

But as with so many other of the important concepts developed by our truly protoscientific Greek ancestors, the wisdom contained in the term "system" did not come into general use. This great dynamic notion faded and 2,000 years had to pass before it was reborn and returned to our language. But as the Middle Ages turned into the Renaissance, the concept returned under different labels. With the introduction of the steam engine, the term "engine" was used, while in the biological and medical sciences equivalent labelings were "organ" and "organism." In politics and in business the most popular labeling was "organization." In manufacturing, the essence of system was called a "factory." In the area of knowledge development, the term used was "university," and the dynamic parts whose integration was being attempted were called "disciplines." One would guess that "system" was not used for new forms of dynamic organization because it had become so attached to those more passive and static forms that are implied by the term "systematic."

Introduction of systems language. Why, then, did the term "system" suddenly burst forth into very active usage in the middle part of the 20th century? Here we must return to the notion of the human brain-mind as an intensely system-forming organ that has produced the increasingly manmade world in which we exist. The most obvious area of system forming that has brought this about is science and technology. As we mentioned in the concluding paragraph of our historical review of the evolution of modern psychiatry, the "problem solutions" that have so long been the aim of our human knowledge efforts have turned out to be illusory. Problem solution, rather, serves to open the door to new and more complex problems, and the technological developments that have resulted from previous problem-solving efforts not only result in largely unforeseen side effects, but also provide us with tools that augment our capacity to see, to hear, and to understand, and thus give us the courage to tackle the new problems of increased complexity that arise.

The Double Origin of Systems Theories

Systems theory and general systems theory have distinct origins. This is of fundamental importance in understanding problems of incompatibility between systems theory and psychiatry. Systems theory is connected with the needs of the increasing complexity of industrial development, and general systems theory with the philosophically oriented work of an outstanding figure of the mid-20th century, Ludwig von Bertalanffy. These led to the rather distinct fields of mechanistic systems theory and humanistic general systems theory.

Mechanistic systems theory. The need to develop methodologies for creating highly complex structures in the field of armaments must be considered one of the origins of the system-theoretical and system-analytical movement. To construct a plant that would produce highly complex submarines or aircraft could no longer be accomplished by existing methods of manufacture. So many new skills were now required, so many consultants from increasing numbers of disciplines, so many new types of building materials, so many varieties of machines, that if they were all delivered to the same building site at the same time they could not be handled. It was obvious that extensive advance planning was required.

Quite suddenly this type of planning was christened "system planning," and our old Grecian word was restored not only to its previous splendor, but greatly enhanced. Soon systems analysis was added, and in order to make sense of what such analysis and planning brought to our attention, the field of systems theory was born. It arose from the needs of technology, was imprinted with its technological origin, and remains primarily active in technological fields.

Technologically oriented systems theory and primarily nontechnologically oriented psychiatry do not mate well, which explains the lack of fruitful collaboration between the two fields. Technologically oriented systems theory has undergone a certain degree of evolution and, in combination with computer systems, has become an integral part of the control and tracking systems of government, business, and management, including the fields of medicine and psychiatry. It has become a central tool in the planning and management of psychiatric clinics and hospitals, and in general this has led to further antagonism on the part of psychiatry.

Cybernetics — an important subdivision. A second forerunner of modern systems theory also arose in World War II from the urgent necessity for accurate antiaircraft weaponry. The resolution of this problem was the result of the work of Norbert Wiener, who developed the concept of negative feedback, which allowed for the installation of error-correcting devices on antiaircraft artillery, markedly increasing its effectiveness. Wiener elaborated the concept of negative feedback into a theory of "governors," christening it with its Greek analog, and so the field of "cybernetics" was born. Rapidly he expanded cybernetics to include all systems in which stability was maintained through error-detecting or negative-feedback mechanisms. This has proved of great value in many fields, including medicine, but its initial promise in psychiatry has not worked out, for human minds and brains are not regulated by the type of control and equilibrial states that result from negative feedback.

Humanistic or general systems theory. The father of the general systems theory field, as distinguished from the more mechanistic systems theory, is the biologist Ludwig von Bertalanffy. His first publications in the 1930s were dedicated to the elaboration of what he initially called "organismic theory" and shortly thereafter expanded into general systems theory. Although Bertalanffy trained as a biologist, it rapidly became apparent to the large group of world-class thinkers who gathered around him that the profundity and expansiveness of his knowledge demanded that he be considered a generalist, or even a genius of Renaissance Man type, for in the Renaissance, specialization and fragmentation of knowledge into disparate disciplines had not taken such a strong hold. I was fortunate enough to have become a close friend and colleague of Bertalanffy. A history of our joint work and the continuing evolution of general systems theory can be found in a number of my own publications (9,10,16).

Bertalanffy was the first to introduce the crucial concept of "nonequilibrial equilibrial states," but it has been hard to find an easily understood name for them. The term "steady state" has become standard, and gradually it is becoming widely understood to differentiate the type of equilibria that one finds in living systems from equilibria at rest, the usual connotation of the term "equilibrium." The same difficulty was encountered by the Belgian Nobel laureate chemist Ilya Prigogine, who chose the equally awkward term "dissipative systems" to indicate that such systems dissipate more entropy than they generate and thus are able to maintain nonrest type of equilibria.

Basic Bertalanffian principles. There is a wide gap between the ideological premise and proposals for use of Bertalanffy's general systems theory and technologically born systems theory, including cybernetics. As might be expected from a Renaissance-type man, Bertalanffy's general systems theory is humanistically oriented (1–4), as exemplified in his insistence that (1) general systems theory must concentrate on the unique characteristics of the human species, (2) it must be antirobotic in character and recognize that the human brain-mind is characterized by primary activity rather than the reactivity implicit in stimulus-response models, and (3) values, ethics, and morals must be included. For Bertalanffy the ultimate precept for general systems theory is the recognition that (4) all of our progress stems from the individual mind. Therefore, systems theory must not serve the leviathan of organization, for if it swallows the individual it will seal its own inevitable doom.

Congeniality between general systems theory and psychiatry. Thus Bertalanffy's general systems theory is in accord with psychiatry's respect for the individual, and so it is somewhat of a mystery as to why a more fruitful marriage between general systems theory and psychiatry has not taken place. In part this is due to the very high standards that Bertalanffy set in his insistence on an adherence to humanistic values and in the intensity of his antirobotic stand, which requires such a strong adherence to the concept of *primary activity* of the brain-mind, to the point that he even saw the strongly individually oriented approach of psychoanalysis as still resting on a reactivity model and therefore flawed. But the primary complaint of psychiatrists about general systems theory has been that it is so abstract that it is unusable in specific situations.

Modern developments in general systems theory. These points are well illustrated in a recent paper by two of our most advanced general systems theorists, Brian R. Gaines and Mildred L. G. Shaw (8). They stress that the need for general systems theory is even greater today than when Bertalanffy wrote his basic works 35 or 40 years ago. What Bertalanffy stressed was that the bringing together of the biological, behavioral, and social sciences with modern technology would necessitate a generalization of basic concepts in science and would imply the need for a new category of scientific thinking. When Bertalanffy first argued for general systems theory, much of the physical world was under the control of technology, but the biological and mental worlds had remained naturalistic. With the development of genetic engineering and fifth-generation computing systems, which processed knowledge rather than information, the areas of life and mind came into the domain of technology. Gaines and Shaw point out the important similarities in the thinking of Bertalanffy and of the psychiatrist Karl Jaspers, who believed that man is mind and is able to change the world to suit his purposes (20). Bertalanffy himself emphasized Heisenberg's insight that the object of our research is no longer nature itself, but man's investigation of nature.

But we will need new modes of thought. Bertalanffy wrote that every symbolic world that man creates, including that most abstract one that we call science, is a construct determined by innumerable biological, anthropological, linguistic, and historical factors, the only limiting condition being that the construct does not conflict too much with reality "as is." Here we run into Jaspers' view that the "as is" is increasingly under our control. Gaines and Shaw stress that this apparent contradiction does not lock us in, in view of Bertalanffy's emphasis on the significance of open systems. This becomes most cogent when we realize that the most open system of all is that of our minds, for the constructs we have made are always open to the formation of construct alternatives.

Gaines and Shaw state that the fundamental significance of Bertalanffy's general systems theory is a metasystemic viewpoint counterbalancing realism with neo-idealism. Nothing prevents the mind from inventing the real world and the laws of nature, or nature from creating systems that exhibit all the phenomena of mind. General systems theory should be able to provide foundations for both these positions. The present roadblock is that scientific training has for so long emphasized positive empiricism that the links between the sciences deriving from the characteristics of the mind in imposing meaning on the world tend to be neglected.

A general systems theory definition of "system." We come now to the matter that is puzzling to most psychiatrists, and yet essential as our technology proceeds and extends our ability to shape and control life and mind as well as the physical world. Gaines has evolved a puzzling and simple definition of system: "What is distinguished is a system" (7). Previously he used this definition to distinguish a general system from specific systems. But now he is more blunt and uses this as the definition of system itself.

To make general systems theory understandable and useful to psychiatry and others it is necessary to elaborate on why Gaines defined "system" in such a way. There are two main precursors to his line of thought. The first is the 1969 publication of G. S. Brown's *Laws of Form* (5), which focuses on distinction making in the function of the human brain-mind and the logical calculus that derives therefrom. Briefly, Brown's argument is that a universe comes into being when a space is severed or taken apart, that is, when a distinction is made. What Brown found was that by tracing the way in which we do such a severance we can reconstruct with an uncanny accuracy and extensiveness the basic forms underlying linguistic, mathematical, physical, and biological sciences and see how the familiar laws of our own experience follow inexorably from the original act of severance. Gaines posits that such a reconstruction of the basic forms underlying any culture from the distinctions it makes can be regarded as the foundations of general systems theory.

The second significant precursor lies in the work of the Boston psychologist G. A. Kelly, in his 1955 publication of *The Psychology of Personal Constructs* (21). Gaines and Shaw emphasize the equivalence of Brown's term "distinction" with Kelly's term "construct." Our present interpretations of the universe are the result, then, of a series of personal constructs (distinctions) that we and our surrounding culture have made. Thus Kelly agrees with Bertalanffy's view that the symbolic worlds in which we live are constructs. By indicating their personal nature, Kelly more strongly emphasizes the role of choice and thus the possibility of revision and replacement, giving his theory the title of "constructive alternativism." No one, therefore, needs to be a victim of his biography or circumstances.

Through analyzing the distinctions made, it is possible to account for the formal and psychological foundations of a culture, including science and technology. A new approach to solving problems ensues from making explicit the systems of distinctions underlying problems and changing them appropriately. From these two positions of distinction making and constructive alternativism, Gaines and Shaw develop a general systems theory that fulfills the requirements suggested by Bertalanffy. They proceed along two pathways, the first dealing with explication of the formal development of the two theories, and the second illustrating the derivation of existing systems theories from them. Gaines explains that whenever we distinguish any set of things as distinct from another set we have, perhaps not realizing it, declared a degree of coherence to exist between those things existing on either side of our line of distinction. Thus we have added a new characteristic and so increased complexity.

My own view is in considerable agreement with that of Gaines and Shaw, but is different from theirs in my belief that a system-forming act must be included as a third feature. Otherwise the coherences on either side of the distinction line leading, with further acts of distinction, to system formings of great complexity will be divisive: the world will divide into nations, cultures, disciplines, sciences, and technologies that never understand each other. Thus it is essential to add system-forming acts between the universes that we have walled off from one another. Without bridging system-forming acts, each of the separated universes will increasingly lock into itself and increasingly lock out universes on the other side of the distinction line, and we will have increasingly dangerous wars and strife, leading to world cataclysm (19).

CONCLUSIONS AND IMPLICATIONS

Psychiatry and General Systems Theory — Distinctions and System Formings

Certainly there is a connectedness in the emphasis of both general systems theory and psychiatry on the central importance of the individual. Certainly also there is recognition in both that the individual exists in a variety of social matrices whose form and shape are and continue to be determined by a large number and variety of distinctions—physical, biological, and mental—some accompanied by system formings and some not, and that there are particular aspects of mental life that link us with others, not only in the present, but extending backward historically in the form of education, traditions, cultures, and national boundaries. There are also physical precursors, natural forces that have, over the centuries, changed the environment in which mankind lives, while in the last thousand years mankind itself has changed the physical environment and produced the increasingly man-made world in which we now live. We are also the result of a long period of biological evolution. Genetic engineering demonstrates our relatedness even to the simplest creatures. The work of Paul MacLean in demonstrating the triune nature of the human brain links our present mentality most clearly to our ancestral brains (22).

Psychiatry is in the process of institutionalizing various sets of precursors. The considerable unity that was present in the psychoanalytic era, with its sharp focus on the individual mind, has given way to a variety of psychiatries under the headings of family, group, community, hospital, behavioral, biological, psychosomatic, child, neurological, addiction, forensic, geriatric, anorexic/bulimic, neuropsychopharmacological, cultural, pastoral, and, most hopefully, social, where attempts at integration are most strongly made. A system-theoretical psychiatry has not yet been born.

In the system-theoretical field, general systems theory remains active, although never institutionalized, and a working relationship with the technologically derived systems theories has not been achieved. The advent and amazingly rapid development of electronic computers has become the primary working tool in systems science and has become institutionalized as a field in itself. It has also spawned separate schools of organizational systems, political systems, natural systems, economic systems, agricultural systems, ecological systems, technology transfer systems, strategic material systems, and so forth.

The splitting paradox. Both psychiatry and general systems theory face a particular dilemma to which I will assign the name of "the splitting paradox." It appears that the more we know, the more we split knowledge into separate and distinct disciplines. This was the problem that faced Bertalanffy and led to the strong emphasis on the interdisciplinary nature of knowledge that is such an integral part of general systems theory. We can be comforted in our present dilemma by the insights of Jerzy Wojciechowski (24,25) to the effect that the human knowledge process is evolutionary in nature, with the result that when we speak of "problem solution" we have introduced an illusory term into our language, for "problem solutions" always result in the appearance of new and more complex problems. This does not make us unhappy, for problems are as necessary to our brains as food to our bodies.

But this should not deter us from focusing our attention on the splitting paradox, for the future of human existence depends on our making progress in this area. It is a paradox because increasing human knowledge cannot be allowed to produce increasing splitting and separateness: nation against nation, tribe against tribe, religion against religion have, in our nuclear age, become the program for extinction. We can accept that increasing human knowledge produces increasing complexity of problems, but we cannot accept that it is doomed to produce increasing splitting.

What I have learned as a psychiatrist and general systems theorist is that this paradox can be overcome and that it is possible to explain in a clear and easily understandable way how this can be done. I agree fully with the emphasis that Gaines and Shaw place on the central importance of making distinctions. If these were not made, we would live in a world of total homogeneity that would render thinking and living impossible. I agree further with their view that making a distinction is a system-forming act since it introduces coherence on either side of the line we draw to create two separate universes. But what Gaines and Shaw neglect is that we have introduced a splitting that is not relieved even by the otherwise valuable concept of constructive alternativism.

Flexibly regulated connectedness. What we need to do is system-form a flexibly regulated connectedness between the two separate universes that our acts of distinction making produce. These can be thought of as doorways with doors whose locks can be open or shut by keys distributed in such a fashion as to fulfill the requirements of both distinctiveness and cross-distinction relatedness. For the psychiatrist this is easy to comprehend, as psychiatrists recognize the human need for both individuality and relatedness. If we do not equip our distinctions with such doorways, we will have reverted to the feudal custom of building impermeable brick walls. Our patients will resort to breaking in and locking in to achieve the intimacy they need, and to locking out and breaking out to achieve the individuality they need. And if we do this we will have contributed to the increasing rates of crime and juvenile delinquency and the increasing danger of wars between nations. These notions are described in greater detail in a number of papers on lock in/break out theory (12,15,17).

The same is true of the relationship between psychiatry and systems theory. The general antagonism of psychiatry toward systems theory results from the use of systems theory as an aid to the leviathan of organization, rendering the psychiatrist a cog in the social machine. But if we shift to a general systems orientation and understand the knowledge-processing base of fifth-generation computers, the carpenter skills that will be required of us to create the necessary doorways of flexible regulation will be quite simple and will be a beginning of the role that the two professions are so admirably suited for in overcoming the splitting paradox. Their work will be transferable to the international scene, aiding the resolution of the many future problems that mankind is bound to encounter.

REFERENCES

1. BERTALANFFY, L. VON (1967). *Robots, men and minds.* New York: Braziller.
2. BERTALANFFY, L. VON (1968). *General system theory.* New York: Braziller.
3. BERTALANFFY, L. VON (1975). *Perspectives on general system theory* (Taschdjian, E., ed.) New York: Braziller.

4. BERTALANFFY, L. VON (1981). *A systems view of man.* (LaViolette, P., ed.) Boulder, CO: Westview Press.
5. BROWN, G. S. (1969). *Laws of form.* London: George Allen and Unwin.
6. CHANCE, M. R. A. (1984). Biological systems synthesis of mentality and the nature of the two models of mental operation: Hedonic and agonic. *Man-Environment Systems, 14,* 143.
7. GAINES, B. R. (1979). General systems research: Quo vadis? *General Systems, 24,* 1.
8. GAINES, B. R., & SHAW, M. L. G. (1986). Hierarchies of distinctions as generators of systems theories. *General Systems, 29,* 33.
9. GRAY, W. (1969). History and development of general systems theory. In W. Gray, F. J. Duhl, & N. D. Rizzo, (Eds.), *General systems theory and psychiatry.* Boston: Little, Brown. (Reprinted 1981.) Salinas, CA: Intersystems Publications.
10. GRAY, W. (1972). Bertalanffian principles as a basis for humanistic psychiatry. In E. Laszlo, (Ed.), *The relevance of general systems theory.* New York: Braziller.
11. GRAY, W. (1977). Systems theory in psychiatry. In B. B. Wolman, (Ed.), *International encyclopedia of psychiatry, psychology, psychoanalysis and neurology.* New York: Van Nostrand Reinhold, Aesculapius Publishers.
12. GRAY, W. (1981). The evolution of emotional-cognitive and system precursor theory. In J. E. Durkin, (Ed.), *Living groups.* New York: Brunner/Mazel.
13. GRAY, W. (1983). Systems theory: Recent developments. In B. B. Wolman (Ed.), *International encyclopedia of psychiatry, psychology, psychoanalysis and neurology. First progress volume.* New York: Van Nostrand Reinhold, Aesculapius Publishers.
14. GRAY, W., DUHL, F. J., & RIZZO, N. D. (Eds.) (1969). *General systems theory and psychiatry.* Boston: Little, Brown. (Reprinted 1981.) Salinas, CA: Intersystems Publications.
15. GRAY, W., & ESSER, A. H. (1979). Hypercycles of criminal system formation and their resolution. *Legal Medical Quarterly, 3,* 101.
16. GRAY, W., FIDLER, J. W., & BATTISTA, J. R. (Eds.) (1982). *General systems theory and the psychological sciences.* Salinas, CA: Intersystems Publications.
17. GRAY, W., & GRAY, L. R. (1977). System specifics in "break-in": A therapeutic approach. *International Journal of Offender Therapy and Comparative Criminology, 21,* 31.
18. GRAY, W., & GRAY, L. R. (1986). Origin and development of system precursor/system forming theory. *American Journal of Social Psychiatry, 6,* 151.
19. GRAY, W., & GRAY, L. R. (1987). Interface problems in social psychiatry and international relations. *American Journal of Social Psychiatry, 7*(3), 153–160.
20. JASPERS, K. (1933). *Man in the modern age.* London: Routledge and Kegan Paul.
21. KELLY, G. A. (1955). *The psychology of personal constructs.* New York: Norton.
22. McLEAN, P. D. (1975). On the evolution of three mentalities. *Man-Environment Systems, 5,* 213.
23. WILSON, E. O. (1986). Letter to the editor. *Science, 231,* 1057.
24. WOJCIECHOWSKI, J. A. (1978). Knowledge as a source of problems. Can man survive the development of knowledge? *Man-Environment Systems, 8,* 317.
25. WOJCIECHOWSKI, J. A. (1986). Social psychiatry in the man-made world. *American Journal of Social Psychiatry, 6,* 167.

4

THE PLACE OF COMPUTERS IN PSYCHIATRY

Juan E. Mezzich, M.D., Ph.D.

Professor of Psychiatry,
Department of Psychiatry, University of Pittsburgh,
Pittsburgh, Pennsylvania

and

Ada C. Mezzich, Ph.D., M.I.Sc.

Clinical Assistant Professor of Psychiatry,
Department of Psychiatry,
University of Pittsburgh,
Pittsburgh, Pennsylvania

INTRODUCTION

To place in perspective the roles of computers in psychiatry it is useful to outline first key phases in the history of computer technology.

The first generation of computers was developed during the 1940s and 1950s following the invention of the vacuum tube. With the creation of the transistors in the late 1950s, the second generation was initiated and lasted until the 1960s. During the late 1960s and early 1970s micro- and mini-computers appeared, highlighting the third generation. The fourth generation is characterized by the use of high-level or user-oriented languages as well as by a flexible application of software.

During the second generation, the application of computers to the field of mental health was mainly geared to research in which statistical analyses and generation of reports were the principal activities.

With the third computers' generation (1960–1970), the development of clinical information systems as well as of some clinical applications in psychiatric diagnosis and psychological assessment (18) were initiated.

Among the clinical information systems often mentioned in the literature are those developed at Camarillo State Hospital (14), Fort Logan Mental Health Center (41), the Institute of Living (8,13), the Veterans Administration Hospital System (20), as well as the Multi-State Information System (MSIS) (22), the Missouri Standard System of Psychiatry (SSOP) (17), and Computer Support in Military Psychiatry (COMPSY) (31). A common feature of these systems was an interest in improving patient care and meeting educational and administrative needs through the systematization and accessibility of medical records. These information systems typically were developed in large hospital settings in which the processor of information was a large mainframe computer. The information gathered centered around mental and physical status examinations, demographic identification, developmental history, and social functioning, all addressed at enhancing patient care.

From the mid-1970s on, there was a trend to develop information systems for specific functions, such as service reimbursement from government programs or insurance companies. With the increased usage of microcomputers and greater sophistication of software, clinical information systems have become more flexible and more easily adaptable to the needs of the user. Word processing, report and graphics generation, and networking are some of the functions that are now readily available. As microcomputers have limited capabilities to perform sophisticated statistics with extensive databases, larger computers are required for this purpose.

Three major areas in the development of psychiatric information will be considered next in some detail: clinical information systems, psychodiagnosis and therapy, and artificial-intelligence applications. The first one constitutes the mainstay of institutional care support, the second deals with key professional activities essential in any clinical setting, and the third constitutes one of the most exciting frontiers in informatics.

CLINICAL INFORMATION SYSTEMS

The complex and intricate nature of comprehensive clinical facilities requires the efficient handling of various types of information. In response to this challenge, various forms of clinical information systems (CISs) have been developed.

To ensure and maximize patient care, the system should capture precise information about the condition of the patient and the various phases of care, using reliable and valid instruments. Moreover, a well-designed database management system should also support research, educational, and administrative activities. This support, in the long run, will also expedite and enhance the main goal of the system, namely caring for a suffering human being.

Early efforts toward design and implementation of computerized CISs were severely hampered by critical inadequacies in the instruments used for the acquisition of information regarding patient evaluation, treatment, and disposition. Some of the instruments were totally structured, allowing no opportunity for the clinician to record examples of behaviors rated and other personalized observations and impressions. It is almost impossible for an instrument to be able to capture through checklists all information significant for the care of a given patient. Other systems relied on fully duplicate forms, one structured and the other allowing for a narrative description of the patient condition. Such duplication did not seem to lead to obtaining complete information; some clinicians tended to see the required effort as offensive or wasteful.

Furthermore, the clinicians who are crucial to the process of obtaining sensitive information from patients with various forms and levels of disorder often display a resistant attitude toward computerized information systems. A mosaic of factors underlies this resistance, including the imposed use of instruments perceived as irrelevant to patient care and concerns about privacy and confidentiality, as well as about the potentially dehumanizing aspects of high technology. These issues are magnified when clinicians are not directly involved in the development of clinical information systems.

To illustrate concrete ways of dealing with these issues and the actual configuration of an operational clinical information system, the one developed at the Western Psychiatric Institute and Clinic (WPIC) of the University of Pittsburgh is outlined below. It was designed by a team of clinicians, researchers, administrators, and computer specialists in order to respond to patient care needs and to support related activities of this comprehensive psychiatric institution (25).

The design of this CIS was modeled to follow the organization of patient care at WPIC. Psychiatric care is offered here to children, adolescents, adults, and geriatric patients, amounting to about 2,000 inpatients and 124,000 outpatient visits per year. Treatment programs are implemented via specialized modules (affective disorders, schizophrenia, special therapies, child, adolescent/young adult, and geriatric psychiatry), each consisting of both an inpatient and an outpatient component.

The basic clinical documents composing the WPIC Clinical Information System are the Initial Evaluation Form, the Brief Evaluation Form, and the Discharge Summary Form. They were developed in close interaction with clinicians and other users at WPIC, and each includes mutually complementary standardized and narrative components. They are sketched in the following sections.

Initial Evaluation Form

The Initial Evaluation Form (IEF) (26,27) is the first component of the Clinical Information System at WPIC. It provides a semistructured format for clinicians to use in their evaluation of the patient's condition. All basic areas and items to be investigated are specified, and definitions and guidelines are furnished on the form and in an accompanying manual. On the other hand, the clinician is expected to exercise experience and judgment regarding the sequence and wording of the questions to be asked. In addition, the format allows the clinician to complete the assessment by making a multiaxial diagnostic formulation along DSM-III lines (1), and to make informed and justified decisions regarding disposition and immediate treatment.

The IEF includes first a standardized demographic and financial questionnaire, which is completed by an administrative interviewer. The major clinical sections (history of present and past psychiatric illnesses, symptom inventory, family history, personal and social history, current social supports network, physical health history and examination, problem list and recommendations, plans for family members, DSM-III diagnostic formulation, and clinical disposition) are the responsibility of well-educated professionals.

Clinicians expected to use the IEF at WPIC are trained through a series of sessions that encompass didactic reviews of diagnostic concepts and the IEF manual, as well as exercises with videotapes and live patients under close supervision. Refreshing training is provided through rating exercises and peer reviews of samples of regularly completed IEFs.

Implementation of the IEF at WPIC involves its administration by a psychiatrist working alone, or more frequently, by a team composed of a primary evaluator (a psychiatric nurse, a psychiatric resident, a psychology intern, or another trained mental health professional) and a supervising faculty psychiatrist.

Before the data are entered into the computer system, they are checked for completeness, consistency, and clarity of coding. Subsequently, information from the IEF can be retrieved both on-line and batch for multiple uses (5).

Implementation of the IEF has led to the development of an extensive database, which is actively used to answer service-planning and clinical-epidemiological research questions (3).

The Brief Evaluation Form

The Brief Evaluation Form (BEF) (28) is an abbreviated version of the IEF, focused on the current psychiatric illness. It is used with patients who have had an IEF completed in the past three years and are initiating a new episode of care.

The BEF is concerned primarily with the current episode of illness, covering generally the preceding 12 months. It has a symptom inventory with an item list identical to that of the IEF, but directed exclusively to the current episode. It ends with a diagnostic formulation and disposition identical in format to the IEF's.

The Discharge Summary Form

The end of a treatment period calls for completion of a Discharge Summary Form (DSF) at WPIC (27). Its goal is to present a synopsis of the patient's clinical status at that point in time.

The DSF displays a sketch of the patient's clinical history (including information uncovered during the course of treatment), documents the assessment procedures and therapeutic interventions implemented during the treatment period, summarizes the patient's condition at discharge time, and finally records his disposition and recommendations for further care.

Of particular importance is the longitudinal relationship between the DSF and the IEF/BEF. The DSF has the same symptom list and functioning assessment scales as the initial evaluation documents, which enhances the opportunity for systematic appraisal of status changes before versus after treatment. Also of interest is that information from the IEF/BEF data banks is automatedly retrieved and printed onto blank DSFs to furnish demographic identification, symptom status, and diagnostic formulation at admission, which facilitates completion of similar appraisals at discharge time and facilitates the comparison of corresponding ratings.

The group that designed the above-mentioned instruments is now considering incorporating additional guidelines for the interview process as well as exploring the possibility of also computerizing the narratives. Meanwhile, the CIS database, amounting to over 15,000 patients (i.e., all those applying for care from August 1980 through the end of 1986), is being extensively used and researched.

In addition to semistructured clinical evaluation procedures, other exciting areas of development in clinical information systems are computer-aided treatment planning (e.g., 10), and computerized reviews of clinical care (e.g., 37).

PSYCHODIAGNOSIS AND PSYCHOTHERAPY APPLICATIONS

One of the first psychological areas to capture the attention of computer specialists was psychological testing, especially in the field of personality appraisal. The MMPI received the greatest attention, and computer-based test interpretations were also developed for the Sixteen Personality Factor Questionnaire (16PF), the Rorschach, the Personality Inventory for Children (PIC), the WAIS, Raven's Progressive Matrices, the Peabody Picture Vocabulary Test, the California Psychological Inventory, the Slosson Intelligence Test, and the Halstead Category Test (9).

It has been acknowledged that there are serious methodological problems for validating computer-based test interpretations (29). The difficulties are related to the problematic and distant relationship between test variables and their interpretive patterns, on one hand, and actual behaviors, on the other hand (30).

Another interesting application is direct computer interviewing of patients. It has been argued (7) that the combination of some of the characteristics of the expert clinician and paper-and-pencil questionnaires has significantly enhanced the promise of this technique.

The development of computer interviews involves similar quality control requirements as the development of any psychological test (7). The computer program has to be evaluated in terms of reliability and validity. For example, the computer interview has to show a close relationship to other pertinent characteristics of the person's behavior and ability to predict future behaviors. Furthermore, the computer interview has to demonstrate that the quality and quantity of the data acquired are adequate and that such data are integrated in an effective clinical or research information system.

From the computer science point of view, the content area of behavior to be covered can be approached either comprehensively or on a small scale. An option for an extensive interview approach is to use expert systems based on principles of artificial intelligence. The expert systems use heuristics to investigate the areas of interest without having to specify a priori the questions that have to be covered. It is to be considered that the development of expert systems represents a formidable expenditure of time and effort. In addition, the resulting flow of questions might be actually problematic and awkward when posed to patients (40). Consequently, the development of smaller-scale interviews tends to be a less riskier venture than that of larger interviews.

Another important issue is the impact of different styles of computer interaction. Currently, computer interviews follow the principle that the use of a program should be either menu driven or command driven. In the menu-driven approach, the user selects an option from a list of possible choices. In the command-driven arrangement, the user must directly enter the command to be executed.

An area crucial to the development of the field is the integration of computer interviews in the clinical setting and the involvement of the clinician in the decision-making process. The work with the Diagnostic Interview Schedule (34) and other psychiatric diagnosis interviewing programs has shown the need for clinician review of the information gathered to reach a final diagnosis (7).

In any case, computer interviews offer significant benefits, such as gathering systematic data without interviewer costs, and the possibility of gaining better understanding of a given substantive area through the process of developing an interview for it (7).

Initially, computer interviews were primarily conducted to gather general psychiatric history information (2,16,24). Later they were used effectively in specific areas such as suicide risk (15), substance use disorders (6), mental status examination (39), and sexual dysfunction (16).

More recently, there have been attempts to have the computer act like a human therapist; computer programs have been developed to perform psychotherapy. For example, Ghosh, Marks, and Carr (12) used an interactive eight-session program based on a self-treatment manual for phobias using in vivo exposure (23). A comparison of the outcome of this computer program to those obtained with a human therapist and the self-treatment manual suggested that these three methods were equally effective for the treatment of phobias.

It should be noted that out of concern for safety, therapy computer programs have tended to be used with the active participation of a clinician.

ARTIFICIAL-INTELLIGENCE APPLICATIONS

This section will describe and discuss expert systems developed by utilizing rule-based paradigms from artificial intelligence in order to aid clinicians in making diagnoses and determining appropriate treatment.

Some General Concepts

According to Winston (43), "artificial intelligence is the study of ideas that enable computers to be intelligent" (p. 1).

However, it is critical to have first a clear concept of intelligence on which there is agreement among professionals of the different disciplines that have to deal with it.

Winston (43) treats intelligence as an amalgam of many information representation and information-processing talents. According to Simon (38), "intelligence is the work of symbol systems" (p. 28). He defines these as "goal-seeking, information-processing systems, usually enlisted in the service of the larger systems in which they are incorporated" (p. 27). He considers that the computer and the human mind and brain belong to the family of symbol systems. An important aspect of Simon's view on intelligence is the concept of adaptability. Both the human being and the computer act intelligently to adapt to an environment.

It can be said that the general goals of artificial intelligence are to make computers more useful to human beings in adapting and mastering a growing environmental complexity and to facilitate our understanding of the principles that make intelligence possible. In this regard, computer metaphors help us to think about thinking. For one thing, computer models force precision, which makes it easier to uncover mistakes when implementing a theory. Also, computers can assess how much information is needed to process a particular task. Furthermore, the computer allows testing that is not possible in human beings or animals. On the other hand, our knowledge of human cognition may help to make computers intelligent. Broadly speaking, it is the hope of many artificial-intelligence specialists that the computer may help people enhance their intelligence and shed light on new principles underlying human cognition.

Problem-Solving Paradigms

Artificial intelligence usually has to deal with a problem-solving situation. It must have access to a set of problem-solving paradigms such as rule-based systems (43).

The rule-based systems paradigm fundamentally involves the use of series of deductions based on specified assumptions. They are the most frequently used in the design of expert systems in medicine. Their use here has been mostly for clinical research purposes.

The rule-based (also called "production") systems are among the most widely used paradigms in knowledge engineering, that part of artificial intelligence specialized in building expert systems. Some rule-based systems do synthesis (e.g., configuring computer systems), and others do analysis (e.g., diagnostic processes). They are briefly explained below.

Rule-based systems for synthesis. These are built around rules that include an *if-part* and a *then-part*. To facilitate work with these rules, forward chaining is used.

An example of instructions for such forward chaining using *if-then* rules, follows (43, p. 168).

> 1 Until a problem is solved or no rule's *if-parts* are satisfied by the current situation:
>
> 1.1 Collect rules whose *if-parts* are satisfied. If more than one rule's *if-parts* are satisfied, use a conflict-resolution strategy to eliminate all but one.
>
> 1.2 Do what the rule's *then-parts* say to do.

When all the conditions in a rule are satisfied by the present situation, the rule is said to be triggered. When the actions are performed, the rule is said to be fired.

Rule-based systems for analysis. One application of this approach is in the area of medical diagnosis systems. Such systems include procedures for answering questions and for calculating answer reliability.

Illustrating the deduction basis of these systems, the *if-parts* of some *if-then* rules specify combinations of known facts and the *then-parts* specify new facts to be deduced directly from the triggering combination. The *if-parts* of the rules are called antecedents and the *then-parts* are called consequences.

The deduction system might run forward or backward. For example, the rule-based system can hypothesize a conclusion and then use the antecedent-consequent rules to work backward toward the facts that led to the conclusion.

The following are characteristics of the rule-based deduction systems for analysis:

1. These systems can explain their reasoning; they can answer questions about why a *fact* was used or about how a *fact* was established. To decide how a given *fact* was concluded, a rule-based system needs to reflect only on the antecedent-consequent rules it has used, looking for those that contain the given *fact* as a consequent. The required answer is just an enumeration of those antecedent-consequent rules, perhaps accompanied by information about the *facts* in their antecedent sets.

2. These systems simplify knowledge transfer. To add a question-answering superprocedure, one has to deal only with rules and rule histories. To add a rule-transfer superprocedure that helps knowledge engineers make new rules is relatively easy.

3. Certainty factors help determine answer reliability. Rule-based systems usually operate in areas where conclusions are infrequently accurate. Thus, rule-based system developers often build some sort of certainty-computing procedure on top of the basic antecedent-consequent apparatus. In general, certainty-computing procedures associate a number between 0 and 1 with each *fact*. This number is called certainty factor and reflects how certain a *fact* is, with 0 indicating that it is false and 1 that it is definitely true.

4. Creation of *and/or* trees is an important part of the process, for in this way networks are developed. They also allow the verification of conclusions.

5. Rule-based systems can model human problem solving. In the human-modeling world, condition-action rules generally are called productions and rule-based systems are called production systems. Hardcore rule-based system specialists believe that humans have productions that are triggered by items in short-term memory. Specific combinations of the short-term memory items trigger the long-term memory's productions. The short-term memory is the key to which procedures are called, what they are given to work with, and how they return results.

Consultation with Experts

This represents the second phase in the development of expert systems. Two critical elements are involved here:

1. What the experts know. This information, complemented by that obtained from books and similar sources, is used for forming the knowledge database of the expert system.

2. How the experts think. Such ways of reasoning, translated into specific rules, are incorporated into the expert system.

Psychiatric Expert Systems

To illustrate the use of the above principles, a preliminary psychiatric expert system, named the Blue Box Project, will be sketched first in this section. Following this, some broader considerations for psychiatry will be offered.

The Blue Box is a psychopharmacological expert system developed by Mulsant and Servan-Schreiber (32) at the Palo Alto Veterans Administration Hospital in California to advise clinicians on the treatment of depression. It uses the rules of the EMYCIN program (42) developed for the field of infectious diseases.

The authors started from the premise that the management of a depressed patient basically requires prescription of medication and evaluation of suicidal risk. First, the program rules out certain organic diseases as well as drugs that may induce depression and other psychiatric illness that might look like depression. In addition, it characterizes the type of depression, using the *Diagnostic and Statistical Manual of Mental Disorders* (DSM-III) (1).

The knowledge box for this expert system was developed using textbooks, publications, and discharge summaries as well as the experience and knowledge of medical students and psychiatric residents.

The Blue Box bases its reasoning on raw data furnished by the user regarding the clinical manifestations, medical history, psychiatric history, drug history, and family history of a given patient. With these data the program: (1) rules out the different causes of depressive mood, (2) determines type of depression and the class of drug it should respond to, (3) assesses level of suicidal risk, and (4) selects an appropriate treatment.

Broadly speaking, the goal of expert systems in psychiatry is to augment the clinician's capabilities regarding diagnosis and treatment of patients through the use of rule-based system paradigms that are the product of artificial-intelligence research. Despite current limitations, many specialists expect the development of sophisticated programs that may deal competently with complex clinical problems. Essential to the task will be advances in the knowledge of the nature of the clinician's cognitive processes (33). It should also be kept in mind that, so far, no system has been used outside the environment in which it was developed (21), which calls for competent efforts within psychiatry itself.

Shortliffe (36) pointed out that diagnosis is basically a classification activity, which is a thought not frequently addressed in the artificial-intelligence literature. The developers of expert systems seem to assume that all problems related to diagnostic systems have been solved, that there is universal agreement on the appropriate structure of a diagnostic system, on the concept of disease, and on diagnostic criteria. In fact, these are real problems in all fields of medicine, more so in some areas than in others. Diagnosis is particularly problematic, and an active area for investigation, in psychiatry. There is not agreement here on the definition of mental disorder. The 200 types of mental disorders recognized in DSM-III have for the most part only limited empirical justification, and there are still severe problems in the way disorders are grouped at various levels of organization.

During the next five years the Tenth Revision of the International Classification of Diseases (ICD-10) will be taking shape (it is due for approval by the World Health Assembly in the early 1990s). At present, it appears that ICD-10 will include two specificity levels for diagnostic definitions, a multiaxial schema and a grouping of syndromes somewhat similar to that of DSM-III. This approach will presumably improve psychiatric nosology and better serve the various purposes of diagnosis (19).

It is certainly important, as artificial-intelligence applications purport to do, to augment the capabilities of adaptation of the human being, but it is also important to understand the domain to which he has to adapt and how information is going to be acquired to be helpful in decision making. It will be useful to keep in mind that key professional tools, such as diagnostic systems, have not only clinical but also social, financial, and policy development implications (35). As an example, we have the Blue Box expert system helping with the diagnosis of depression and offering recommendations for drug therapy. This system will also appraise suicidal risk. We are talking here about dangerousness, a complex and controversial issue with very serious clinical, social, and legal ramifications.

COMMENTS

There seems to be a broad gap between progress in computer technology and its applications to the medical field, especially psychiatry. The closer the matter is to the human mind, the more difficult it is to grasp and formulate effectively.

Before sophisticated procedures such as expert systems are used in every-day clinical work, the issues related to understanding and assessing the event (4), in this case the mental disorders presented by the patient, need to be approached and discussed.

It is also important to consider ethical issues. We have to remember that we are dealing here not with the complaints of an automobile that needs to be repaired, but with the lives and futures of human beings, their families, and communities.

REFERENCES

1. American Psychiatric Association (1980). *Diagnostic and statistical manual of mental disorders* (3rd ed.) (DSM-III). Washington, DC: American Psychiatric Press.
2. CARR, A. C., & GHOSH, A. (1983). Accuracy of behavioral assessment. *British Journal of Psychiatry, 142,* 66–70.
3. COFFMAN, G. A., MEZZICH, J. E., & RUDISIN, S. M. (1986). Uses of a psychiatric information system. In J. E. Mezzich (Ed.), *Clinical care and information systems in psychiatry.* Washington, DC: American Psychiatric Press.
4. DEBONS, A., & CAMERON, W. J. (1975). *Perspectives in information science.* Leyden, The Netherlands: Noordhoff International Publishing.
5. DOW, J. T., & STRIEGEL, D. (1986). Computer functions in a clinical information system. In J. E. Mezzich (Ed.), *Clinical care and information systems in psychiatry.* Washington, DC: American Psychiatric Press.
6. ERDMAN, H. P., KLEIN, M. H., & GREIST, J. H. (1983). The reliability of a computer interview for drug use/abuse information. *Behavior Research Methods and Instrumentation, 15,* 66–68.
7. ERDMAN, H. P., KLEIN, M. H., & GREIST, J. H. (1985). Direct patient computer interviewing. *Journal of Consulting and Clinical Psychology, 53,* 760–773.
8. ERICSON, P. R. (1986). An integrated medical information system. In J. E. Mezzich (Ed.), *Clinical care and information systems in psychiatry.* Washington, DC: American Psychiatric Press.
9. FOWLER, R. D. (1985). Landmarks in computer-assisted psychological assessment. *Journal of Consulting and Clinical Psychology, 53,* 748–759.
10. FOWLER, D. R., FINKELSTEIN, A., PENK, W., ITZIG, B., & BELL, W. (1986). Problem tracking by computer: The Dallas Problem Rating Interview. In J. E. Mezzich (Ed.), *Clinical care and information systems in psychiatry.* Washington, DC: American Psychiatric Press.
11. GHOSH, A., MARKS, I. M., & CARR, A. C. (1983). *Self-exposure treatment for phobics: A controlled study (preliminary).* Paper presented at the Royal Society Meeting, Psychiatry Section, London.
12. GHOSH, A., MARKS, I. M., & CARR, A. C. (1984). Controlled study of self-exposure treatment for phobics: Preliminary communication. *Journal of the Royal Society of Medicine, 77,* 483–487.
13. GLUECK, B. C. (1974). Computers at the Institute of Living. In J. L. Crawford, D. W. Morgan, & D. T. Gianturco (Eds.), *Progress in mental health information systems: Computer applications.* Cambridge, MA: Ballinger.
14. GRAETZ, R. E., AGAN, M. L., ARNSFIELD, P. J., JACOBUS, J. H., & WELLS, W. S. (1965). *Psychiatric data automation project: Final report (National Institute of Mental Health Grant R-11MH889).* Unpublished manuscript. Camarillo State Hospital, Camarillo, CA.
15. GREIST, J. H., GUSTAFSON, D. H., STAUSS, F. F., ROWSE, G. L., LAUGHREN, T. P., &

CHILES, J. A. (1973). A computer interview for suicide risk prediction. *American Journal of Psychiatry, 130*, 1327–1332.

16. GREIST, J. H., & KLEIN, M. H. (1980). Computer programs for patients, clinicians, and researchers in psychiatry. In J. B. Sidowski, J. H. Johnson, & T. A. Williams (Eds.), *Technology in mental health care-delivery systems*. Morewood, NJ: Ablex.

17. HEDLUND, J. L., SLETTEN, I. W., EVENSON, R. C., ALTMAN, H., & CHO, D. W. (1977). Automated psychiatric information systems: A critical review of Missouri's Standard System of Psychiatry (SSOP). *Journal of Operational Psychiatry, 8*, 5–26.

18. HEDLUND, J. L., VIEWEG, B. W., & CHO, D. W. (1985). Mental health computing in the 1980's: II. Clinical applications. *Computers in Human Services, 1*, 1–31.

19. KENDELL, R. E. (in press). Priorities for the next decade. In J. E. Mezzich & M. von Cranach (Eds.), *International classification in psychiatry*. Cambridge, England: Cambridge University Press.

20. KOLODNER, R. M. (1986). Computer applications for mental health treatment in the Veterans Administration. In J. E. Mezzich (Ed.), *Clinical care and information systems in psychiatry*. Washington, DC: American Psychiatric Press.

21. KUNZ, J. C., SHORTLIFFE, E. H., BUCHANAN, B. G., & FEIGENBAUM, E. A. (1984). Computer assisted decision making in medicine. *Journal of Medicine and Philosophy, 9*, 135–160.

22. LASKA, E. M., & BANK, R. (1975). *Safeguarding psychiatric privacy: Computer systems and their uses*. New York: Wiley.

23. MARKS, I. M. (1978). *Living with fear*. New York: McGraw-Hill.

24. MAULTSBY, M. C., & SLACK, W. V. (1971). A computer-based psychiatry history system. *Archives of General Psychiatry, 25*, 570–572.

25. MEZZICH, J. E., DOW, J. T., & COFFMAN, G. A. (1981). Developing an efficient clinical information system for a comprehensive psychiatric institute: I. Principles, design and organization. *Behavior Research Methods and Instrumentation, 7*, 459–463.

26. MEZZICH, J. E., DOW, J. T., RICH, C. L., COSTELLO, A. J., & HIMMELHOCH, J. M. (1981). Developing an efficient clinical information system for a comprehensive psychiatric institute: II. Initial Evaluation Form. *Behavior Research Methods and Instrumentation, 13*, 464–478.

27. MEZZICH, J. E., DOW, J. T., GANGULI, R., MUNETZ, J. R., & ZETTLER-SEGAL, M. (1986). Computerized initial and discharge evaluations. In J. E. Mezzich (Ed.), *Clinical care and information systems in psychiatry*. Washington, DC: American Psychiatric Press.

28. MEZZICH, J. E. (in press). The Brief Evaluation Form: Semi-structured assessment of current psychiatric illness. In J. E. Mezzich & B. Zimmer (Eds.), *Emergency psychiatry: A University of Pittsburgh reader*. New York: International Universities Press.

29. MITCHELL, J. V. (1984). Computer-based test interpretation and the public interest. In I. M. Matarazzo (Ed.), *Use of computer-based test interpretations, prospects, and problems*. Symposium conducted at the Annual Meeting of the American Psychological Association, Toronto, Ontario, Canada.

30. MORELAND, K. L. (1985). Validation of computer-based test interpretations: Problems and prospects. *Journal of Consulting and Clinical Psychology, 53*, 816–825.

31. MORGAN, D. W., & FRANKEL, S. I. (1974). Computer support in military psychiatry. In J. L. Crawford, D. W. Morgan, & D. T. Gianturco (Eds.), *Progress in mental health information systems: Computer applications*. Cambridge, MA: Ballinger.

32. MULSANT, B., & SERVAN-SCHREIBER, D. (1984). Knowledge engineering: A daily activity on a hospital ward. *Computers and Biomedical Research, 17*, 71–91.

33. PAUKER, S. G., GORRY, G. A., KASSIRER, J. P., & SCHWARTZ, W. B. (1976). Toward the simulation of clinical condition: Taking a present illness by computer. *American Journal of Medicine, 60*, 981–995.

34. ROBINS, L. N., HELZER, J. E., CROUGHAN, J., & RATCLIFF, K. S. (1981). The National

Institute of Mental Health Diagnostic Interview Schedule: Its history, characteristics and validity. *Archives of General Psychiatry, 38*, 381–389.

35. SCHACHT, T. E. (1985). DSM-III and the politics of truth. *American Psychologist, 40*, 513–521.
36. SHORTLIFFE, E. H. (1976). *MYCIN: Computer-based medical consultation*. New York: Elsevier.
37. SIEGEL, C., & ALEXANDER, M. J. (1986). Computerized review of clinical care. In J. E. Mezzich (Ed.), *Clinical care and information systems in psychiatry*. Washington, DC: American Psychiatric Press.
38. SIMON, H. A. (1984). *The science of the artificial*. Cambridge, MA: MIT Press.
39. SLACK, W. V. (1971). Computer based interviewing system dealing with nonverbal behavior as well as keyboard responses. *Science, 8*, 84–87.
40. SZOLOVITS, P., & PAUKER, S. G. (1978). Categorical and probablistic reasoning in medical diagnosis. *Artificial Intelligence, 11*, 115–144.
41. TRUITT, E. I., & BINNER, P. R. (1969). The Fort Logan Mental Health Center. In C. Taube (Ed.), *Community mental health center data systems: A description of existing programs*. Washington, DC: USPHS publication no. 1990.
42. VAN MELKE, W., & CARLISLE, S. (1981). *The EMYCIN Manual*. Technical Report. Stanford, CA: Stanford University.
43. WINSTON, P. H. (1984). *Artificial intelligence*. Reading, MA: Addison-Wesley.

5

LIAISON PSYCHIATRY

James J. Strain, M.D.

Professor/Director of Consultation/Liaison Psychiatry,
The Mount Sinai School of Medicine,
New York City, New York

and

Jeffrey W. Strain, B.A.

Case Western Reserve University School of Medicine,
Cleveland, Ohio

INTRODUCTION

Liaison psychiatry is positioned at the interface of psychiatry and medicine. It includes not only the traditional psychiatric consultation on an individual patient, but goes beyond this essential task to establish psychiatry as a bona fide member of the medical–surgical team. Establishing a liaison relationship means that the psychiatrist will be in contact with all the psychiatric and medical comorbidity on a unit or ward, and not only be consultant to those identified and referred. In epidemiological terms, liaison psychiatry attempts to deal with the denominator of the prevalence of psychiatric morbidity in the medical setting, whereas consultation psychiatry, by the very nature of the referral process, is involved only with the numerator.

Although consultation psychiatry is routine in most teaching hospitals, the sampling bias imposed by the referral method means that a skewed population is available on which to establish pedagogical and clinical needs. Research efforts are similarly hampered for either prevalence, mind-body interaction, intervention, or mechanism studies, since the referred consultation population is only a small subset of those with psychiatric and medical comorbidity in the general hospital setting.

Psychiatry's attempt to examine psychiatric and medical comorbidity has gained momentum in the United States during the last half century because of several ongoing developments: the establishment of departments of psychiatry within medical schools, the creation of psychiatric inpatient units in general hospitals, the unfolding understanding of the interrelationships and mechanisms of mind and body interactions in health and disease (Psychosomatic Medicine-Transduction), and the awareness that large numbers of patients with mental illness are seen exclusively in the medical setting.

Although liaison psychiatry employs the conceptual formulations and data from psychiatry, it also draws on those from medicine, public health, systems theory, and epidemiology. Finally, the psychiatrist in the medical setting examines how existing psychiatric precepts are altered by the co-morbidity of medical and psychiatric dysfunction. Accordingly, this chapter will review liaison psychiatry from several perspectives: historical, rationale, models of mental health training, and the critical issues that differentiate consultation psychiatry per se from the liaison approaches.

HISTORICAL PERSPECTIVES

The First Decade: The 1930s

Even though the term "liaison" was not coined by Billings until 1936 (1), a clear indication of the problems that psychiatry was to encounter in its relations with medicine had been formulated by Henry in 1929: "When psychiatry is first introduced into a general hospital there is likely to be indifference or even resistance on the part of the hospital staff" (2, p. 481). Henry stressed the fact that there was inadequate teaching of psychiatry in the medical school and concluded what was to become one of the major tenets of liaison psychiatry: "Relegating this work [psychiatric diagnosis and treatment] to specialists is futile for it is doubtful whether there will be a sufficient number of psychiatrists to respond to all requests for consultations" (2, p. 491), i.e., to deal with the vast numbers of patients with psychiatric and medical comorbidity.

Psychiatry in the 1930s was primarily preoccupied with the care of chronic mentally ill patients deposited in asylums. Furthermore, society was sufficiently skeptical of psychiatry's role that Henry warned that the psychiatrist should not reveal his identity when called into the medical setting, but rather acknowledge only that he is one of the medical staff. Even when the psychiatrist's interventions permitted medical and surgical efforts to proceed with the reluctant or the noncompliant patient, the reception to the seemingly beneficial procedure was cold. Finally, this early liaison psychiatrist stressed the paramount importance of avoiding the confusion between psychiatry and psychoanalysis and the necessity of the psychiatrist to be eclectic in his approach.

Medicine was becoming aware of the necessity of incorporating psychological components into the care of the medically ill, but poor linkages prevailed because of the psychiatrist's tendency to emphasize the social and environmental aspects and not to incorporate the biological concepts of disturbed behavior. However, Rappleye, the Dean of Columbia's College of Physicians and Surgeons in New York, recognized the contributions that could be made by psychiatry and called for the transition from a custodial position (even in the care of the chronic inpatient population) to an empirically scientific one (3). He also understood the need for medicine to be more receptive and to encourage the former "alienists" to assume a larger role in patient care. "What obviously is needed is an infiltration of the training in general medicine with a much greater appreciation than now exists of the role which environmental, social, emotional, and psychological factors play in the general health and well being of the individual . . ." (3, p. 243).

One of the key events in the development of liaison psychiatry in this early era was the support of the Rockefeller Foundation under the leadership of Alan Gregg, which in 1933 established full-time psychiatric faculty positions in six medical schools (4,5). This served to promote and expand the number of liaison programs in the United States. The Rockefeller Foundation had been influenced by Ebaugh of Colorado, who reported in 1932 that only 58 percent of the 68 medical schools had developed clinical facilities for teaching general psychiatry and only eight had any liaison program. Ebaugh also emphasized that 35 to 75 percent of the general physicians' caseload were patients with psychiatric morbidity.

Supported by a Rockefeller grant, the University of Colorado liaison program was formulated by Billings, who provided the first broad definition of liaison psychiatry (1):

1. To sensitize physicians and students to the opportunities offered by every patient and teach them a common sense psychiatric approach for the patient to handle both somatic and personality problems.
2. To include psychobiology as a part of professional thinking.
3. The prevention of false thinking and making the public aware of both personality and psychiatric disorders.

And one of the important contributions from Colorado to enhance liaison psychiatry was moving the center of its focus from the inpatient to the outpatient departments. "The Department of Psychiatry purposely had no hospital beds assigned to it and no specific niche in the outpatient clinic" (6, p. 30). Patients on medical, surgical, and pediatric wards were the focus for psychiatry's clinical, teaching, and research programs. Billings stated that doing so was much like unmasking the shaman or witch doctor, since other physicians could observe the liaison psychiatrist and, upon finding his techniques useful, could employ them in their own patient evaluation.

Part II: The 1940s to 1960s

Numerous advances in medicine occurred as a result of World War II, but for psychiatry, one of the greatest accomplishments was the recognition by medicine that it had something useful to contribute to patient care. Cobb's *Borderlands of Psychiatry* is indicative of this "new psychiatry," which had dichotomized into at least two subspecialties — biological and psychological (7).

But before psychiatry had to champion its own cause, one was thrust upon it: Since one-third of World War II casualties were psychiatric, it became an unavoidable medical profession! A dramatic example is given by Bond, who describes the trauma that flyers underwent during combat missions (8). Even when they could still function as pilots, many were no longer reliable. After Pentothal injection, the trauma could be reenacted and explored, thus returning the pilots to the front line quicker than any known medical treatment.

Although in 1948 Kaufman and Margolin (9) reported a policy of "indoctrination and infiltration," clearer evidence of a more secure foothold in medicine is found in the literature by 1950 with the advent of psychosomatics and the pioneering efforts of Flanders Dunbar and Franz Alexander (10,11). In this period, "psychiatrists, concurrently, had stopped being preoccupied with a search for physiologic causes for emotional balance and had become interested in the physiological concomitant of emotional maladjustment" (12, p. 103).

This early psychosomatic atmosphere supported the furthering of liaison goals, as greater concern was placed on the adjustment of the patient to his illness. Also, the idea of the medical team to complement education, improve medical care, and study the role of emotions in the "causation" of disease was gaining significance. Attention to personality factors was regarded as a critical factor in making medical treatment possible or effective (13).

By 1953, Kaufman reported that: "Psychiatry had come back into medicine as a co-equal member in a scientific discipline and is making a significant contribution. However, this new relationship is confronting the psychiatrist with the necessity for reorientation of some of his basic concepts toward a dynamic psychobiological point of view" (14, pp. 380–381). Kaufman established a ward for psychosomatic patients at the Mount Sinai Hospital in New York City and espoused a more holistic biopsychosocial point of view that was to encompass all medically ill persons throughout the hospital.

The liaison psychiatrist was also assuming the role of drug specialist, and this move from a purely psychological focus to a biological or drug perspective encountered less resistance from the ardent practitioner of a medical model where drugs were the daily fare. Psychopharmacological approaches offered a greater biological and scientific basis and thereby made psychiatry more acceptable to medicine.

In 1959, Schiff and Pilot portrayed a further shift in psychiatry's involvement with medicine (15). Orientation of the consultation moved to the consultee instead of being exclusively patient centered. Focusing on the idea that the concerns of the referring physician are not always explicitly stated, the liaison psychiatrist found himself in a position of assisting the consultee to improve his skills of psychological management instead of taking complete control of the case, which would quickly solve the problem, but teach very little. By 1962, Bernstein and Kaufman described the liaison officer at the Mount Sinai Hospital in New York City as a full-fledged member of the medical team whose advice was continually sought out (16). The Mount Sinai liaison effort demonstrated that a greater variety of patients were being referred from medicine, that they seldom had to be transferred to an inpatient psychiatry unit, and that medical doctors were curious about the use of psychotropic medication and other psychiatric modalities.

Part III: The 1970s to the Present

The period of the 1970s to the present marked a greater acceptance of liaison psychiatry by medicine. Training grants supplied by the National Institute of Mental Health supported much of the teaching effort. Engel's "The Need for a New Medical Model: A Challenge for Biomedicine," published in *Science* in 1977, attests to the climate of the times, although its impact on medical care and the training of physicians is still to be evaluated (17). Finally, several studies were implemented to evaluate the cost effectiveness of liaison work as further proof to administration and departmental heads of the need for a biopsychosocial approach and for funds to teach and practice this concept. These studies, however, were also in response to the increase of social work and nonmedical behavioral scientists seeking to provide the same services and competing for the same scarce resources.

According to Greenhill, the decade of the 1970s saw four shifts in the role of liaison psychiatry (4). First liaison nursing assumed more responsibilities for the psychological care of the patient since physicians continued to specialize and reduce their contact time with patients. Second, because there was a reduction in the average length of stay (this problem is intensified in the 1980s with the implementation of Diagnostic Related Groupings—DRGs), traditional forms of psychotherapy were not suitable in the medical–surgical inpatient setting, thereby resulting in a greater emphasis on outpatient treatment. Third, the development of bioethics as a result of malpractice suits and patients' rights groups forcefully sensitized physicians to the needs of patients. Consequently, resistance to the psychological components in medicine was reduced and requests for liaison psychiatry assistance, including participation in bioethics deliberations, increased.

The fourth important change in the 1970s was the advent of the critical-care model in which physicians and nurses who are specialized in critical care need the support of the liaison staff to manage the more difficult cases and the pressures upon themselves (4). In this setting the liaison psychiatrist is viewed as a psychobiologist, neuroscientist, and psychopharmacologist with a behavioral science emphasis.

There is no doubt that the psychiatric consultation is the *sine qua non* for clinical care of the individual patient and the cornerstone for general hospital psychiatry. Nevertheless, depending on the support available, *additional* approaches exist to augment the consultation and impact on: (1) nonconsult patients (the unreferred hospital patient population), (2) staff, and (3) administration, in order to move toward a more inclusive public-health-based population model.

Finally, in 1979 Hackett and Cassem, of the Harvard Medical School, elegantly described some of the differences between a consultation and liaison service and pointed to the broader and more poignant role available to psychiatry in the general hospital (18, p.5):

> A distinction must be made between a consultation service and a consultation liaison service. A consultation service is a rescue squad.

It responds to requests from other services for help with the diagnosis, treatment, or disposition of perplexing patients. At worst, consultation work is nothing more than a brief foray into the territory of another service, usually ending with a note written in the chart outlining a plan of action. The actual intervention is left to the consultee. Like a volunteer firefighter, a consultant puts out the blaze and then returns home. Like a volunteer fire brigade, a consultation service seldom has the time or manpower to set up fire prevention programs or to educate the citizenry about fireproofing. A consultation service is the most common type of psychiatric-medical interface found in the departments of psychiatry around the United States today.

A liaison service requires manpower, money and motivation. Sufficient personnel are necessary to allow the psychiatric consultant time to perform services other than simply interviewing troublesome patients in the area assigned to him. He must be able to attend rounds, discuss patients individually with house officers, and hold teaching sessions for nurses. Liaison work is further distinguished from consultation activity in that patients are seen at the discretion of the psychiatric consultant as well as the referring physicians. Because the consultant attends social service rounds with the house officers, he is able to spot potential psychiatric problems.

RATIONALE FOR LIAISON PSYCHIATRY

From the recent Epidemiological Catchment Area (ECA) study, Regier and his co-workers report that 19 percent of American adults in any six-month period experience the following disorders: anxiety (8.3 percent), affective (6 percent), alcoholic (5 percent), drug abuse (2 percent) (19). Alcohol, drug abuse, and mental disorders (ADM) result in at least 108,000 deaths per year: 69,000 are secondary to alcohol (up to one-half of all motor vehicle crash deaths involve alcohol); 6,000 are drug related; and 33,000 are associated with mental-health causes (20).

In 1983, ADM disorders cost 50.4 billion dollars in direct and 200 billion dollars in indirect treatment (21). More than one-half of all hospitalized and medically ill patients manifest significant psychological dysfunction, either as a result of or in conjunction with medical illness, and such dysfunction inevitably interferes with the effectiveness of treatment (22). It is also estimated that between 15 and 50 percent of all patients encountered in the ambulatory medical setting have psychological dysfunction that is either primary in nature or secondary to physical illness (22).

Finally, at the international level, the World Health Organization has declared that the only way to provide mental health care in developing countries is by way of the primary-care physician (PCP) and his or her physician extenders (23). And even in the most developed country in the world, the United States, 54 to 60 percent of mental health care delivered by doctors is via PCPs (19,24,25). However, primary care providers have a low recognition rate for ADM disorders: Only 10 percent of all ADM disorders were appropriately identified in one study and 25 to 50 percent of all major depressions in other investigations (20,26–28). On the other hand, Balter, at the National Institute of Mental Health, found that 70 percent of tricyclic antidepressants and 90 percent of anxiolytics are administered by PCPs (29).

Critical barriers impede the PCP from administering mental health care, in addition to the problem of nonrecognition, including:

1. The PCPs' inadequate training, knowledge, and negative attitudes toward their delivery of mental health care.
2. Patients' denial of their problems and their negative attitudes about seeking mental health care and/or accepting referral.
3. Constraints within the health care systems, e.g., cost, availability of psychiatrists and the impediments between the general health and mental health systems (30, p. 316).

With regard to the availability of psychiatrists, several considerations prevail to keep mentally ill patients within the domain of the PCP. The number of graduating medical students who entered the specialty of psychiatry declined significantly from 1970 to 1981 (31). Through the 1990s psychiatry will continue to be a shortage specialty, with insufficient numbers to deal with even the major psychiatric syndromes, despite a projected abundance of other physicians (32).

Since studies find that 15 to 50 percent of all patients who visit PCPs evidence some emotional or cognitive disorder, psychiatry's role in the general health sector needs to be defined (30). The question of psychiatry's role is further emphasized by other studies which describe the effect of behaviorial factors on the development, onset, course, and treatment of physical disorders (33–36). Furthermore, investigators report that psychological interventions in general health care settings not only improve overall care, but reduce total health care costs as well (37–39). For example, Levitan and Kornfeld demonstrated the cost benefits of a liaison psychiatrist on an orthopedic ward, i.e., $10,000 expended for a liaison psychiatrist's salary resulted in a savings of $190,000 in hospital charges and health-related-facilities costs upon discharge (39).

Mumford et al. similarly demonstrated, from their metaanalysis of several psychosocial interventions in the general hospital setting, that hospital length of stay can be shortened, especially in the over-65 population (40). Although the American Board of Internal Medicine, the American Medical Association, and the American Academy of Pediatrics have taken positions on mental health training for their respective members, the place of psychiatry in these training programs remains uncertain (41–44).

Finally, from the Hospital Utilization Cost Program currently underway at the National Institute of Mental Health (NIMH), it has been shown that the psychiatric consultation rate among a random sample of general hospitals in the United States ranged from .2 to .8 percent (45). This indicates that the consultation is not a widely employed vehicle to evaluate patients in the general health inpatient sector and is an infrequently used teaching vehicle to convey psychiatric and psychological knowledge by the consultant to nonpsychiatric consultees.

In addition to presenting the conceptual framework and data that argue the need for liaison psychiatry, it is important to consider psychiatry's role with regard to mental health care in the United States. What should psychiatry's role be with the nonpsychiatric physician in regard to the identification, diagnosis, and treatment of alcohol and drug abuse and mental disorders? What are medicine and surgery's goals in these domains? What does a particular medical milieu lend itself to? And what resources are available for mental health care and training?

In summary, it is apparent that if the large numbers of mentally ill patients presenting themselves in the general health sector are to be adequately cared for by nonpsychiatric physicians, their doctors must possess a comprehensive and clinically relevant body of mental health knowledge and skills.

MODELS OF MENTAL HEALTH TRAINING FOR PCP

In order to develop a taxonomy and to understand the models of mental health training currently extant for residents in three specialties regarded as primary care—internal medicine (IM) (7,000 trainees), family practice (FP) (4,000 trainees), and primary-care internal medicine (PC) (1,000 trainees) — three research contracts were awarded by the National Institute of Mental Health to the senior author. Initially, Strain, Gise, Houpt, and Pincus reviewed the literature, examined NIMH grant proposals, interviewed funding agency personnel, and made 35 site visits to IM, PC, and FP residency training programs supported by the NIMH and the Health Resources Services Administration (HRSA) (46,47). Based on this survey, the authors described six models of mental health training for the nonpsychiatrist physician (Figure 1) (48). Although the following descriptions focus more on the administrative organization of each model and its relationship to psychiatry than on the content taught and the form of teaching used, they illustrate ways in which consultation programs differ from other, more formal liaison teaching structures.

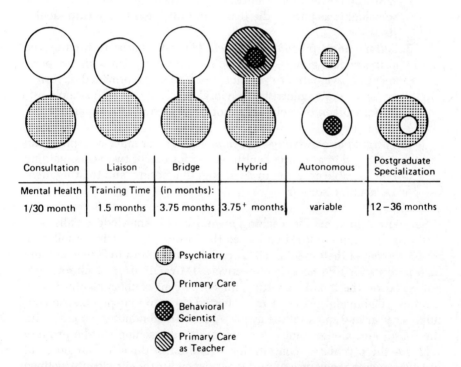

Consultation	Liaison	Bridge	Hybrid	Autonomous	Postgraduate Specialization
Mental Health	Training Time	(in months):			
1/30 month	1.5 months	3.75 months	3.75⁺ months	variable	12–36 months

Psychiatry

Primary Care

Behavioral Scientist

Primary Care as Teacher

Figure 1. Models of primary care training in mental health (Bridge, hybrid, autonomous, and postgraduate are variants of the liaison model.) (Reprinted with permission from Strain et al., in the *Journal of the American Medical Association*, *249*, p. 3066, 1983. Copyright 1983, American Medical Association.)

1. *Consult model*: The standard medical consultation approach is based on the case method, the need for the consultee to initiate the consult, and uses no formal, structured teaching methods, e.g., didactic sessions, seminars, precepting, and so forth.
2. *Liaison model*: In addition to the use of the consultation, formal, structured pedagogical exercises are employed to teach basic knowledge and skills. A psychiatrist–teacher often becomes part of a medical or surgical unit and team.
3. *Bridge model*: The psychiatrist–teacher is connected with a formal department of psychiatry. The psychiatrist is assigned to one primary-care teaching site (often an ambulatory training site) for a major portion of his or her time, and teaching is structured.
4. *Hybrid model*: Psychosocial teaching is provided by (1) a psychiatrist, (2) a behavioral scientist (e.g., psychologist, social worker, or sociologist) as part of the team, and (3) the primary-care faculty itself.
5. *Autonomous, psychiatric model*: The psychiatrist is hired by the primary-care group and has no formal connection with a department of psychiatry, or psychosocial teaching is provided exclusively by a nonpsychiatrist behavioral scientist (e.g., a psychologist, social worker, or sociologist) not connected with a department of psychiatry.
6. *Postgraduate specialty-trained model*: The primary-care physician is trained in a mental health setting for one or two years, gaining considerable expertise in detecting, diagnosing, and treating mental health disorders.

Several mechanisms for teaching mental health knowledge, skills, and attitudes were reported: IM employed the formal psychiatric consultation for 68 percent of their mental health training in contrast to 30 percent and 22.5 percent for FP and PC, respectively. IM rarely used block rotation, but relied on the inpatient setting for 80 percent of their mental health training. The modal IM resident requested three to four psychiatric consults per year and spent on the average less than 15 minutes per case with the consultant. Consequently, the accumulated teaching via the primary vehicle — the psychiatric consultation — resulted in three to four hours of instruction over the course of an IM residency for those residents inclined to initiate a consultation. And some IM residents never requested a psychiatric consultation during their entire training.

Furthermore, that specialty relying on the consult mode as the primary vehicle of teaching—IM—was less likely to: (1) emphasize sociocultural issues, use communication skills, utilize complex psychosocial management or simple pharmacotherapy; (2) evaluate trainees' performance as a result of pedagogical efforts; or (3) pay for the mental health instruction of their trainees. Seventy-one percent of the funds for mental health training in IM programs was paid exclusively by psychiatry, in contrast to 15 percent in PC and 1.6 percent in FP. All in all, the consult method of relating with medicine was the weakest pedagogical model that psychiatry offered. When it was employed with PC and FP, it was relegated to a minor role, as these specialties relied primarily on nonpsychiatric behavioral scientists for the bulk of their teaching, declaring that they preferred a liaison relationship with the teacher, rather than with an intermittent, itinerant consultant.

Another classification program was presented by Greenhill, in which he described five variations of liaison psychiatry (4):

1. *Basic liaison model*: Typically, in this model, a psychiatrist is assigned, from a department of psychiatry, to a medical-surgical unit for the express purpose of teaching.
2. *Critical-care model*: The critical-care model provides for the assignment of mental health personnel to critical-care units rather than to clinical departments. The goal is patient care and staff consultation, with the psychiatrist as a participating member of the unit team. Teaching combines behavioral and psychodynamic models as well as the model of biological psychiatry.
3. *Biological model*: The biological model is a more exacting variation of the critical-care model that emphasizes neuroscience and psychopharmacology as well as psychological management. The psychiatrist acts as a member of diagnosis-centered treatment units (e.g., dysphoria clinic, pain center, psychopharmacology clinic) and through psychological, psychopharmacological, and environmental manipulation serves as a member of the team.
4. *Milieu model*: The milieu model emphasizes the group aspects of patient care group process, staff reactions and interactions, interpersonal theory, and creation of a therapeutic environment on the ward.
5. *Integral model*: The integral model is emerging as a result of social pressure on medicine. It relies more on hospital governance than on triage by physicians. The aforementioned models of liaison programs depend in the main on consultation with patients and

staff and on working relationships with physicians. This model emphasizes the inclusion of psychological care as an integral component and the availability of the psychiatrist to function openly at the point of administrative and clinical need.

Hammer et al., at Northwestern University, have taken the integral alliance model of liaison psychiatry to its most developed form in an innovative Human Services Department (49,50). Moving well beyond the consult and referral model, Hammer and his colleagues have in place an administrative organization for the delivery of psychological care in the contemporary teaching hospital. This model takes an evolutionary step beyond multidisciplinary team approaches, by combining core psychosocial service delivery disciplines under centralized medical leadership: consultation/liaison psychiatry, social work services, pastoral care, home care, supportive care, and patient representatives. "The long range goal of this organization is to provide cost-effective psychosocial services. . . while maintaining the unique role contributions of the participating disciplines" (49, p. 189).

Reading states that (51, p. 187) "consultation/liaison (C/L) psychiatry is one of the only forms of psychiatric care provided in an organized service setting in which the psychiatrist works alone, rather than as a leader of the team. . . . As a consequence, the various services (including C/L) have generally been provided in a disjointed, unrelated, and often competitive manner." Finally, Reading asks (51, p. 187): "Should C/L psychiatrists get involved in the politics of the general hospital in order to help catalyze . . . change? There are many advantages to the patient in providing such coordination and integration as well as potential cost efficiencies."

The integrated human services model of liaison psychiatry remedies the isolation and lack of integrated formal structure that characterize the traditional consultation mode.

CONSULTATION IN COMPARISON WITH LIAISON PSYCHIATRY

Although consultation remains the cornerstone of the liaison process, the emphasis of the latter on certain issues distinguishes these two models of psychiatric intervention. The pedagogical thrust of liaison psychiatry and the attempt at formalizing patient care versus the "catch-as-catch-can" format of the consultation model is underscored by the following aims (52):

1. To practice primary, secondary, and tertiary prevention.
2. To foster case detection and triage techniques.
3. To clarify the status of the caretaker.
4. To provide continuing education to the nonpsychiatric staff in order to promote autonomy.
5. To develop basic biopsychosocial knowledge.
6. To promote structural changes in the medical setting.

The practice of liaison psychiatry differs from consultation in yet another way: it cannot charge third-party payers for its efforts and instead depends on support from a host department, hospital administration, federal grants, or innovative funding procedures. Finally, a systematic attempt at "liaison" occurs in no other specialty of medicine. For example, radiology, surgery, and internal medicine all rely on the consultation method for the primary exchange of information and patient care on a host service. What makes the liaison model particularly appropriate in the medical setting is the fact that the psychosocial model dictates that every illness and every patient require the inclusion of psychological and social considerations in assessment, treatment, and follow-up (17).

Primary, Secondary, and Tertiary Prevention

By using Caplan's model of prevention, that is, by anticipating and preventing the development of psychological symptoms (primary prevention), by treating such symptoms after they have become manifest (secondary prevention), and by forestalling their recurrence (tertiary prevention), liaison psychiatry enhances the quality of psychological care of the medically ill (53).

Secondary prevention tactics attempt to reduce the factors — biological, psychological, social — that have initiated disease; attend to the stress of illness; and manage acute symptoms such as anxiety, depression, and exaggeration of character traits that may enhance stress and impede recovery. As Hackett and Cassem stated, consultation psychiatry is primarily a secondary prevention effort (18).

Finally, the liaison psychiatrist strives to alter, through tertiary prevention, the psychological sequelae that may follow an acute episode: for example, psychological conflicts that result in mood disturbance, depression, anxiety, inhibitions, and phobias about returning to work or resuming sexual activity despite a physiological competence to do so. Psychological intervention in the tertiary phase will facilitate patients' adaptation to their physiological limitations, consequently lessening the possibility of recurrent illness, but frequently requires skilled ambulatory follow-up postdischarge from the general hospital for maximal effectiveness (54).

Detection and Diagnosis

Case detection in the medical setting is a major skill of the liaison psychiatrist and goes well beyond the consultant's waiting to be called by colleagues who have difficulties in detecting psychosocial dysfunction and who may be resistant to psychiatric intervention. In fact, the rate-limiting aspect of the consultation mode that keeps it a secondary prevention intervention is its dependence on referral from poorly motivated and/or poorly informed consultees. Specifically, for the physician, diagnosis proceeds along a continuum: (1) understanding the stated reason for the patient's visit (e.g., problems, complaints, signs, symptoms), (2) assessing the reason for contact (e.g., establishing the disorder, disease, syndromes), and (3) formulating, if possible, a diagnosis with a known etiology and prognosis. Management can flow from any point on this continuum. For example, a patient who has acute chest pains will be "managed," that is, hospitalized, even before the underlying problem and diagnosis are established.

The nature of the diagnostic process also varies as a function of the setting in which the patient is seen: (1) primary-care ambulatory office practice; (2) ambulatory hospital outpatient clinic; or (3) acute hospital inpatient medical or surgical unit. For 50 percent of the patients seen in the primary-care ambulatory setting, neither physiological, psychological, social, nor combined diagnoses are achieved (55). Rather, these patients remain at the "reason for visit" or "problem" level of diagnosis (56).

Several factors contribute to the patient's remaining at the "reason for visit," "presenting complaint," or "problem" level of diagnosis:

1. The patient's problem may be subclinical.
2. The biological, psychological, social, and/or cultural determinants that underlie the patient's complaint may not reach diagnostic criteria.
3. The physician may be unable to alternate hierarchial levels of conceptualization, that is, to move from the physical, to the psychological, to the social.
4. The physician may not take into account the interrelationship among physiological, psychological, and social factors.

In a formal manner, the liaison psychiatrist attempts to familiarize prospective consultees about how to acquire and synthesize data to enhance awareness, detection, diagnosis, and/or referral of psychological deficits and syndromes, in contrast to the consultant psychiatrist, who awaits the consultee to seek him out. The organic mental syndromes are the prototype of the psychophysiological disorders frequently present, but often undetected, in the medical–surgical setting (57).

If potential consultees are unaware that their patients have a dysfunction, how can they request a consultation? Strategies and tactics for case detection and triage are essential in the medical/surgical setting and constitute a "hallmark" of liaison psychiatry. Diagnostic screening devices for the disorders of organicity (58,59), depression, anxiety, and substance abuse are currently available if the structure can be altered from a consultation model to one that incorporates triage methodology (60).

Assessment of Medical Care Providers

The alliance model of liaison psychiatry incorporates the proposition that responsibility for the psychological care of the medically ill hospitalized patient cannot be relegated solely to the psychiatrist. Rather, this responsibility belongs jointly to doctors, nurses, social workers, important family members, and others who create the psychological climate of the ward (50). A crucial function of the liaison psychiatrist is to assess the degree of stress that patients produce in their medical care providers and in their families; the capacity of the providers and family members to adapt to patients and to their illnesses (and to the interventions of psychological care); and, above all, the capacity of staff and family to engage in psychological care.

Development of Autonomy in Nonpsychiatric Staff

Burns et al. have described several domains of mental health knowledge and skills that can be used as a schema for teaching and assessment (44) (Figure 2). This grid allows educators and evaluators to establish goals for their training programs or for particular disciplines: psychiatrists, primary-care physicians, psychologists, social workers, clinical nurse specialists, pastoral counselors, discharge planners, patient advocates, and even village health care workers in developing countries (46). The question to be asked, guided by the grid, is what competencies should the modal trainee be expected to have? The training program director or the disci-

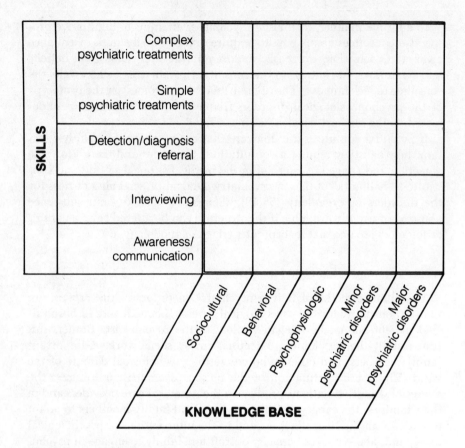

Figure 2. A model of domains of knowledge and skills. (Reprinted with permission of the publisher from Burns et al. [44], p. 160. Copyright 1983 by Elsevier Science Publishing Co., Inc.)

plines *themselves* establish the competencies they feel their practitioners should possess. The knowledge and skill base for other disciplines is *not* established by the psychiatrist.

For example, two-year fellow trainees in the University of Rochester liaison program (Engel) and their teachers do not expect their candidates to know or practice complex psychiatric skills. For such issues they refer to psychiatry. On the other hand, social workers at the Mount Sinai Hospital (New York City) are involved with sociocultural, behavioral risk issues and simple psychiatric disorders from awareness through simple treatments. They refer complex psychiatric problems and psychophysiological disorders, e.g., organic mental syndromes and endocrinopathies, to the psychiatrist. The pure consultation model promoted by Hackett focuses on detection, diagnosis, and/or referral of simple and complex psychiatric disorders. It eschews emphasizing awareness, communication skills, interviewing, or teaching about psychiatric treatment. Its major objective is direct patient care, preferably by the psychiatrist.

Liaison psychiatry expands the goal of the psychiatrist to include teaching awareness, interviewing, and knowledge of simple psychiatric interventions. The liaison goal is based on the fact that the majority of the mentally ill will be seen in the ambulatory general health sector in which a consulting psychiatrist will not always be at hand to take over the patient's mental health care.

Therefore, liaison psychiatry attempts to structure and formalize its teaching of the nonpsychiatric staff at morning rounds, weekly nurses' conferences, combined ward-staff meetings (61), staff-run patient groups, and grand rounds presentations. The liaison psychiatrist is asked to evaluate specific patients in the presence of the house staff and nurses, so that in time the latter will become more skilled in eliciting, interpreting, and applying psychosocial data to biopsychosocial treatment and management plans (61). Consequently, when physicians leave the arena of the teaching hospital and the consulting psychiatrist awaiting at the end of his beeper, they may — at the least — be aware of, able to interview, and competent to detect/diagnose and/or refer patients with mental disabilities.

Development of New Knowledge

Until recently, consultation and liaison psychiatry lacked both a systematic method for accumulating a database and suitable models for processing it. A computerized database schema for needs assessment, learner appraisal, systems analysis, and a measure of the impact of liaison teaching on the consultation-referral process has been developed (62). This field-tested instrument incorporates information as to the source of patient referral, demographic data, history of recent stress, use of psychotropic medicines, mental status, relevant DSM-III diagnoses, and recommendations. It includes significant biological data (e.g., EEG, computer-assisted tomography [CAT] scan) and social issues (e.g., family constellation, social class, living situation). The instrument has a termination section that organizes follow-up data: diagnostic tests, medical drugs (dosage and reaction), who terminated the consult, number of follow-up visits, presence of a social service note in the chart, follow-up DSM-III diagnoses, and the physical and mental outcome of the patient, as well as the fate of the recommendations made by the consultant.

Hammer, using the database schema of Strain et al., has created a microcomputer software package—MICROCARES—with report writing, literature searching, variable analyses, and billing functions for Clinical, Administrative, Research and Education (CARES) pursuits in the consultation and liaison setting of the general hospital (63,64) (Figure 3). Administrative uses include the ability to track the function of the consultation/liaison service over time (65). Patterns of consultation use and misuse may be studied along with the over- or underutilization of services. Workloads of staff can be monitored. Because consultation/liaison psychiatry serves the hospital, the availability of accurate records satisfies administrators who need to know what services are being provided to whom. Research paradigms using the database have been developed to study common problems encountered in the consultation/liaison setting: organicity, depression, anxiety, substance abuse, noncompliance, the elderly, behavioral management, and the use of psychopharmacology in the medically/surgically ill.

By noting the problem stated by the consultee versus the problem assessed by the consultant, it is possible to detect the nonpsychiatric physician's view of "labeling" of the patient (64). With regard to the organic mental disorders (OMD), 239 of 1,065 (22.4 percent) consultations in one teaching hospital did not indicate the presence of an OMD by the consultee (66). It is also possible to note that the incidence of erroneous labeling increases with age, thereby suggesting policy interventions with regard to mandatory screening. Organic mental screening devices would be appropriate for those inpatients in the general hospital who are over 65 years of age.

The database and computer management system permit the study of liaison ward versus nonliaison ward (67). Liaison ward consultees were more likely to detect an OMD than those from nonliaison wards ($p = <.01$). The biopsychosocial database encourages multiple and complex research studies, including those of cost-effectiveness and the "substitutability" of mental health workers in the consultation/liaison setting.

The MICROCARES system encourages trainees and faculty with minimum computer skills to examine their own data and to generate a continuous profile of the caseload carried over a training rotation—the

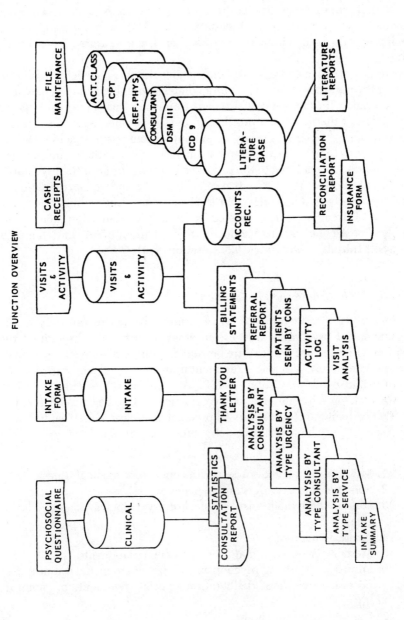

Figure 3. Reprinted with permission of the publisher from Hammer, Lyons, & Strain (63). Copyright 1985 by Elsevier Science Publishing Co., Inc.

"CONDAT" (68). In addition, the system makes it possible to compare current cases with those in the databank. With a microcomputer in the liaison office, the clinician or researcher is not separated from his/her data.

Four incentives encourage the resident consultants to participate in completing the database form: (1) an immediately available printed chart note to place in the hospital medical record from their own data; (2) ongoing assessment of their caseload profile that can be augmented in the rotation if certain care problems, e.g., dying patient, chronic pain, machine dependency, and so forth, have not yet been seen; (3) pertinent and current literature citations affixed to the printed chart note for both the psychiatric consultant and the nonpsychiatric consultee (67); and (4) participation in research efforts that can result in student or resident publication, e.g., "Refusal of Treatment: The Role of Psychiatric Consultation" (69), "The Problem of Alcohol in the Medical/Surgical Patient" (70), and "Patients Who Self Initiate a Psychiatric Consultation" (71).

Structural Changes in the Medical Setting

Liaison psychiatry strives to effect structural changes not only in the department of psychiatry, but also in other departments throughout the hospital, changes that will endure beyond the tenure of a given individual. For example, several interface treatment units have been established at the Mount Sinai Medical Center (NYC). A Psychiatry-Medicine Inpatient Unit, which cares for patients too psychiatrically ill to be on medicine, but too medically ill to be on a standard psychiatric inpatient service, has been established (72). The unit is especially interested in the following:

1. Major psychiatric disorders with concurrent medical illness.
2. Somatization disorders and hypochondriasis.
3. Illness where diagnosis — physical or psychological or both — is unclear.
4. Anorexia nervosa.
5. Medical illness with major psychosocial components.
6. Disorders requiring psychotropic drugs where medical illness may necessitate caution, deliberation, special treatment, or monitoring.
7. Drug-induced psychoses.

The concept of an ambulatory liaison clinic permits the follow-up of consultations after discharge, of patients discharged from the psychiatry-medicine unit, and of ambulatory patients from the medical and surgical clinics who have psychological dysfunction (54). Since psychiatric outpatient departments in most hospitals are often unable to accommodate psychologically dysfunctional, medically ill patients, an ambulatory clinic under liaison auspices offers an important addition to the psychiatric armamentarium in the general hospital.

Within a department of medicine, liaison psychiatry can establish in the ambulatory medical clinics psychosocial teaching rounds and principles of direct observation precepting to enhance mental health skills and knowledge in the nonpsychiatric physicians. In this setting it is also possible to establish, as Hossenlopp and Holland described, the concept of a special medical clinic whereby medically ill patients with psychiatric disorders can be treated by the psychiatrist in conjunction with medical trainees in order to expose the latter to their diagnosis and management in contrast to the traditional consultation-referral model, operative in the standard general medical clinic (73).

After it became apparent at one teaching hospital that psychological factors were responsible for a failure to maintain patients in the "life island" (the complete isolation technique for immunosuppressant therapy of leukemia and aplastic anemia), psychiatric clearance became mandatory for all life island candidates. Similarly, psychiatric clearance is now standard for all drug overdose patients before they are discharged from the intensive-care unit. The next logical step would be to make psychiatric clearance mandatory for high-risk patients, such as candidates for open-heart surgery, those who present as diagnostic problems, those whose need for surgery is in doubt, and patients who have repeated hospital admissions, apparently as the consequence of self-abuse through neglect.

One hundred and twenty-nine (35%) of the 372 patients referred by hospital mandate to assess the patient's capacity to execute a consent form for a medical or surgical procedure were given psychiatric diagnoses (DSM-II) by the consultant and received recommendation for primary psychiatric treatment (74). The "judgment" group had significantly more organic mental disorder and psychoses associated with central nervous system conditions ($p = <.001$) whereas the "nonjudgment" group was diagnosed as exhibiting significantly more neurosis, alcoholism, psychophysiological disorders, transient situational reactions, and personality disorders ($p < .001$). Psychological assessment of these patient groups and other groups yet to be identified should be regarded as an intrinsic part of liaison psychiatry patient evaluation and management in the contemporary teaching hospital.

CONCLUSION

Authentic liaison services accommodating formal pedagogical pursuits are not feasible in many medical-surgical settings. Unless a liaison contract can be written with a chief of service, it may be better to offer consultation. Specifically, if the psychiatrist cannot by negotiation obtain teaching time and adequate coteaching representation by attending physicians; if mandatory attendance, as at any other medical conference, cannot be ensured; if the psychiatrist cannot have access to medical patients for teaching purposes and cannot take up the subject of financial support, the consultation model should be relied upon.

Consultation psychiatry has been found sufficiently wanting by FP and PC so that these specialties have turned to psychologists, social workers, sociologists, and clergy for their mental health training and psychosocial research (46). On the other hand, IM uses psychiatry to "educate" through the consultation, but usually pays little from its resources for mental health training.

Liaison psychiatry offers a viable alternative to enhance clinical care, education, and research for psychiatric and medical comorbidity, by its reliance upon the public health model which emphasizes strategies to interact with the population (denominator) rather than a selected referred consultation cohort (numerator). Furthermore, the objective of liaison psychiatry to approach the psychological and psychiatric morbidity of the medically ill by an effective alliance with primary care physicians will enhance the capacity of the "de facto mental health service" to more optimally care for the majority of the mentally ill who are primarily seen in the general health sector (75).

REFERENCES

1. BILLINGS, E. G. (1936). Teaching psychiatry in a general hospital. *Journal of the American Medical Association, 107*, 635.
2. HENRY, G. W. (1929). Some modern aspects of psychiatry in general hospital practice. *American Journal of Psychiatry, 86*, 481–499.
3. RAPPLEYE, W. C. (1934). Comments on psychiatry. *American Journal of Psychiatry, 91*, 241–246.

4. GREENHILL, M. H. (1977). The development of liaison programs. In G. Usdin (Ed.), *Psychiatric Medicine*. New York: Brunner/Mazel.
5. GREGG, A. (1944). A critique of psychiatry. *American Journal of Psychiatry, 101.*
6. BILLINGS, E. G. (1966). The psychiatric liaison department of the University of Colorado Medical School and Hospital. *American Journal of Psychiatry, 122* (Supplement), 28–33.
7. COBB, S. (1943). *Borderlands of psychiatry.* Cambridge, MA: Harvard University Press.
8. BOND, D. D. (1952). *Love and fear of flying.* New York: International Universities Press.
9. KAUFMAN, M. R., & MARGOLIN, S. G. (1948). Theory and practice of psychosomatic medicine in a general hospital. *Medical Clinics of North America*, 611–616.
10. DUNBAR, F. (1952). *Emotions and bodily changes.* New York: Columbia University Press.
11. ALEXANDER, F. (1950). *Psychosomatic medicine.* New York: Norton.
12. LINDZ, T., & FLECK, S. (1950). Integration of medical and psychiatric methods and objectives on a medical service. *Psychosomatic Medicine, 12,* 103.
13. GREENHILL, M. H., & KILGORE, S. R. (1950). Principles of methodology in teaching the psychiatric approach to medical house officers. *Psychosomatic Medicine, 12,* 38–48.
14. KAUFMAN, M. R. (1953). The role of the psychiatrist in a general hospital. *Psychiatric Quarterly, 27,* 367–381.
15. SCHIFF, S. K., & PILOT, M. L. (1959). An approach to psychiatric consultation in the general hospital. *Archives of General Psychiatry, 1,* 349–357.
16. BERNSTEIN, S., & KAUFMAN, M. R. (1962). The psychiatrist in the general hospital: His functional relationship to the nonpsychiatric services. *Journal of Mount Sinai Hospital, New York, 29,* 385–394.
17. ENGEL, G. L. (1977). The need for a new medical model: A challenge for biomedicine. *Science, 196,* 129.
18. HACKETT, T., & CASSEM, N. (1979). *The Massachusetts General Hospital handbook of psychiatry.* St. Louis: Mosby.
19. REGIER, D. A., MYERS, J. K., KRAMER, M., ROBINS, L. N., BLAZER, D. G., HOUGH, R. L., EATON, W. W., & LOCKE, B. Z. (1984). The NIMH Epidemiologic Catchment Area (ECA) program: Historical context, major objectives, and study population characteristics. *Archives of General Psychiatry, 41,* 934–941.
20. HOEPER, E. U., et al. (1979). Estimated prevalence of RDC mental disorder in primary medical care. *International Journal of Mental Health, 8,* 6–15.
21. Health Care Financing Administration 1983 figures. Quoted in the *Washington Post*, Oct. 17, 1984.
22. LIPOWSKI, Z. J. (1967). Review of consultation psychiatry and psychosomatic medicine I and II. *Psychosomatic Medicine, 29* (2,3).
23. International Conference on Primary Health Care, WHO and UNICEF, Alma Ata, Russia, September, 1978.
24. REIGER, D. A., GOLDBERG, I. D., & TAUBE, C. A. (1978). The "de facto" U.S. mental health services system: A public perspective. *Archives of General Hospital Psychiatry, 35,* 685–693.
25. *Report to the President from the President's Commission on Mental Health,* Vol. 1. Washington, DC, 1978.
26. GOLDBERG, D. (1979). Training family physicians in mental health skills: Implications of recent research findings. In *Mental Health Services in General Health Care* (pp. 114–166). Institute of Medicine, National Academy of Sciences, Washington, DC.
27. WHEATLY, D. (1973). *Psychopharmacology in medical practice.* New York: Appleton-Century-Crofts.
28. GOLDBERG, D. (1978). Mental health priorities in a primary care setting. *Annals of the New York Academy of Sciences, 310,* 65–68.
29. BALTER, M. B. (1973). An analysis of psychotherapeutic drug consumption in the United States. In R. A. Bowen (Ed.), *Proceedings of the Anglo-American Conference on*

Drug Abuse: Etiology of Drug Abuse, Vol. 1 (pp. 58–65). London: London Royal Society of Medicine.

30. PINCUS, H. A. (1980). Linking general health and mental health systems of care: Conceptual models of implementation. *American Journal of Psychiatry, 137*, 315–320.

31. TAINTOR, Z., & NIELSON, A. C. (1981). The extent of the problem: A review of the data concerning the declining choice of psychiatric careers. *Journal of Psychiatric Education, 3*, 63–100.

32. Graduate Medical Education National Advisory Committee. (1981). *Report to the secretary, Department of Health and Human Services*, Vol. I–VIII, DHHS, PHS, Health Resources Administration; Office of Graduate Medical Education. DHHS publication no. (HRA) 81-651-658, Hyattsville, MD.

33. Institute of Medicine (1981). *Research on stress and human health: Report of a study*. Washington, DC: National Academy Press.

34. Healthy People (1979). *The Surgeon General's report on health promotion and disease prevention*, DHEW (PHS), publication no. 79-55071. Washington, DC.

35. SACKETT, D. L., & HAYNES, R. B. (Eds.) (1976). *Compliance with therapeutic regimens*. Baltimore: Johns Hopkins University Press.

36. LEY, P., WHITWORTH, M. A., SKILBECK, C. E., et al. (1976). Improving doctor-patient communication in general practice. *Journal of the Royal College of General Practitioners, 26*, 720–724.

37. JONES, J. R., & VISCHI, T. R. (1979). Impact of alcohol, drug abuse and mental health treatment of medical care utilization: A review of the research literature. *Medical Care, 17* (Suppl.), 1–82.

38. MUMFORD, E., SCHLESINGER, H. J., & GLASS, G. V. (1982). The effects of psychological intervention on recovery from surgery and heart attack: An analysis of the data. *American Journal of Public Health, 72*, 141–151.

39. LEVITAN, S., & KORNFELD, D. (1981). Clinical and cost benefits of liaison psychiatry. *American Journal of Psychiatry, 138*, 790–793.

40. MUMFORD, E., SCHLESINGER, H. J., GLASS, G. V., PATRICK, C., & CUERDON, T. (1984). A new look at evidence about reduced cost of medical utilization following mental health treatment. *American Journal of Psychiatry, 141*(10), 1145–1158.

41. WILDER, R. (1979). American Board of Internal Medicine: Clinical competence in internal medicine. *Annals of Internal Medicine, 90*, 402–411.

42. American Academy of Pediatrics (1977). *The future of pediatric education. A report by the Task Force on Pediatric Education*. Evanston, IL: American Academy of Pediatrics.

43. American Medical Association. (1984). Essentials of accredited residencies. In *Directory of Graduate Medical Education Programs*. Chicago: American Medical Association.

44. BURNS, B., SCOTT, J., BURKE, J., & KESSLER, L. (1983). Mental health training of primary care residents: A review of recent literature (1974–1981). *General Hospital Psychiatry, 5*, 157–169.

45. WALLEN, J., PINCUS, H. A., GOLDMAN, H. H., & MARCUS, S. E. (1987). Psychiatric consultations in short term hospitals. *Archives of General Psychiatry, 44*, 163–168.

46. STRAIN, J. J., GISE, L. H., HOUPT, J. L., PINCUS, H. A., & TAINTOR, Z. T. (1985). Models of mental health training in primary care. *Psychosomatic Medicine, 47*, 95–110.

47. PINCUS, H. A., STRAIN, J. J., HOUPT, J. L., & GISE, L. H. (1983). Models of mental health training in primary care. *JAMA, 249*, 3065–3068.

48. STRAIN, J. J., GEORGE, L. K., PINCUS, H. A., GISE, L. H., & HOUPT, J. (1987). Models of mental health training for primary care. *Psychosomatic Medicine, 49*, 88–98.

49. HAMMER, J. S., LYONS, J. S., BELLINA, B., STRAIN, J. J., & PLAUT, F. A. (1985). Toward the integration of psychosocial services in the general hospital. The human services department. *General Hospital Psychiatry, 7*, 189–194.

50. STRAIN, J. J., & GROSSMAN, S. (1975). *Psychological care of the medically ill: A primer in liaison psychiatry* (pp. 208–209). New York: Appleton-Century-Crofts.

51. READING, A. (1985). Editorial: The human services department. *General Hospital Psychiatry, 7*, 187–188.
52. STRAIN, J. J., & GROSSMAN, S. (1975). *Psychological care of the medically ill: A primer in liaison psychiatry* (p. 9). New York: Appleton-Century-Crofts.
53. CAPLAN, G. (1964). *Principles of preventive psychiatry.* New York: Basic Books.
54. ROWAN, G., STRAIN, J. J., & GISE, L. H. (1984). The liaison clinic: A model for liaison psychiatry funding, training and research. *General Hospital Psychiatry, 6*, 109–115.
55. MARLAND, D. W., WOOD, M., & MAYO, F. (1976). A data bank for patient care, curriculum and research in family practice: 196 problems. *Journal of Family Practice, 3*, 25.
56. STRAIN, J. J. (1981). Diagnostic consideration in the medically ill. *Psychiatric Clinics of North America, 4*, 287–300.
57. ENGLE, G. (1967). Delirium. In A. M. Freedman & H. I. Kaplan (Eds.), *The comprehensive textbook of psychiatry* (pp. 711–716). Baltimore: Williams & Wilkins.
58. FOLSTEIN, M. F., FOLSTEIN, S. E., & McHUGH, P. R. H. (1975). Mini-mental state. *Journal of Psychiatric Research, 12*, 189–198.
59. JACOBS, J., BERNHARD, M. R., DELGADO, A., & STRAIN, J. J. (1977). Screening for organic mental syndromes in the medically ill. *Annals of Internal Medicine, 86*, 40–46.
60. GEHL, M., STRAIN, J. J., WELTZ, N., & JACOBS, J. (1980). Is there a need for an admission and discharge cognitive screening for the medically ill? *General Hospital Psychiatry, 2*, 186–191.
61. STRAIN, J. J., & HAMERMAN, D. (1978). Ombudsmen (medical-psychiatric) rounds. An approach to meeting patient-staff needs. *Annals of Internal Medicine, 88*, 550–555.
62. TAINTOR, Z., GISE, L., SPIKES, J., & STRAIN, J. J. (1979). Recording psychiatric consultations. *General Hospital Psychiatry, 1*, 139–149.
63. HAMMER, J., LYONS, J., & STRAIN, J. (1985). Microcomputers and consultation psychiatry in the general hospital. *General Hospital Psychiatry, 7*, 119–127.
64. STRAIN, J. J., NORVELL, C. M., STRAIN, J. J., MUEENUDDIN, T., & STRAIN, J. W. (1985). CLINFO: A mini computer approach to consultation/liaison data basing: PEDAGOG ADMINISTRATIVE CLINFO. *General Hospital Psychiatry, 7*, 113–118.
65. POPKIN, M., MacKENZIE, T., & CALLIES, A. (1983). Consultation liaison outcome evaluation system. *Archives of General Psychiatry, 40*, 215–219.
66. HAMMOND, D., STRAIN, J. J., & MELONOVICH, T. (In preparation). Detection of organic mental syndromes in the medical setting.
67. STRAIN, J. J., & BARNARD, W. (In preparation). Liaison versus non-liaison wards in a general hospital.
68. STRAIN, J. J., FULOP, G., STRAIN, J. J., HAMMER, J., & TAINTOR, Z. (1986). Use of the computer for teaching in the psychiatric residency. *Journal of Psychiatric Education, 10*, 178–186.
69. STAM, M., & STRAIN, J. J. (1985). Refusal of treatment: The role of psychiatric consultation. *Mount Sinai Medical Journal, 52*, 306–310.
70. DULIT, R. A., STRAIN, J. J., & STRAIN, J. J. (1986). The problem of alcohol in the medical/surgical patient. *General Hospital Psychiatry, 8*, 81–85.
71. FULOP, G., & STRAIN, J. J. (1985). Patients who self initiate a psychiatric consultation. *General Hospital Psychiatry, 7*, 267–271.
72. GOODMAN, B. (1985). Combined psychiatric-medical inpatient units: The Mount Sinai model. *Psychosomatics, 26*.
73. HOSSENLOPP, C. M., & HOLLAND, J. C. B. (1978). Ambulatory patients with medical and psychiatric illness: Care in special medical clinics. *International Journal of Psychiatry in Medicine, 8*, 1–12.
74. STRAIN, J. J., TAINTOR, Z., GISE, L., & SPIKES, J. (1985). Informed consent: Mandating the consultation. *General Hospital Psychiatry, 7*, 228–233.
75. REIGER, D. A., GOLDBERG, I. D., & TAUBE, C. A. (1978). The "de facto" U.S. Mental Health Services System: A public perspective. *Archives of General Hospital Psychiatry, 35*, 685–693.

6

BRAIN IMAGING TECHNIQUES

ROBERT M. COHEN, M.D., PH.D.

and

THOMAS NORDAHL, M.D., PH.D.

*Section on Clinical Brain Imaging,
NIMH, Bethesda, Maryland*

INTRODUCTION

Progress in medical research is usually measured in terms of incremental additions in our knowledge of the pathophysiology of an illness. This is because frequently each such addition of knowledge not only advances our understanding of the etiology of the studied illness, but is often accompanied by improved treatment. A pathophysiology for traditional mental or functional illnesses, e.g., schizophrenia or manic-depressive illness, however, is yet to be delineated.

If we assume that clinical researchers in this field (mental or functional illnesses) attend as assiduously and creatively to their work as their colleagues, we must conclude that the reason for this relative lack of success lies in the difficulty in measuring the pertinent physiology of the brain. For example, it is "relatively" easy to assess the normal and abnormal functioning of the kidney or pancreas through measurements of plasma and urinary levels of hormones, metabolites, electrolytes, and glucose. These observations can then be correlated with morphological data obtained through biopsy or postmortem examination of the organs of interest.

Psychiatric researchers, however, face the difficult prospect of attempting to examine the morphology and physiology of the brain. The human brain, located within the cranium and behind the blood-brain barrier, presents significant and special challenges to *in vivo* measurement. As a result, even the principles of normal brain morphology and physiology have only begun to be elucidated.

Fortunately, however, recent technical developments may presage an era of rapid advancement in the understanding of psychiatric illness. These technical advances, on occasion, lumped together under the rubric of *brain imaging*, not only have aided in the advancement of our understanding of the biology of the brain, but promise to become important tools for assessing the morphology and physiology of the *functioning* human brain.

As the advances in "brain imaging" are complex and multidimensional, we decided that this review would better serve the reader by concentrating on three of the newest of these technologies which appear most promising in this regard, namely, positron emission tomography (PET), single-photon-emission tomography (SPECT), and nuclear magnetic resonance imaging (NMRI). We shall delineate the principles and assess the findings and potential of each of these methodologies for relevance to our understanding of mental illness. (See Table 1.)

POSITRON EMISSION TOMOGRAPHY

Methodology and General Importance of PET

What makes PET a technology uniquely suited to psychiatric research is its current standing as the best available methodology for the quantitative study of tracers in humans. A tracer is a chemical substance that is both (1) perceived by the body to be similar to an important endogenous component and (2) effectively "visualized" by researchers at such low concentra-

Table 1
Summary of Differences Between PET, SPECT, and NMRI

Technique	Invasive	Irradiation	CBF/CMR	Expense	Spatial Resol.	Staff
PET	Art/ven puncture	+ +	CBF & CMR	Very	5 mm	+ + +
SPECT	Ven puncture	+	CBF	Not	10 mm	+ +
NMRI	None	None	GMR (?)	Moderate	1 mm	+

Art/ven = arterioventricular; ven = ventricular.

tions that the substance itself does not alter the physiological process it is intended to measure. Its "visibility" allows researchers to follow (or "trace") the "life course" of this substance (tracer) and as a result discover important information about the resembled endogenous component and thereby the physiology of the organ(s) of study.

PET is unique in its capacity to visualize tracers because of the extreme sensitivity and high spatial resolution with uniform quantification that can be obtained with a PET scanner. This results from the use of positron-emitting radionuclides as tags for identifying tracers. A positron-emitting radionuclide decays by emitting a positron as a proton is converted to a neutron. The emitted positron travels only a few millimeters before it meets its antiparticle, the electron. This results in annihilation of both particles and production of two 511-kiloelectron-volt photons at a 180-degree angle. By creating a scanner that makes use of the simultaneous detection of photons in this specific geometrical arrangement (antipodal), one achieves the quantitative imaging power possible only with PET.

The image acquired is a representation of the spatial location of isotope as reconstructed in x-ray computerized tomography (CT) scanning from the decay events that have been measured by a ring (or several rings) of detectors that are positioned around the human head.

Modeling, or the Marriage Between Imaging and Tracer Technologies

The location of the isotope, however, is not sufficient for the measurement of a physiological process. What must be measured is the time-dependent change in both concentration and chemical form of the tracer. By scanning at different times, the time dependence of the tracer's spatial distribution can be measured. The scanner, however, is indifferent to the exact chemical form that the radioactive isotope it measures exists in.

Thus, the life course of the tracer cannot be directly measured by PET. One must know the amount of isotope that is contained within the various chemical structures that the tracer can be converted to. For example, after administration of a radioactively labeled amino acid, the amount of isotope recorded by PET could include the original amino acid, its metabolites, and proteins containing this amino acid. Therefore, a model must be derived that converts the raw PET data to information concerning a physiological process, e.g., protein synthesis.

Since the usefulness of PET in biomedical research is dependent on the tracer methodology available, the development of the physics and engineering of positron scanning would only be of theoretical interest to medical researchers if it were not for *two fortuitous properties* of positron-emitting radionuclides, as discussed below.

Availability of positron-emitting radionuclides. The ease of substitution of a positron-emitting radionuclide for a natural element is reflected in a recent review of positron emitter-labeled compounds, where Fowler and Wolf (28) tabulated well over 250 positron-emitting tracers that have been synthesized to date.

For example, ^{11}C can frequently be substituted for ^{14}C, the natural constituent of all organic compounds (e.g., leucine), with minimal change in the properties of the compound. Alternatively, ^{11}C can frequently replace ^{1}H to form a substituted compound (e.g., spiperone to form methylspiperone) with minimal alteration of biological properties. When positron emitters are substituted for natural elements, there is the additional bonus of rapid agency approval for human use by primarily satisfying radioactive dosimetry problems and the assurance of quality control. Also, ^{18}F can frequently substitute for hydrogen in organic compounds with minimal steric hinderance problems, although the change in electronegativity of the compound may make for quite different chemical and biochemical properties. This consideration frequently causes investigators not only to have to perform sophisticated studies of the biological and toxicological properties of these new compounds, but also to adequately correct for these differences from the endogenous compound in the kinetic model.

Short half-lives and high specific activity. Positron-emitting isotopes, in general, have short half-lives and high specific activities. This allows for maximum resolution and specificity for the tracers with a minimum of ionizing radiation exposure for the subject. For example, the four most commonly used positron-emitting radionuclides in biomedical applications and their half-lives are ^{15}O (2 min), ^{13}N (10 min), ^{11}C (20 min), and ^{18}F (110 min).

The Marriage Itself

We shall illustrate with a specific example, the *marriage* that must take place between the *imaging technology* and *tracer methodology*, if better methods for the understanding and evaluation of brain physiology are to be developed. The example involves the evolution of the most commonly used PET tracer, 18F-2-fluoro-2-deoxy-D-glucose (FDG). The extraordinary usefulness of the deoxyglucose model for the measurement of glucose metabolic rate in both autoradiographic studies of animals and PET studies of humans derives from the close association or tight coupling of brain function (activity) and metabolism and blood flow.

The initial nitrous oxide studies of Kety and his colleagues (37,38) used these principles to address a number of important biomedical questions, but were hampered by the technology available in the 1940s and 1950s. The methodology created was only sufficient to address scientific questions with respect to global or, at most, hemispheric metabolism and blood flow. Despite this limitation, however, the concept of tight coupling between metabolism and blood flow and functional activity was basically confirmed. This was usefully applied to diffuse alterations of brain function as observed in dementia, anesthesia, and seizure and cerebrovascular disorders.

More sophisticated scanning techniques did permit increases in the spatial resolution of blood flow methods (SPECT), but it has been with the development of PET, that the best spatial resolution has become possible. Perhaps even more important, the advent of PET made possible the use of FDG for the measurement of regional brain glucose metabolic rate. As explicated by Sokoloff et al. (72,73), who developed the autoradiographic FDG model adapted for use in PET modeling of metabolism, the brain, perhaps unique in the extent of its heterogeneity as an organ or tissue, would be expected to require appropriate relationships among all the various functional brain regions or units (e.g., neuronal pathways) to function properly.

Nor is it sufficient to study these integrated relationships at rest. These relationships require examination with respect to the various task requirements of the brain in mind. It was therefore quickly recognized that despite impressive developments in electrophysiology and histochemistry, a method that could simultaneously examine an entire set of brain regions could make unique contributions toward the understanding of brain function.

Mapping Normal Functional Activity

Task relevance in defining normal functional activity. Clearly, the most important problem to be resolved in the application of PET in order to understand mental illness is a determination of PET parameters of normal brain function. Normal brain function can, however, only be defined or evaluated with respect to a particular task that the organism is addressing.

Thus, one should expect different PET images when the subject is pleasantly daydreaming compared to when that individual is directing his attention to the perception and discrimination of sensory stimuli.

Evidence from the vast literature of behavioral studies suggests that any task ideally must be viewed with respect to information concerning the specific environmental stimuli, the response set of the individual, and the rewards for the subject. Although a large number of variables might result from such an analysis, the likelihood is that there would exist for any task a small subset of "indicator" variables whose range of values would be sufficient for the differential description of normal functioning (18).

PET studies of stimulated states. One of the more obvious types of indicator variables with respect to such considerations might take the form of the glucose metabolic rate (GMR) of a specific anatomical region as observed either when an individual is at rest or when engaged in a specific task. For example, determination of a range of resting GMRs for a large number of anatomical sites is consistent with normal brain function and sufficient for defining normality with respect to some demented patients whose values dip significantly below the range of these values (59,60).

Visual stimulated states. The normal variation in the regional GMR values in response to light was sufficiently narrow to observe abnormalities in the visual cortex of individuals with lesions in the visual pathway (58,59). Furthermore, using a range of visual tasks, investigators have demonstrated an apparent differential recruitment of brain regions with the increasing complexity of visual stimuli as reflected in observably greater increases in GMR in the higher-order associative visual cortex (Brodmann areas 18 and 19) than those observed in primary visual cortex.

Auditory stimulated states. Similarly, auditory stimulation studies have suggested that cortical site and extent of activation depend not only on the nature of the stimulus, but also on the subject's analysis strategy. Some of these studies, principally those by Mazziotta et al. (51), demonstrated frontal cortical and subcortical responses in addition to the temporal and parietal cortex responses expected to auditory stimuli. Furthermore, somatosensory stimulation appears to activate those cortical areas previously ascertained as topographical to specific dermatomes (52).

Whether this type of indicator variable (mean GMR or change in mean GMR with respect to rest) will be sufficient to fully describe normal function (as it has been in defining regional involvement in specific tasks, as illustrated above) and the pathophysiology of mental illnesses is at present unknown. However, a number of investigators in this area have felt that *regional* mean values for GMRs are insufficient. Essentially, such variables do not emphasize the presumably important relationships that must exist between and among various brain regions that are part of normal brain function (14).

Problems with different resting states. Several groups have looked for such relationships by means of both correlational analyses and factor analytical approaches. Unfortunately, these studies have utilized different "resting" conditions, e.g., eyes patched, ears plugged compared to eyes open, ears unplugged, so that it is not possible to know whether the relationships observed in these studies are replicable.

For example, all investigators observed substantial associations among homologous regions in the right and left hemispheres. However, whereas Metter et al. (53) observed substantial positive relationships among the superior frontal cortex and parietal and occipital cortices, and a second set of positive relationships among the inferior frontal cortex, the posterior temporal, and Broca's and Wernicke's areas, Horwitz et al. (34), using the eyes patched, ears plugged condition, were more impressed by the positive associations they found between the temporal and occipital regions and between the frontal and parietal regions. Such discrepancies could be accounted for by the nature of the two resting states or the amount of error introduced by analyses that look for relationships among a large number of anatomical regions.

Nevertheless, this approach has already begun to yield important information as patients with chronic neurological diseases apparently show metabolic defects of symmetry. This is observed through loss of effective association strength among homologous cortical regions (31,53) or through other more commonly used laterality measures, e.g., L-R/L, that are more robust than those one observes by comparing regional changes in GMRs. In principle, these types of approaches may be useful in *subtyping* or "profiling" psychiatric disorders, as abnormalities have been observed in both biological and functional studies of laterality in psychiatric patients.

Metabolic PET in Psychiatric Disorders

Schizophrenia. To date the psychiatric illness most extensively studied with PET has been schizophrenia. The fundamental finding from these studies has been the confirmation of the subtlety of this illness! PET scans of schizophrenic subjects much more closely resemble normal scans than they do the scans of neurologically impaired individuals. One must be struck by this finding in view of the tendency during the last few years to view schizophrenia as a neurological disorder. The scans of these patients do not at all resemble dementia, as might be suggested by the terminology of "dementia precox."

There are, however, some hints of positive differences to be observed in this population. The most important, perhaps, of these differences is that concerning "relative hypofrontality." Hypofrontality is a concept that was derived from the idea that deficits in schizophrenia are primarily observed in the "higher" cortical functions. As observed initially by Ingvar and Franzen (35) and others, the *normal* resting pattern of "functional" activity in resting humans demonstrates greater activity in the frontal cortex as opposed to other, more posterior areas that are more closely associated with the receiving and initial processing of sensory stimuli. It is the attenuation of this pattern in schizophrenia that has been observed by a number of investigators (9,10,27,81), but not by all (39,69,79).

Hypofrontality does not appear to relate directly to symptomatology or cerebral atrophy as ascertained with CT (21). It is "apparently" more easily observed in patients with chronic illness and or those who have received neuroleptic treatment in the past. As the human frontal cortex is extremely large and consists of a number of functionally somewhat independent entities, it should not be surprising that the evidence in favor of hypofrontality has been dependent on the anatomical regions chosen for evaluation and the statistical analysis attempted to demonstrate it. As the studies often do not adequately control for psychological set and frequently demonstrate greater differences in the "functional" values of the parietal or occipital cortices, no firm conclusions can as yet be drawn about the importance of the hypofrontality hypothesis and its inference of the implication of disordered "executive" function.

Issues of laterality differences in schizophrenia have been incompletely examined and inconsistently observed (17). The number of subjects examined to date is quite small, and laterality findings are likely to be quite dependent on task during the PET procedure. Similarly, basal ganglia and temporal cortex differences have been inconsistently observed and found to be affected by neuroleptic treatment (17,20,23). Furthermore, data have been reported suggesting a different coupling or linkage of anatomical regions in schizophrenics compared to normals in the handling of somatosensory stimuli (15). These data, however, are also in need of replication.

PET in affective illness. In the largest study of major depressive disorder patients, Buchsbaum and his associates (10,20) found relative hypofrontality, as defined by the anterior-posterior analysis of variance approach, similar to that observed in schizophrenic patients under similar task conditions, somatosensory stimulation. As in the instance of the schizophrenic patients, no relationship was observed between symptomatology or medication on the anterior-posterior gradient.

In contrast to the above study, Baxter et al. (2) observed a significant change in the whole-brain or global GMR in depressed bipolar patients in comparison to bipolar manic patients, unipolar depressed patients, or controls. As in the study of Buchsbaum et al. (10), the unipolar patients showed no global differences from controls, although Baxter et al. did observe a reduced caudate GMR when standardized to hemispheric GMR. These investigators also did *not* observe their variant of hypofrontality in their patient group. However, these studies are somewhat marred by the small number of patients and the unusually small global metabolic variation (compared to most reports) in their small control sample.

In contrast to both the above studies, Raichle et al. (63) found, again in a very small sample, decreased blood flow and metabolism in a group of mostly unipolar depressed subjects compared to controls. This study is also complicated by medication issues and diagnostic heterogeneity.

Finally, in another small study of chronic major depression and chronic schizophrenia, by Kling et al. (39), hypofrontality was not observed nor were significant changes in global metabolism, although a trend was apparent for both schizophrenic and depressed patients with enlarged ventricles and widened Sylvian fissures.

PET in anxiety disorders. In a study of 10 pure panic disorder patients, Reiman et al. (65) compared left-to-right rCBF ratios of seven preselected regions thought to mediate symptoms of panic, anxiety, and vigilance, namely, hippocampus, parahippocampal gyrus, inferior parietal lobule, anterior cingulate gyrus, hypothalamus, orbitoinsular gyri, and the amygdala. They found that patients who were positive lactate responders had significantly lower ratios in the parahippocampal gyrus in comparison to normals and non-lactate responders.

The issue of medication is not fully addressed in the report. A larger follow-up study by this group (66) with one additional lactate responder, five additional non-lactate responders, and 19 additional controls was recently published. Reiman et al. continue to report a significantly lower left-to-right ratio of parahippocampal blood flow for lactate responders as compared to normals and non-lactate responders. They actually report higher blood flow to both parahippocampal regions in comparison to normals. In addition to the parahippocampal abnormalities, lactate responders had significantly higher global cerebral blood flow and metabolism than the controls and non-lactate responders. Because of the global changes noted, the specificity of the observed parahippocampal asymmetry is uncertain. Increases in cerebral blood flow would be expected to accompany anxiety, in particular right hemisphere greater than left. Lactate-responding patients are noted to be more highly anxious than non-lactate responders and normals. Clearly, continued work is needed to clarify the significance of the parahippocampal asymmetry.

Baxter et al. (3) reported preliminary findings in a study comparing seven obsessive compulsives with 13 normal controls and 12 patients with unipolar depression. They report that the left and right orbital gyri showed significantly higher metabolic rates in the obsessive compulsive patients, while the unipolar depressed patients did not differ from controls on this measure. The activity of the left orbital gyri, when normalized to the ipsilateral hemisphere, was also significantly higher in obsessive compulsive patients than normals and tended to be higher than in the unipolar depressed patients. The heads of the caudate nuclei also showed significant metabolic elevation for obsessive compulsives in comparison to normals and unipolar depressed patients.

Studies of Neurotransmitter-Dependent Tracers

Historical or developmental issues. FDG PET or, for that matter, PET studies with tracers that measure oxygen metabolism and blood flow allow us to examine brain function with respect to the anatomy of this function. Additional tracer methods are required if we are to develop anatomical images from the perspective of the neurotransmitter pathway dependence of this function.

This progression in PET studies in some sense would then recapitulate the developments that occurred in neuroscience. Neuroscience progressed from an initial interest in the heterogeneity of the anatomy of the brain as the overriding explanation of behavior, to an overriding concern with a "pure" neurochemical explanation of behavior, to the present-day concern with neurotransmitter pathway approaches, combining both the anatomical and chemical approaches.

Relevance to psychiatry. We would like to have the ability to measure physiological processes relevant to specific neurotransmitter pathways. Just as earlier views of brain function were driven by the techniques available for brain study, PET explanations of brain function will progress with the development of new techniques. Although it is possible to imagine that certain psychiatric illnesses will be associated with a very specific finding that will be revealed by one specific PET tracer, it is more likely that definitions of both normal and abnormal states will require the assignment of precise ranges of values for a host of biological or neurochemical "indicator" variables some of which hopefully can be defined by using different PET tracers (18). That is, a complete set of indicator variables would be sufficient to predict other nonindicator variables and thereby function as a basis for diagnosis. For example, no one phenomenological variable is sufficient to define schizophrenia; hallucinations may occur in schizophrenia, organic psychosis, manic-depressive illness, and so forth.

Measurement strategies. In principle, PET studies of neurotransmitter function can be approached by two fundamentally different, but complementary methods. The first, the *pharmacological challenge approach*, is to use the available tracers, FDG, for example, to look at the differential effects of neurotransmitter-selective drugs on patient populations to imply differences in neurotransmitter pathway function, indirectly. The second is the *development of a new tracer* that will provide information about physiological processes that are directly translatable into an understanding of the functioning of a specific neurotransmitter pathway, because the tracer's localization is dependent on a physiological process that is selective for that transmitter.

The former approach suffers from the lack of selectivity of known agonists and the complex feedback systems that exist in the brain that muddy the interpretation of the altered FDG PET findings; the latter suffers because you can generally obtain only one specific measure of neurotransmitter function at a time, and therefore although you obtain data on one neurotransmitter-specific physiological process, you may miss the forest for the trees; i.e., the functioning of a neurotransmitter pathway is dependent on both presynaptic and postsynaptic variables. The new tracer approach is also divisible into two complementary approaches, the presynaptic approach of looking at the uptake, synthesis, and turnover of tracers related to specific neurotransmitters and the postsynaptic approach, i.e., the study or evaluation of the physiological processes that form the molecular mechanism whereby the information conveyed by the neurotransmitter is set into motion in the receiving neuron.

Several groups have conducted preliminary work with the pharmacological challenge strategy using methylphenidate and amphetamine to differentiate FDG-PET responses of normals compared to manic-depressive and schizophrenic patients, respectively. Findings, to date, do not appear impressive.

With regard to neurotransmitter-dependent tracer studies, investigators have concentrated on studying receptor-dependent phenomena (19,25,29,36,56). Measurements of receptor-dependent physiological processes would appear to be good candidates for assessment by PET. Alterations in these processes appear to result from an integration over time of neurotransmitter occupancy. Receptor-dependent measurements have been observed to change in animal models of psychiatric and neuropsychiatric conditions, at postmortem in humans, and upon psychotropic drug treatment, as observed in animals by direct measurement and in humans through indirect measurements of selective agonist challenge studies. Although receptor adaptation is a clearly complex process that is dependent on the specific receptor type, it appears to be of specific interest for psychiatry in that receptor changes have been observed to relate to brain location and animal behavior and be both environmentally and genetically influenced, just as psychiatric illness appears to be (18).

D_2 *receptor tracers.* The receptor-dependent tracer that has received the most attention to date and appears to be of most interest to psychiatry is that of the dopamine (D_2) receptor-dependent tracers. Under the leadership of Dr. Henry Wagner, the Johns Hopkins PET group has scanned the largest number of individuals with a D_2-dependent tracer, (^{11}C)-labeled 3-N-methylspiperone (NMSP). To differentiate NMSP binding that is related to D_2 receptor from nonspecific uptake, kinetic measurements of cerebellar (the cerebellum being an area relatively bereft of D_2 receptors) NMSP uptake are used to standardize striatal (D_2-rich) uptake measurements. The appropriate kinetic model to use with NMSP is still in need of verification in animal models where D_2 changes have been established.

A second ligand, ^{11}C-raclopride, has recently been developed in Sweden (25) that offers some theoretical advantages over NMSP in terms of its specificity and its ability to reach steady state much faster than NMSP. Neither isotope has shown differential uptake with respect to schizophrenia so far. The use of ^{11}C-raclopride, however, has demonstrated that

schizophrenic patients receiving neuroleptics have their D_2 receptors sufficiently occupied that uptake of raclopride is substantially diminished, and
upon withdrawal of the neuroleptic, there is an increase in the uptake of
^{11}C-raclopride (Ref. 26 and personal communication per L. Farde).

6-Fluoro-dihydroxy-phenylalanine (6-18F-L-DOPA). With regard to the
presynaptic approach, Garnett et al. (30) have visualized dopamine-con-
taining regions in the monkey and human brain with 6-18F-L-DOPA. The
uptake of this isotope has been demonstrated to reflect the loss of dopamine
neurons in MPTP (1-methyl-4-phenyl-1,2,3,6-tetrahydropyridine)-lesioned
monkeys (Figure 1). Distinctly different uptake of 6F^{18}-L-DOPA has also
been observed in patients with idiopathic and MPTP-induced Parkinson's
disease in comparison to normals. The use of this ligand for the study of
psychiatric illness, however, must be based on whether or not this ligand will
usefully reflect the "functional" qualities of the dopamine system, as opposed to lesions, which eliminate the neurons in that pathway.

Benzodiazepine receptor tracers. Similarly, substantial progress has
been made in the visualization of the benzodiazepine receptors. The best
apparent tracer is the benzodiazepine antagonist RO 15-1788, which has
now been studied both in monkey and in humans (60). The uptake of this
compound is consistent with the localization of benzodiazepine receptors
from neuroanatomical studies. However, two patients receiving chronic
benzodiazepine therapy who were administered ^{11}C-RO 15-1788 did not
show the expected loss of accumulation that was observed with ^{11}C-raclo-
pride uptake in schizophrenic subjects treated with neuroleptics. Persson et
al. (56) speculated on the possibility of receptor adaptation due to chronic
benzodiazepine exposure or a difference in benzodiazepine receptors being
associated with the illness itself. Since the benzodiazepines are, as a class of
drug, the most selective for the treatment of anxiety, our increased understanding of its mode of action and the study of these receptors as they
might be modulated by genetics, environment, and drug treatment should
prove to be of great importance for psychiatry.

SINGLE-PHOTON-EMISSION COMPUTED TOMOGRAPHY (SPECT) IN PSYCHIATRY

The mainstay of clinical nuclear medicine is the in vivo measurement of
the regional uptake of gamma-emitting radionuclides. There is wide availability of diverse instruments for the recording of the number and direction of the origin of gamma rays emerging from the body.

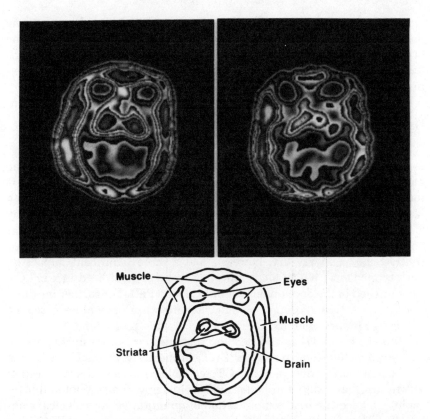

Figure 1. The use of 6[18]F-L-DOPA as a PET tracer. (Left) PET scan reconstructed horizontal slice through the striata of a normal Rhesus monkey following 6[18]F-L-DOPA intravenous administration, demonstrating the preferential accumulation of the tracer in the striata. (Right) Scan obtained on an animal following MPTP lesion. Little, if any, preferential accumulation of tracer is visible. We are indebted to Dr. Chiueh and his colleagues for providing the photographs.

The term single-photon-emitting radioisotope refers to the commercially available and widely used photon-emitting isotopes that emit only one photon per disintegration, such as ^{131}I, ^{99m}Tc, or [133]Xe. The term single-photon-emitting isotope distinguishes these radionuclides from the dual-emitting isotopes used in positron emission tomography, discussed earlier. As the dual-photon (positron) emitters are, however, short-lived, and the technology is cumbersome and expensive, there is interest in developing the more practical single-photon radioisotopes for imaging blood flow in the brain. In this section we shall discuss the development of SPECT, similarities and differences between SPECT and PET, limitations of SPECT, blood flow studies, and their applications to psychiatry.

Development and Methodology of SPECT

Prior to the introduction of x-ray CT in 1973, radionuclide brain imaging (particularly technetium) for the detection of abnormalities in the blood-brain barrier (BBB) or blood pool was the most commonly performed procedure in a nuclear medicine laboratory. X-ray CT led to a large decrease in the number of radionuclide scans performed, since x-ray CT could reveal more precise anatomical detail (with resolution of 1 mm) and abnormalities of the BBB could be detected with the use of iodinated contrast media. X-ray CT, however, had a more significant impact on nuclear medicine, as the algorithms and technology utilized in x-ray CT were utilized in the development of SPECT and PET. For further information on blood flow studies of psychiatric patients prior to SPECT, see the survey by Mathew et al. (50).

Kuhl et al. (40,41) introduced the first scanner-based, single-photon, transverse section tomography (SPECT) in the early 1960s. However, the subsequent application of x-ray CT technology, such as backprojection algorithms, has resulted in better SPECT imaging. Single-photon tomography provided the first demonstration of quantitative physiological studies (42). Through the work of Lassen et al. (46) and others, SPECT has been shown to be a practical tool for the measurement of cerebral blood volume and flow.

Similarities and Differences Between PET and SPECT

Both PET and SPECT measure the same parameter, namely, radionuclide concentration. Both PET and SPECT have similar medical applications, namely, to study metabolism, receptor site concentration, and blood flow. One advantage of PET over SPECT is its much greater sensitivity for detecting radiopharmaceuticals. This is because in SPECT, the technique of physical collimation results in the loss of many available photons. The ability to label compounds with positron-emitting isotopes of carbon, nitrogen, fluorine, and oxygen is the basis for great expectations for PET (see previous section), but this requires that one has a cyclotron nearby for the production of radiopharmaceuticals. In contrast, single-photon emitters, e.g., ^{99m}Tc, ^{123}I, can be obtained from noncyclotron or remote sources, and because they have longer half-lives than the positron-emitting isotopes, they are easier to work with.

Limitations of SPECT

The spatial resolution for single-photon devices can be 11-mm FWHM with good sensitivity (12). Increased sensitivity, however, is obtained at the cost of resolution. Scanner systems (PET, SPECT) are a tradeoff between resolution and sensitivity. This is more of an issue for SPECT than PET. Adequate tradeoffs for SPECT (PET) have been accomplished for as low as 10-mm (5-mm) resolution. The major impact of poor resolution is a loss of the ability to accurately measure the concentration of isotope in regions whose size is less than two times the dimension of the resolution of the system. System resolution defined as the "full width at half-maximum" (FWHM) will not capture the true concentration of an object with similar or smaller dimensions. Thus, an instrument with a resolution of 20-mm FWHM has only limited ability to give data representative of the true concentration for many of the structures of clinical relevance, because regions of interest, such as the basal ganglia, are less than that dimension.

Sensitivity/resolution comparison of PET and SPECT. A single-photon system having four detector banks around the head has a sensitivity that is not much less than that of a positron system if its resolution is in the range of 20-mm FWHM (12). However, at a resolution of 10-mm FWHM or better, the positron tomography sensitivity advantage is as high as 10-fold better than that of single-photon tomography.

An important design aspect of a single-photon tomograph is the ability to perform dynamic studies. Dynamic SPECT is the use of a time sequence of transverse sections from which uptake and washout kinetics can be deduced. The two major limitations to the application of dynamic computed tomography are the low statistics (counts) obtained and the necessity for rapid angular sampling. Uptake kinetics might not be practical for single-photon tomography.

Clinical Applications

After an isotope has been introduced into brain, continuous external measurement of its persistence can provide an index (and often a fairly accurate absolute number) defining regional blood flow. The various techniques developed to this end have introduced the isotope intravenously, by inhalation, and by intracarotid injection. At present the main interest in brain imaging is focused on the use of two approaches to the measurement of blood flow. One approach involves rapidly sampling the change in activity using [133]Xe (6,46). The second approach came as a result of the development of iodinated phenylalkylamines, which accumulate in the brain (44,68,80). The static measurement of the relative accumulation of these compounds can be used to infer local cerebral metabolism (33,43). The possibility for revival in brain imaging appears to be great because the new compounds concentrate in the brain in proportion to flow and can be imaged over short periods of time (5 min) with a resolution of 11–12 mm FWHM by appropriate SPECT instrumentation.

Applications of Brain Blood Flow Imaging in Behavioral Neurophysiology

Roland (67) notes that one observation which has been made again and again since the first high-resolution studies with regional cortical blood flow (rCBF) measured during physiological brain work always increases in fields of the size of 3 cm² to 6 cm². This holds for physiological activation of the cortical motor areas as well as for the primary sensory areas and the sensory association areas. It would be of interest to see whether these large activated fields persist when studied with instruments with increased resolution.

Some SPECT and Pre-SPECT Findings in Schizophrenia

There have been many "two-dimensional" (pre-SPECT) ^{133}Xe blood flow studies of schizophrenia and other psychiatric disorders. The articles by Weinberger, Berman, et al. (4,77) are among the latest of such reports. They compare performance on automated Wisconsin Card Sort (WCS) versus regional and absolute blood flow. They found that the only cortical region that distinguishes their 20 chronic medication-free schizophrenics from 25 normal controls was the dorsolateral prefrontal cortex, which had significantly lower blood flow in schizophrenics performing the WCS. The pre-SPECT works, however, are marred by large contributions from regions outside the region of interest. Because of this problem, researchers are utilizing tools such as SPECT and PET.

Preliminary findings of Dr. Joachim Raese (62) of the Schizophrenia Research Center, University of Texas, Dallas, were reported in the October

1985 issue of *Psychiatry*. Raese's group studied 29 chronic schizophrenics versus 19 mixed psychiatric controls with dynamic SPECT. Their analysis of regional cerebral blood flow abnormalities in schizophrenia subtypes showed that 80 percent of the paranoid schizophrenic patients had "hypo-frontal" flow compared to 29 percent of the nonparanoid schizophrenic patients. They noted that for the nonparanoid schizophrenic patients, 43 percent had hypotemporal cerebral blood flow compared to 10 percent of paranoid schizophrenic patients. They add that in the paranoid group, "hypofrontality" was demonstrated within the context of increased hemispheric flow bilaterally.

Left (frontal) hypoperfusion was significantly related to performance deficits on three neurophysiological measurements of frontal function. The report did not comment on medication or whether the subjects were scanned at rest.

NUCLEAR MAGNETIC RESONANCE IMAGING (NMRI) IN PSYCHIATRY

NMRI imaging rivals x-ray CT scan of the brain in terms of neuroanatomical detail, and NMRI allows imaging along any axis instead of only along a single axis, as in x-ray CT. NMRI imaging of the brain may also in the future be important for investigating metabolic and/or neurotransmitter defects of the brain. An important feature of NMRI is that it involves no ionizing radiation for the subject being imaged, though tissue heating is a potential risk when more powerful magnets are used, especially if the subject being imaged has prosthetic devices (11).

NMRI involves the electromagnetic generation of information from specific nuclei (most scanners in operation image the ubiquitous hydrogen proton ^{1}H). The NMRI apparatus consists of a static magnet, gradient magnets, radiofrequency (RF) transceivers, preamplifier, signal mixer, a computer, and image displayers.

Molecular Spin and External Magnetic Fields

The nuclei of atoms (such as ^{1}H, ^{13}C, ^{31}P, ^{15}N, ^{19}F) with an odd number of protons or neutrons have "spin." Since nuclei are electrically charged and movement of electrical charges has an associated magnetic field, nuclei with spin act like extremely small magnets. In the absence of any external magnetic field, the magnetic fields of the nuclei are oriented randomly and not subject to measurement.

For the energy of the nuclear spins (again generally ¹H spins) to be detected, the system of nuclei must be subjected to external electromagnetic forces. The primary force is the static magnet. Typically this involves a superconducting cryomagnet with field strengths up to 2.5 Tesla currently and actually as high as 4.5 Tesla for animal studies. The stronger the field (up to a point), the finer the resolution.

The nuclei in the static field tend to align with that field ("parallel alignment"), adding a small net increment of magnetism in the direction of the field applied. Individual nuclei may also exist in a slightly higher energy state, which corresponds to an "antiparallel" alignment to the field. The stronger the static magnetic field applied, the greater the proportion of nuclei that will align with it.

In addition to spinning, the nuclei also precess (wobble) about the axis of the applied field, tracing out a cone-shaped path. The rate (Larmor frequency) of this precession is determined by the strength of the static field and the "magnetogyric ratio" of the nuclei, which is the ratio of the magnetic moment to the angular momentum of the nuclei.

These spinning, precessing nuclei exist in a less random state because of the static magnet but still do not produce a signal appropriate for imaging. Pulsed signals from an RF transmitter system must be applied to the nuclei (of interest) in order to image them.

Gradient Magnets and Spatial Position

The NMRI signal obtained from a sample placed in a uniform static field and excited by a sequence of RF pulses would be an average of contributions from different locations within the sample and would contain no inherent spatial information. To obtain an image, spatial information needs to be encoded into the NMRI signal.

In the method originated by Lauterbur (48), this is done by superimposing a linear magnetic field gradient on the uniform static field. When this is done, the resonance frequencies of the precessing nuclei will depend primarily on their position along the direction of the gradient field. As a consequence, one essentially obtains a one-dimensional projection of the three-dimensional object. By taking three orthogonal projections, one can obtain a three-dimensional image of the object. The mathematics involved in constructing images from these one-dimensional projections is similar to the method of constructing images obtained by x-ray CT. Various alternative methods for spatial imaging have also been developed.

Radiofrequency Transmitter System

As noted earlier, the nuclei being imaged can be changed from the lower to the higher energy state by applying a second field of oscillating RF electromagnetic waves to the nuclei. In the NMRI apparatus, saddle-shaped coils are placed in such a way that bursts of RF will act at right angles to the direction of the static field. The imaged nuclei absorb the RF energy only at a certain frequency, the Larmor frequency, described above. This property of absorbing energy at a specific frequency is called resonance.

Following RF stimulation, the magnetic energy of the nuclei is now greater, and the nuclei leave their approximate parallel alignment with the static field and take on an antiparallel alignment to the static field. An RF pulse inducing this new alignment would be called a 180-degree pulse. A shorter RF pulse can be generated which causes the nuclei being imaged to rotate only 90 degrees, called a 90-degree pulse. Following the (say 90-degree) RF pulse, the stimulated nuclei will again begin to precess about the axis of the static field.

A signal is generated upon terminating each RF pulse. The imaging process involves information generated from a sequence of 90- and/or 180-degree RF pulses. This information in part reflects the physical relationships among molecules, depicting information derived from the density and from the different times required for the nuclei, which have been "oriented" and "excited" by the NMR imaging process, to return to the original parallel alignment with the static field. The time differences noted above are used to compute time constants T_1 and T_2, which depend on the microenvironment of the tissue.

Measuring the Relaxation Times and the Imaging Process

Saturation recovery (SR) images or proton density. The strength of the NMR signal is a function of the density of the nuclei being imaged and the microenvironment of the nuclei. This density is denoted spin density (and if hydrogen is being imaged, proton density).

The SR image exhibits little contrast. Areas of increased proton density (fat, blood, brain) appear white or gray while the lower proton density areas (skull) are dark. Cerebrospinal fluid (CSF) is an exception to this rule and appears dark because of its long T_1, which gives an incomplete recovery between pulses.

Inversion recovery to calculate T_1. Inversion recovery refers to techniques involving RF pulses that are used to compute an estimate of the T_1 time constant. T_1 is also called "spin-lattice" relaxation, as it depends on how well the "lattice" or environment can absorb energy. T_1 is also called "longitudinal relaxation" time as T_1 is a rate constant that describes the time required (post-RF stimulation) for the nuclei being imaged to become aligned with the static field.

The inversion recovery of T_1 weighted images give an excellent contrast between white and gray matter. The white matter and fat appear white, the gray matter and muscle appear gray, and CSF, blood vessels, air, and cortical bone appear black.

Spin echoes to calculate T_2. In addition to the longitudinal (T_1) relaxation, there is transverse (T_2) relaxation, which is also known as "spin-spin relaxation." The exponential decay of the NMRI signal (post-RF pulse) involves transference of energy among nuclei with the same spin (and so the name spin-spin relaxation). T_2 depends on the arrangement of the other nuclei in the molecular environment. In particular, prolonged T_2 tends to correlate with increased fluidity and molecular size.

Following the initial RF impulse, a series of RF "echoes" are applied. The amplitudes to these echoes decay exponentially with time constant T_2. Longer T_2 tissues (gray matter) usually appear white while shorter T_2 tissues (white matter) are usually darker. CSF appears darker than brain.

Some NMR Imaging Findings in Psychiatry

Findings in bipolar affective disorder. Rangel-Guerra et al. studied T_1 weighted images of the frontal and temporal cortices of 20 bipolar patients, mostly in the depressed phase, in comparison to 18 controls (64). Both groups were evaluated prior to and following lithium administration. The patients were off lithium and had a T_1 in the frontal-temporal region of 277 ± 10.5 msec, which was significantly greater than control values. Ten days after treatment with 900 mg of lithium per day, the T_1 weighted values (frontal-temporal) of the patients were changed significantly to 208.9 ± 6.6 msec. There was no significant change in the control group post-lithium treatment. The authors hypothesize that bipolar patients may have too high a proportion of "free" cellular water which is reduced by lithium. Unfortunately, a breakdown of ages and sex for controls was not given, nor is it stated how long the patients were off medication prior to beginning the study. Furthermore, the reliability of T_1's obtained with the imaging instrument used in this study is not as good as one would hope for.

Findings in schizophrenia. Robert C. Smith et al. studied 23 psychotic patients, mostly chronic schizophrenic patients, versus a comparison group consisting of 17 normals (71). Multiple linear and area measurements were made, including bifrontal ratio, bicaudate ratio, and a variety of ventricular to brain ratios. No significant differences were found on these measures between schizophrenics and the comparison group. Schizophrenic patients had, however, significantly higher image intensity values in both gray and white matter as measured from coronal slices of anterior and anterior temporal regions which were imaged in a T_1 weighted mode.

Thus schizophrenic patients appear to have longer T_1 weighted values, as was seen in the bipolar patients off medication. However, a more precise calculation of T_1 relaxation times is needed. The authors note that their findings of higher image intensity of white matter in the T_1 weighted mode are consistent with similar x-ray CT findings of higher pixel density of white matter in the brains of schizophrenics as compared to normals, and may indicate abnormal increased fibrosis or gliosis in these areas (45). We remark that it is not noted whether the patients were on medication or not.

Andreasen et al. studied 38 schizophrenic patients versus 49 normal controls (1). Nearly all of the patients (95 percent) had been on neuroleptics at some time and most were on neuroleptics at the time of scanning. All subjects received a single midsagittal cut and eight coronal slices, utilizing an inversion recovery pulse sequence. In addition, 16 transverse cuts were obtained using a spin echo sequence. It was found that schizophrenic patients had smaller cranial, cerebral, and frontal cortex sizes or volumes. It is somewhat difficult to evaluate the importance of these findings in the absence of corroborating data from other groups that have used CT data.

Findings in alcoholism. Besson et al. studied six chronic alcoholics, during acute intoxication and in subsequent withdrawal (5). T_1 weighted measurements were taken from gray and white matter in the parietooccipital and frontal regions above the corpus callosum on a horizontal plane. They found that T_1 values of both gray and white matter seemed to be reduced during the acute intoxification phase and increased during withdrawal (three to nine days of abstinence) and during abstinence (values at sixth week of abstinence). They state that these findings would be consistent with decreased free water during intoxication and an increase in free brain water during alcohol withdrawal. This latter notion has led authors to suggest the use of lithium in alcohol withdrawal.

Findings utilizing tracers. Jeffrey Coffman et al. (16) at Ohio State University are currently investigating benzodiazepine receptors in rabbits comparing clonazepam labeled with the nitroxide-stable free-radical TEMPO in rabbits, versus vehicle and unlabeled clonazepam. They are studying the animals with a 0.5-Tesla Picker NMRI system, using T_1 weighted pulse sequences. Although this approach appears promising, we are not aware of any studies in humans using a neurotransmitter pathway-dependent tracer and NMRI.

Future and Limitations of NMRI

Currently NMRI is primarily utilized to visualize endogenous components of the organism. Tracer methodology has played a negligible role. It should be emphasized that the image obtained in NMRI of protons (or other nuclides), although produced by the density of the signal-generating nuclei, is modulated by chemical and physical variables that affect their relaxations, T_1 and T_2. It should be kept in mind, therefore, that NMRI provides information about the chemical-physical state of the imaging-forming nuclide.

In this regard, the normal composition of living tissues includes, in addition to hydrogen, several other nuclides capable of generating NMRI signals, including ^{31}P, ^{23}Na, ^{13}C, ^{19}F, and therefore of potential use in NMRI. Unfortunately, because of their low concentration in soft tissue and their lower NMRI sensitivity as compared to hydrogen, the imaging of these nuclides yields a dismal signal-to-noise ratio as compared to hydrogen. Nevertheless, highly promising images of ^{31}P and ^{23}Na have been achieved, though with lower spatial and temporal resolutions than achievable with protons.

Moving fluids, particularly blood, can be imaged by NMRI by utilizing the property that NMRI-excited nuclides in a moving medium may be swept out, or, under certain circumstances, swept into, the plane of signal observation. This property offers promise in NMRI angiography. Van J. Wedeen et al. (76) point out that a 0.6 Tesla power machine is capable of visualizing flow in vessels as small as 1 to 2 mm in diameter.

Tracer methodology has been used and is being used in NMR by introducing, into the sample being analyzed, compounds labeled with nuclides capable of producing NMRI signals, such as ^{13}C, which exhibits a low natural isotopic abundance compared to ^{12}C. One would like to extrapolate the use of tracer to NMRI. Unfortunately, the applications of tracer methodology in NMRI are severely impeded by the relatively low signal-to-noise ratio, which leads to the requirement of large concentrations of NMRI radionuclides to achieve useful resolution in a tolerably short time.

This requirement of large concentrations of NMRI-sensitive isotopes makes it unlikely that NMRI (tracers) will be significantly useful in the immediate future in the study of local metabolic processes or in the investigation of neurotransmitters, although ^{31}P images appear promising for studying global metabolic changes. Still, the possibility of new coils, new tracers, further development of paramagnetic contrast material, and so forth may open the doors to NMRI's usefulness in the study of local metabolic changes and in the study of neurotransmitter pathways.

CONCLUSIONS

Despite the remarkable progress in the last 10 years in the application of brain imaging techniques to the study of psychiatric illness, we remain fundamentally uncertain that this application will lead to a breakthrough in our understanding of "functional" illness. Needless to say, the brain imaging methods outlined are not yet at the stage of psychiatric clinical trials. During the next decade, however, we can look forward to more methods producing detailed anatomical and neurochemical analyses of some of the "networks" involved in the fundamental processes of normal and abnormal cognition and emotion.

REFERENCES

1. ANDREASEN, N., NASRALLAH, H., et al. (1986). Structural abnormalities in frontal system schizophrenia. *Archives of General Psychiatry, 43*, 136.
2. BAXTER, L. R., PHELPS, M. E., MAZZIOTTA, J. C., et al. (1985). Cerebral metabolic rates for glucose in mood disorders, studies with PET and fluorodeoxyglucose F 18. *Archives of General Psychiatry, 42*, 441.
3. BAXTER, L. R., PHELPS, M. E., MAZZIOTTA, J. C., et al. (1985). Local cerebral metabolic rates in patients with obsessive-compulsive disorder, compared to unipolar depressives and normal controls. Abstract presented at the 1985 ACNP meeting. (Updated in *Archives of General Psychiatry, 44*, 211, 1987.)
4. BERMAN, K. F., ZEC, R. F., & WEINBERGER, D. R. (1986). Physiologic dysfunction of dorsolateral prefrontal cortex in schizophrenia: II. Role of neuroleptic treatment, attention, and mental effort. *Archives of General Psychiatry, 43*, 126.
5. BESSON, J. A. O., GLEN, A. I., & FOREMAN, E. I. (1981). Nuclear magnetic resonance

observations in alcoholic cerebral disorder and the role of vasopressin. *Lancet, 2,* 923.
6. BONTE, F. T., & STOKELY, E. M. (1981). Single-photon tomographic study of regional cerebral blood flow after stroke. *Journal of Nuclear Medicine, 22,* 1049.
7. BRODIE, J. D., CHRISTMAN, D. R., CORONA, J. F., et al. (1984). Patterns of metabolic activity in the treatment of schizophrenia. *Annals of Neurology, 15,* s166.
8. BROWNELL, G., BUDDINGER, T. F., LAUTERBUR, P. C., & McGEER, P. L. (1982). Positron tomography and nuclear magnetic resonance imaging. *Science, 215,* 619.
9. BUCHSBAUM, M. S., INGVAR, D. H., KESSLER, R., et al. (1982). Cerebral glucography with positron tomography. *Archives of General Psychiatry, 39,* 251.
10. BUCHSBAUM, M. S., DELISI, L. E., et al. (1984). Antero posterior gradients in cerebral glucose use in schizophrenia and affective illness. *Archives of General Psychiatry, 41,* 1159.
11. BUDDINGER, T. F. (1981). Nuclear magnetic resonance (NMR) in vivo studies: Known thresholds for health effects. *Journal of Computer Assisted Tomography, 5,* 800.
12. BUDDINGER, T. F. (1985). Quantitative single-photon emission tomography for cerebral flow and receptor distribution imaging. In M. Reivich & A. Alari (Eds.), *Positron emission tomography.* New York: Alan R. Liss.
13. BURNETT, K. R., & WOLF, G. L. (1984). NMR contrast media. *Resident and Staff Physician, 30,* 23.
14. CLARK, C., CARSON, R., KESSLER, R. et al. (1985). Alternative statistical models for one examination of clinical PET/FDG data. *Journal of Cerebral Flow Metabolism, 5,* 142.
15. CLARK, C., KESSLER, R., BUCHSBAUM, M. S., et al. (1984). Correctional methods for determining regional coupling of cerebral glucose metabolism: A pilot study. *Biological Psychiatry, 19,* 663.
16. COFFMAN, J. A., BARFKNECHT, C. F., NEFF, N., et al. (1985). Benzodiazepine receptor site imaging by magnetic resonance techniques. Abstract presented at the 1985 ACNP meeting.
17. COHEN, R. M., SEMPLE, W. E., & GROSS, M. (1986). Positron emission tomography. *Psychiatric Clinics of North America, 9,* 63.
18. COHEN, R. M., & CAMPBELL, I. C. (1984). Receptor adaptation in animal models of mood disorders: A state change approach to psychiatric illness. In R. M. Post & J. C. Ballenger (Eds.), *Neurobiology of mood disorders* (p. 572). Baltimore: Williams & Wilkins.
19. COMAR, D., MAZIERE, M., et al. (1979). Visualization of 11C-flunitrazepam displacement in the brain of a live baboon. *Nature, 280,* 329.
20. DELISI, L. E., & BUCHSBAUM, M. S. (1986). Positron emission tomography (PET) of regional cerebral glucose in psychiatric patients, Monograph. In M. Tremble (Ed.), *New brain imaging techniques in psychopharmacology.* New York: Oxford University Press, pp. 49–62.
21. DELISI, L. E., BUCHSBAUM, M. S., HOLCOMB, H. H., et al. (1985). Clinical correlates of decreased anteroposterior metabolic gradients in positron emission tomography of schizophrenic patients. *American Journal of Psychiatry, 142,* 78.
22. DELISI, L. E., BUCHSBAUM, M. S., HOLCOMB, H. H., et al. (In press). Increased temporal lobe glucose activity with PET in schizophrenic patients. *Biological Psychiatry.*
23. DELISI, L. E., HOLCOMB, H. H., COHEN, R. M., et al. (1985). Positron emission tomography in schizophrenic patients with and without neuroleptic medication. *Journal of Cerebral Blood Flow, 5,* 201.
24. DEMYER, M., HENDRIE, H. C., GILMOR, R. L., et al. (1985). Magnetic resonance imaging in psychiatry. *Psychiatric Annals, 15,* 262.
25. FARDE, L., EHRIN, E., ERICKSON, L., GREITZ, T., HALL, H., HEDSTROM, C. G., LITTON, T. E., SEDVALL, G. (1985). Substituted benzamides as ligands for visualization of do-

pamine receptor binding in the human brain by positron emission tomography. *Proceedings of the National Academy of Science, 82*, 3863.

26. FARDE, L., HALL, H., EHRIN, E., & SEDVALL, G. (1986). Quantitative analysis of D_2 dopamine receptor binding in the living human brain by PET. *Science, 231*, 258.

27. FARKAS, T., WOLF, A. P., JAEGER, J., et al. (1984). Regional brain glucose metabolism in chronic schizophrenia. *Archives of General Psychiatry, 41*, 293.

28. FOWLER, J. S., & WOLF, A. P. (1986). Positron emitter-labelled compounds: Priorities and problems in positron emission tomography and autoradiography. In M. Phelps, J. Mazziotta, & H. Schelbert (Eds.), *Principles and applications for the brain and heart* (p. 391). New York: Raven Press.

29. FROST, J. J., WAGNER, H. N., DANNALS, R. F., et al. (1985). Imaging opiate receptors in the human brain by positron tomography. *Journal of Computer Assisted Tomography, 9*, 231.

30. GARNETT, E. S., FIRNAU, G., & NAHMIAS, G. (1983). Dopamine visualized in the basal ganglia of living man. *Nature, 305*, 137.

31. HAXBY, J. V., DUARA, R., GRADY, C. L., et al. (1985). Relations between neuropsychological and cerebral metabolic asymmetries in early Alzheimer's disease. *Journal of Cerebral Blood Flow and Metabolism, 5*, 193.

32. HERHOLZ, K., PAWLIK, G., WAGNER, R., & WIENARD, K. (1985). *Atlas of positron emission tomography of the brain.* Berlin: Springer-Verlag.

33. HILL, T. C., HOLMAN, B. L., LOVETT, R., et al. (1982). Initial experience with SPECT (single photon computerized tomography) of the brain using *n*-isopropyl I-123-*p*-iodoamphetamine. *Journal of Nuclear Medicine, 23*, 191.

34. HORWITZ, B., DUARA, R., & RAPOPORT, S. I. (1984). Intercorrelations of glucose metabolic rates between brain regions: Application to healthy males in a state of reduced sensory input. *Journal of Cerebral Blood Flow and Metabolism, 4*, 484.

35. INGVAR, D. H., & FRANZEN, G. (1974). Abnormalities of cerebral blood flow distribution in patients with chronic schizophrenia. *Acta Psychiatrica Scandinavica, 50*, 425.

36. INOUE, Y., WAGNER, H. N., WONG, D. F., et al. (1985). Atlas of dopamine receptor images (PET) of the brain. *Journal of Computer Assisted Tomography, 9*, 129.

37. KETY, S. D., WOODFORD, R. B., HARMEL, M. H., et al. (1948). Cerebral blood flow and metabolism in schizophrenia. *American Journal of Psychiatry, 104*, 765.

38. KETY, S. D. (1950). Circulation and metabolism of the human brain in health and disease. *American Journal of Medicine, 8*, 205.

39. KLING, A. S., METTER, E. J., RIEGE, W. H., & KUHL, D. E. (1986). Comparison of PET measurement of local brain glucose metabolism and CAT measurement of brain atrophy in chronic schizophrenia and depression. *American Journal of Psychiatry, 143*, 175.

40. KUHL, D. E., & EDWARDS, R. Q. (1963). Image separation radioisotope scanning. *Radiology, 80*, 653.

41. KUHL, D. E., & EDWARDS, R. Q. (1964). Cylindrical and section radioisotope scanning of liver and brain. *Radiology, 83*, 926.

42. KUHL, D. E., REIVICH, M., et al. (1975). Local cerebral blood volume determined by three dimensional reconstruction of radionuclide scan data. *Circulation Research, 36*, 610.

43. KUHL, D. E., BARRIO, J. R., HUANG, S. C., et al. (1982). Quantifying local cerebral blood flow by *n*-isopropyl-*p*-^{123}I-iodoamphetamine (IMP) tomography. *Journal of Nuclear Medicine, 23*, 196.

44. KUNG, H. F., & BLAU, M. (1980). Regional intracellular pH shift: A proposed new mechanism for radiopharmaceutical uptake in brain and other tissues. *Journal of Nuclear Medicine, 21*, 147.

45. LARGEN, J. W., SMITH, R. C., CALDERON, M., et al. (1984). Abnormalities of brain structure and density in schizophrenia. *Biological Psychiatry, 19*, 991.

46. LASSEN, N. A., HENRIKSEN, L., & PAULSON, O. (1981). Regional cerebral blood flow in stroke by 133-xenon inhalation and emission tomography. *Stroke, 12,* 284.
47. LASSEN, N. A. (1985). Measurement of regional cerebral blood flow in humans with single photon emitting radioisotopes. In L. Sokoloff (Ed.), *Brain imaging and brain function.* New York: Raven Press.
48. LAUTERBUR, P. C. (1973). Image formation by induced local actions: Examples employing NMR. *Nature, 242* 190.
49. MATHEW, R. J., DUNCAN, G. C., WEINMAN, M. L., & BARR, D. L. (1982). Regional cerebral blood flow in schizophrenia. *Archives of General Psychiatry, 39,* 1121.
50. MATHEW, R. J., MARGOLIN, R. A., & KESSLER, R. M. (1985). Cerebral function, blood flow and metabolism: A new vista in psychiatric research. *Integrative Psychiatry, 3,* 214.
51. MAZZIOTTA, J. C., PHELPS, M. E., CARSON, R. E., & KUHL, D. E. (1982). Tomographic mapping of human cerebral metabolism: Auditory stimulation. *Neurology, 32,* 921.
52. MAZZIOTTA, J. C., & PHELPS, M. E. (1986). Positron emission tomography studies of the brain. In M. E. Phelps, J. C. Mazziotta, & H. Schelbert (Eds.), *PET and autoradiography: Principles and applications for the brain and heart* (p. 493). New York: Raven Press.
53. METTER, E. J., RIEGE, W. H., KUHL, D. E., & PHELPS, M. (1984). Cerebral metabolic relationships for selected brain regions in healthy adults. *Journal of Cerebral Blood Flow and Metabolism, 4,* 1.
54. METTER, E. J., RIEGE, W. H., KAMEYAMA, M., et al. (1984). Cerebral metabolic relationships for selected brain regions in Alzheimer's, Huntington's, and Parkinson's diseases. *Journal of Cerebral Blood Flow and Metabolism, 4,* 500.
55. OLDENDORF, W. (1981). Nuclear medicine in clinical neurology: An update. *Annals of Neurology, 10,* 207.
56. PERSSON, A., EHRIN, E., ERIKSSON, K. L., FARDE, L., HEDSTROM, C. G., LITTON, J. C., MINDUS, P., & SEDVALL, G. (1985). Imaging of [^{11}C]-labelled RO 15–1788 binding to benzodiazepine receptors in the human brain by positron emission tomography. *Journal of Psychiatric Research, 19,* 609.
57. PHELPS, M. E., HOFFMAN, E. J., MULLANI, N. A. & TER-POGOSSIAN, N. M. (1975). Application of annihilation coincidence detection to transaxial reconstruction tomography. *Journal of Nuclear Medicine, 16,* 210.
58. PHELPS, M. E., KUHL, D. E., & MAZZIOTTA, J. C. (1981). Metabolic mapping of the brain's response to visual stimulation: Studies in man. *Science, 211,* 1445.
59. PHELPS, M. E., MAZZIOTTA, J. C., & HUANG, S. C. (1982). Review: Study of cerebral function with positron computed tomography. *Journal of Cerebral Blood Flow, 2,* 113.
60. PHELPS, M. E., & MAZZIOTTA, J. C. (1985). Positron emission tomography: Human brain function and biochemistry. *Science, 228,* 799.
61. PYKETT, I. L. (1982). NMR imaging in medicine. *Scientific American, 246,* 78.
62. PAULMAN, R. G., DEVOUS, M. D., SR., BONTE, F. J., CHEHABI, H., GREGORY, R. R., RUSH, A. J., & RAESE, J. D. (1985). Neuropsychological correlates of regional cerebral blood flow in schizophrenia. *International Journal of Clinical Neuropsychology, 7,* 58.
63. RAICHLE, M. E., TAYLOR, J. R., HERSCOVITCH, P., & GUZE, S. B. (1985). Brain circulation and metabolism in depression. In T. Greitz, et al. (Eds.), *The metabolism of the human brain studied with positron emission tomography* (p. 335). New York: Raven Press.
64. RANGEL-GUERRA, R. A., PEREZ-PAYAN, H., MINKOFF, L., et al. (1983). Nuclear magnetic resonance in bipolar affective disorders. *American Journal of Neuroradiology, 4,* 229.
65. REIMAN, E. M., RAICHLE, M. E., BUTLER, F. K., HERSCOVITCH, P., & ROBINS, E. (1984). A focal brain abnormality in panic disorder, a severe form of anxiety. *Nature, 310,* 683.

66. REIMAN, E. M., RAICHLE, M. E., ROBINS, E., & HERSCOVITCH, P. (1986). The application of positron emission tomography to the study of panic disorder. *American Journal of Psychiatry, 143,* 469.

67. ROLAND, P. E. (1985). Applications of brain blood flow imaging in behavioral neurophysiology: Cortical field activation hypothesis. In L. Sokoloff (Ed.), *Brain imaging and brain function* (p. 87). New York: Raven Press.

68. SARGENT, T., BUDDINGER T. F., et al. (1978). An iodinated catecholamine congener for brain imaging and metabolic studies. *Journal of Nuclear Medicine, 19,* 71.

69. SHEPPARD, G., GRUZELIER, J., MANCHANDA, R., et al. (1983). ^{15}O positron emission tomographic scanning predominantly never treated acute schizophrenic patients. *Lancet, 2,* 1448.

70. SMITH, F. W. (1983). Review: Nuclear magnetic resonance in the investigation of cerebral disorder. *Journal of Cerebral Blood Flow and Metabolism, 3,* 263.

71. SMITH, R. C., BAUMGARTNER, R., CALDERON, M. D., et al. (1985). Brain imaging in psychiatry: New developments. *Psychopharmacology Bulletin, 2,* 588.

72. SOKOLOFF, L., REIVICH, M., KENNEDY, C., et al. (1977). The [14C] deoxyglucose method for the determination of local cerebral glucose utilization: Theory, procedure, and normal values in the conscious and anesthetized albino rat. *Journal of Neurochemistry, 28,* 897.

73. SOKOLOFF, L. J. (1981). Localization of functional activity in the central nervous system by measurement of glucose utilization with radioactive deoxyglucose. *Journal of Cerebral Blood Flow and Metabolism, 1,* 7.

74. TER-POGOSSIAN, M. (1985). PET, SPECT, and NMRI: Competing or complementary disciplines. *Journal of Nuclear Medicine, 26,* 1487.

75. WAGNER, H. N., BURNS, H. D., DANNALS, R. F., et al. (1983). Imaging dopamine receptors in the human brain by positron emission tomography. *Science, 221,* 1264.

76. WEDEEN, V. J., MEULI, R. A., EDELMAN, R. R., et al. (1985). Projective imaging of pulsatile flow with magnetic resonance. *Science, 230,* 946.

77. WEINBERGER, D. R., BERMAN, K. F., ZEC, R. F. (1986). Physiologic dysfunction of dorsolateral prefrontal cortex in schizophrenia: I. Regional cerebral blood flow evidence. *Archives of General Psychiatry, 43,* 114.

78. WIDEN, L., BERGSTROM, M., BLOMQUIST, G., et al. (1983). Positron emission tomography studies of brain energy metabolism in schizophrenia. In W. D. Heiss & M. E. Phelps (Eds.), *Positron emission tomography of the brain* (p. 192). New York: Springer-Verlag.

79. WIDEN, L., BLOMQUIST, G., DEPAULIS, T., et al. (1984). Studies of schizophrenia with positron CT. *Journal of Clinical Neuropharmacology, 7*(suppl.), 538.

80. WINCHEL, H. S., HORST, W. D., BRAUN, L., et al. (1980). N-Isopropyl [^{123}I]p-iodoamphetamine single-pass uptake and washout: Binding to brain synaptosomes and localization in dog and monkey brain. *Journal of Nuclear Medicine, 21,* 947.

81. WOLKIN, A., JAEGER, J., BRODIE, J. D., et al. (1985). Persistence of cerebral metabolic abnormalities in chronic schizophrenia as determined by positron emission tomography. *American Journal of Psychiatry, 142,* 564.

82. WONG, D. F., WAGNER, H. N., DANNALS, R. F., et al. (1984). Effects of age on dopamine and serotonin receptors measured by positron tomography in the living human brain. *Science, 226,* 1393.

83. PHELPS, M. E., MAZZIOTTA, J. C., SCHELBERT, H. R., HAWKINS, R. A., & ENGEL, J., JR. (1985). Clinical PET: What are the issues? *Journal of Nuclear Medicine, 26,* 1353.

7

FROM MENTAL HOSPITALS TO ALTERNATIVE COMMUNITY SERVICES

MICHELE TANSELLA, M.D.

Professor of Medical Psychology and Director of the
South-Verona Mental Health Centre, Institute of Psychiatry,
University of Verona, Verona, Italy

and

CHRISTA ZIMMERMANN-TANSELLA,
DIPL.PSYCH., M.SC., PH.D

Associate Professor of Medical Psychology, Institute of Psychiatry,
University of Verona, Verona, Italy

INTRODUCTION

In the last three decades the organization of psychiatric care in the community has attracted increasing interest and concern from psychiatrists and other professionals, administrators and planners, as well as from lay people. In many countries a gradual shift from hospital-centered to community-based psychiatry has been observed, with more patients being treated in ambulatory facilities whenever possible, rather than in remote bed-care institutions. This shift is proceeding at different speeds in the various countries and regions, but in most of them it appears to be a slow process characterized by a growth in outpatient care as well as by the organization of psychiatric wards in general hospitals and day-care facilities and, to a lesser extent, by a decrease in the number of beds in mental hospitals and by the provision of decentralized residential facilities for

130

long-term patients. In other words, often new outpatient and community services are being added to the old, hospital-based system of care instead of replacing it. It has been noted, for example, that in Britain, where a full community care policy was officially adopted in 1959, despite the considerable reduction in the number of inpatients, not even one mental hospital had closed since (24).

Many critical views on the possibility for community services to be alternative and to replace mental hospitals have also been voiced (5,27,51).

The aims of this chapter are first to present a brief review of the main features of mental hospitals and then to discuss community psychiatry and alternative community services, the rationale for the suggested shift from the hospital-based to the community-based system of care, together with some critical views on this trend expressed so far, and to present the Italian experience of moving toward a comprehensive, integrated, alternative system of community care without mental hospitals. Finally the South-Verona Community Psychiatric Service (CPS) will be described, and some data and material relevant to clinical practice, derived from our experience in coping with the problems that emerge when treating the whole range of psychiatric patients in the community, will be presented.

THE MENTAL HOSPITAL

First, we would like to address the title of our chapter by defining *mental hospital* as well as *community psychiatry* and *alternative services*.

According to the conclusions reached by the WHO Working Group on *The Future of Mental Hospitals* (72), "there is no definition of a mental hospital" (p. 3). In an early WHO meeting on *Trends in Psychiatric Care* (71) the main features of the mental hospital were identified. These were "its large size, its usually remote location from the population to be served, the custodial rather than rehabilitative approach by staff, and the lack of therapeutic contact between staff and patients" (p. 2).

Mental hospitals have also been defined as "the antithesis of the general hospital psychiatric unit, which is small in size, is located in a health facility which is accepted by the community as a focus of medical expertise, and promotes continued contact between the patient and his relatives" (37, p. 26). The WHO Working Group quoted above (72) stated that probably the most satisfactory definition of a mental hospital would be a modification of the definition of a specialized hospital, as given in the Regional Office for Europe's *Glossary of Health Care Terminology* (30):

"A hospital admitting primarily patients suffering from mental disorder, where clinical and administrative responsibility rests predominantly or exclusively with psychiatrists" (quoted by WHO [72], p. 4).

A radical view has been expressed by Franco Basaglia, an eminent Italian psychiatrist, and Ongaro-Basaglia, who in 1971 (9), considering the function and the role that the mental hospital (*manicomio*) has had in many Western countries, defined it as

> a deposit where people believe the mad (*i pazzi*) are sent, where intellectuals believe the lunatics (*i folli*) are sent and where doctors believe mental patients are looked after and treated. For the mad, the lunatic and the mental patient it is a locked, oppressive and total institution where punitive, prison-like rules are applied, in order to slowly eliminate its own contents. Its role is to explicitly isolate and control socially disturbing subjects, the illness being only a very marginal element. (p. 12)

This definition could be considered appropriate only for the mental hospitals in some "backward" regions or countries, for example Italy, where Basaglia, at the time this definition was written, was acting as a catalyst of a movement for radical change of a highly unsatisfactory system of psychiatric care. However, also in other Western countries, at that time, the model of the "best mental hospital" as a "collection of hostels and sheltered workshops, far from being cut off from its community, encouraging unrestricted visiting as well as arranging for many patients to work outside the hospital" (67, p. 209) was probably rather rare. In fact, a 1974 report of the Royal College of Psychiatrists, defining "the average standard of psychiatric care in Britain as abysmally low," states: "In the average mental hospital, a long-stay patient is likely to see a doctor for only ten minutes or so every three months. Even a recently admitted patient is seen by a doctor for an average of only 20 minutes each week. Scandals about the ill-treatment of patients in mental hospitals, including those of relatively good reputation, occur with monotonous regularity" (52, quoted by Clare [19], p. 370). A few years later a leading English psychiatrist declared "such conditions can still be found in many psychiatric hospitals at the present time" (19, p. 371). Similar views were expressed later by Professor Kathleen Jones, who in 1979 wrote, "We have plenty of evidence that such institutions [i.e., mental hospitals] can be damaging" (34, quoted by Ramon [48], p. 209), and by a WHO Working Group in 1978 in Cologne. In the conclusions of its final report it may be read, "The Group considered it a matter of great regret that in some countries large new mental hospitals are still under construction and was of the opinion that no more such institutions should be built . . . " (73, p. 46).

COMMUNITY PSYCHIATRY

A wide range of definitions of community psychiatry and of community mental health services may be found in the literature.

Rehin and Martin (49) considered community mental health services as "any scheme directed to providing extramural care and treatment . . . to facilitating the early detection of psychiatric illness or relapse and its treatment on an informal basis, and to providing some social work service in the community for support or follow-up" (quoted by Freeman, p. 354). On the other hand, Caplan (18) regarded community psychiatry as being primarily concerned with applying techniques of prevention, at different levels, and with achieving "positive mental health." Bennett (12) expressed the view that

> according to Sabshin (53), it is possible to reformulate community psychiatry as a use of the techniques, methods and theories of social psychiatry, as well as those of the other behavioural sciences, to investigate and treat the mental health needs of a functionally or geographically defined population over a significant period of time. According to this definition, community psychiatry is concerned with the mental health needs not only of the individual patient but of the district population, not only of those who are defined as sick, but those who may be contributing to that sickness and whose health or well-being may, in turn, be put at risk. (p. 214)

In the United States Serban (55) described community psychiatry as having three aspects — first, a social movement; second, a service delivery strategy, emphasizing the accessibility of services and acceptance of responsibility of the mental health needs of a total population; and third, provision of best possible clinical care, with emphasis on the major psychiatric disorders and on treatment outside total institutions. All these three aspects are nowhere better exemplified than in the Italian model of community psychiatry, as suggested by the 1978 psychiatric reform. We will report on this model later in this chapter. However, an attempt to clarify the meaning of "social movement" as applied to Italian community psychiatry is relevant here.

The rapid political, social, and cultural change that occurred in Italy from the 1960s onward provided a fertile background for the development of a movement for psychiatric reform, the focus of which was the work of Franco Basaglia and his associates. Participation in this development was not, however, confined to those professionally involved, and concern with psychiatric reform became an issue of general interest.

On the basis of practical experience of implementation of the Italian reform, one of us has recently defined community psychiatry as

> a system of care devoted to a defined population and based on a comprehensive and integrated mental health service, which includes outpatient facilities, day and residential training Centres, residential accommodation in hostels, sheltered workshops and inpatient units in general hospitals and which ensures with multidisciplinary team work, early diagnosis, prompt treatment, continuity of care, social support and a close liaison with other medical and social community services and, in particular, with general practitioners. (58, p. 664)

COMPLEMENTARY OR ALTERNATIVE COMMUNITY SERVICES?

It has been often stated that "the reduction in the numbers of mental hospital beds and admissions should proceed in pace with the creation of alternative services, such as psychiatric units in general hospitals, day hospitals, outpatient clinics, after-care hostels and rehabilitation workshops" (73, p. 6). The success of such a program depends on both the quantity and the quality of the resources made available and by the effective organization, integration, and coordination at the local level of the community services that should allow them to function as "alternative" services, instead of being additional or complementary to the mental hospital. Case-register studies conducted both in the United Kingdom (25) and in mainland Europe (26,27) have demonstrated that increases in outpatient care made according to a complementary model do not automatically lead to a reduction in the use of mental hospital beds. On the contrary, it has been found that such increases in care either bring about an increase in the number of admissions to hospital or shift the focus of attention toward a different and much less disturbed category of patients, with an increase in the total "treated prevalence."

This also applies to outpatient services started by mental hospitals (32). Data from the Groningen Psychiatric Case Register demonstrate that such services do not provide more continuity of care (from one type of service to another and also from one illness episode to another) for patients discharged from hospital. Such patients are referred to the independent and community-based social psychiatric services which, with few exceptions, have failed over the years to develop programs for continuous care and support (27). On the other hand, Häfner (29), in a study on schizophrenic patients in Mannheim, reported a relatively small and not statistically significant reduction of the probability of readmission to hospital as an effect of extensive utilization of complementary care.

This discouraging outcome of expanding community services can be expected in all situations in which inpatient treatment is planned as the principal component of the system of care, and in which community care is considered and planned (and often also defined) as complementary or additional. On the other hand, community services are alternative when they prove to be able to provide care and support to *all* groups of patients in the at-risk population, including long-term patients, and to develop new patterns of treatment and management, while decreasing the average duration of hospital stay and with it the total number of persons occupying psychiatric beds, and while gradually dismantling mental hospitals and similar closed and custodial institutions.

To build up alternative community services it appears to be necessary to reverse the above-stated rank order and to consider and organize community care as the principal component of the system (the so-called "community priority") (58).

TRANSFERRING CARE FROM MENTAL HOSPITALS TO ALTERNATIVE COMMUNITY SERVICES

The Rationale for a Shift

The reasons for a shift from psychiatric care centered in the mental hospital to care in a comprehensive mental health service have been extensively discussed elsewhere (22,56). It has been stated that "if properly conceived and executed, this changed, or changing, pattern of care offers much more flexible, and it is hoped, more effective help to the patient and his family" (72, p. 15). The aim of community care is to reverse the long-accepted practice of isolating mental patients in large institutions, to promote their integration in the community enabling them to keep ties with family and friends and offering them an environment that is socially stimulating, while avoiding exposing them to excessive social pressures (58). The hospital is *not* a natural social environment; hospital-based treatment therefore cannot provide the full range of opportunities that enable the patient to acquire confidence and self-esteem through success in social roles. On the contrary, hospitals are often places where excessive emphasis continues to be placed on physical treatments. The harmful aspects of prolonged institutional life and of segregation of patients have been stressed (7,28,69), and the higher risk of those patients who stay in the hospital for long periods of time to remain in hospital or to be readmitted after discharge has been demonstrated in a number of studies (31,47,63). Moreover, as Bennett stated (12), "it is not illogical to try to tackle a person's difficulties in the first instance in the place where they occur" (p. 214). This possibility has many advantages in offering useful and unique therapeutic opportunities. Mosher (45), after reviewing recent studies comparing the outcome of community treatment versus hospitalization, concludes: "By making available alternatives to hospitalization . . . it is possible to provide cheaper, more effective care to many of our seriously disturbed patients" (p. 1580). Tantam (62), discussing this subject, has recently declared,

> The consequences of hospital admission have changed considerably during the span of time covered by the studies that Mosher cites. Brief, informal admission to a ward in a general hospital is a very different experience from the prolonged, often involuntary incarceration in a large mental hospital so vividly described by Goffman (28). . . . The perils of decarceration now claim equal attention with the perils of institutionalism, and both should be taken into account in future research and clinical practice. (p. 4)

Critical Views

In spite of the general consensus on the superiority of community-based care, the development of community services has remained inadequate in many countries. In 1978 a WHO Working Group (72), reviewing the situation of 16 European countries, concluded that progress toward comprehensive community-based mental health care was disappointingly slow in all these countries and that the reasons were to be found in a complex group of problems, financial, organizational, political, and attitudinal. Similar observations had also been made in regard to the situation of community services in the United States (57), where the attempt to reduce mental hospital beds or to close psychiatric hospitals has not been accompanied by adequate provision of alternative resources in the community.

Among the more frequently mentioned factors which, apart from insufficient funds, inhibited further development of community services and explain why hospitals have remained the center of mental health care are:

(1) *The persistence of the "medical model,"* which is locked into the concept of the central position of hospital. The continued use of the hospital relieves the pressure from community agencies to develop alternatives, which in turn reinforces the utilization of hospitals. Mendel and Allen (40) discussed the social, economic, and professional difficulties that make it impossible within the medical model to change the traditional mental health intervention from hospital treatment to community care.

(2) *The social and political context of community care* (39,54), which is in large part beyond the control of mental health professions. Moving a large number of patients into the community has met often the resistance of communities and neighborhoods. Bachrach (1) observed that evidently neither the success of model programs in serving psychiatric patients nor the active concern of patients' advocacy groups has succeeded in bringing about the expected change in public opinion and prejudices against the mentally ill. One consequence of this failure to modify the public attitude, according to Bachrach (1), has been the drying up of funds and federal support for the development of community alternatives.

In more recent years criticisms have shifted more and more from quantitative issues, such as insufficient implementation of community services, to examination of the functioning of community services themselves, whose exclusive superiority has increasingly come under question (5,27,41,62). There is general agreement that it is no longer sufficient to equate progress in service delivery with shifts in the locus of care (2,13,68). It is evident that the institutionalism syndrome caused by a socially understimulating and undemanding environment not only is a feature of large institutions but can occur in the community setting as well. In particular the shift to a community setting has not led to improved conditions for psychiatric patients who are severely disordered for a long time (5,41). It has been observed that the basic needs of these chronic patients in community-oriented systems of care tend to be overlooked or subordinated to the needs of the less seriously ill, who appear to be the new target population of the community services (2,4,36,57,68).

Serious problems, predicts Bachrach (2), will arise whenever a community lacks adequate equivalence for the full range of functions traditionally served by psychiatric hospitals. These functions include material resources (food, shelter, clothing, medical care, and so forth) and the provision of "asylum" offering protection and security, which in particular for ex-mental hospital patients continues to represent a temporary or enduring need (3).

This issue is of particular concern in those countries, such as the United States, where many chronic long-stay patients have been discharged from mental hospitals into the community, and community services have to face the many practical difficulties of meeting the special problems and needs of these patients for total, comprehensive, and continuous care. When all services can be delivered within a single physical setting, providing total care is relatively simple, but to provide comprehensive care and continuity in a context characterized by fragmented service systems presents almost insurmountable problems. It has been stated that, without the necessary continuity of care, many patients will return to the chronic patient's role, with a pattern of frequent hospitalization and poor community adjustment between admissions (57).

Another frequent criticism regards the issue that the community approach shifts the burden from the hospital to the family. The burden of families with severely ill members living at home has been investigated by several authors (20,21,23), who concluded that the quality of life of the family was heavily compromised by the presence of a psychiatrically ill member. However, these families were not at all aided, or felt poorly assisted, by community services. When patients instead are intensely assisted and special attention is given to the needs of the families, it has been shown that the family burden is less than under the traditional hospital approach (64).

The answer to the question of whether it is possible to provide adequate and effective alternatives to the mental hospital depends, therefore, on the evaluation of community services, which should be characterized by comprehensiveness and continuity of care provided for a total patient population and its families, and in which facilities for evaluation should be available.

Following is an account of the organization of psychiatric community services in Italy after the psychiatric reform. It will be seen that the prescribed organizational features of these services avoid the above-cited possible structural deficiencies of community services in other countries. We shall then describe the community psychiatric services of South-Verona, in which we both work, including what has been achieved so far and what evaluation shows.

THE ITALIAN MODEL OF COMMUNITY PSYCHIATRY WITHOUT MENTAL HOSPITALS AND THE 1978 PSYCHIATRIC REFORM

It has been suggested (72) that "there are two ways for replacing mental hospitals by alternative services. The *first* is to divert patients to the alternative services thus reducing, and eventually stopping, admissions to the mental hospital altogether. Thus, the mental hospital population would slowly decline as long-term residents were discharged or died. The *other* method would be to close the mental hospital and evacuate or transfer its residents" (p. 17). Italy chose the first way.

In May 1978 the Italian Parliament passed Law 180, the main aims of which were *gradually* to dismantle the mental hospitals (closing their doors—to first admissions after May 1978 and to all admissions after December 1981—without encouraging abrupt deinstitutionalization) and to institute a comprehensive and integrated system of community psychiatric care in each Unitá Sanitaria Locale (100,000 to 200,000 inhabitants). This new psychiatric law is part of legislation that reformed the health services in Italy and introduced the National Health Services (NHS). The implementation of this legislation is still incomplete and has varied so far both regionally and in different parts of the system (50,61). In general, the northern regions are better provided as compared with the central-southern regions.

The major provisions of Law 180 have been extensively reported elsewhere (60,75). The distinctive features of the Italian model of community psychiatry are shown in Table 1. As may be seen, this model differs considerably from the American community mental health experience, where an abrupt deinstitutionalization of chronic patients occurred (16,44) (feature no. 1), and differs also from most European programs for community psychiatry, considering it as "complementary" to hospital treatment (feature no. 3), i.e., set up in places where admissions to the mental hospital are still possible. Under these circumstances, as Basaglia (8) noted, "the community services work merely because only the cases they are likely to succeed with get sent to them, and this is only possible as long as the asylum is in the background as a repository for intractable suffering" (p. 192).

It is important to point out that the new Italian law was introduced after the successful outcome of several long-term pilot studies that took place in Gorizia, Arezzo, Trieste, Perugia, and Ferrara between 1961 and 1978. It was demonstrated that it was possible to replace old-fashioned custodial care in mental hospitals with alternative patterns of care (10). In-depth evaluations, made by experts, of the psychiatric services provided after the psychiatric reform in a specific locality (14,33), as well as quantitative evaluations of the reform and its effects, have already appeared in the English language literature (11,15,42,43,61,65,66).

The evidence collected so far shows that currently there are essentially three styles of psychiatric services in Italy (38). First, there are districts, predominantly in the South, which have managed to ignore the law.

Table 1

Distinctive Features of the Italian Model of Community Psychiatry

1. The phasing out of mental hospitals is intended to be a gradual process (by means of a block on admissions rather than an abrupt deinstitutionalization of chronic patients).
2. The new services are designed to be alternative, rather than complementary or additional to mental hospitals.
3. It is hospital psychiatry which is considered complementary to community care, and not vice versa.
4. Integration is intended between the various facilities within the geographically based system of care, the same team providing domiciliary, outpatient, and inpatient care, an approach that facilitates continuity of care and long-term support.
5. There is special emphasis on multidisciplinary teamwork, domiciliary visits, and crisis intervention, and on easy access to the community mental health centers.

Second, there are districts in which there has been, and still is, a slow transfer from psychiatric hospital to community-based care. The third pattern is that of the districts where comprehensive community services have been developing and are actually functioning, and where the reform can be regarded as having been fully implemented. Data from these places indicate that the Italian model of alternative community care is able to cope with the problems presented by the whole range of psychiatric patients resident in the catchment area.

Evaluative follow-up studies of cohorts of patients treated in the new community-based system of care and epidemiological large-scale inquiries are currently underway, conducted under the aegis of the Italian National Research Council (CNR).

AN EXAMPLE OF A COMMUNITY-BASED SYSTEM OF CARE: THE SOUTH-VERONA CPS

The aim of this section is to give an example of the organization of a standard community service, set up in South-Verona after the Italian psychiatric reform.

Verona is a city of about 260,000 inhabitants, located in Northern Italy, halfway between Milan and Venice. South-Verona is an area of 75,000 inhabitants which includes part of the city of Verona and three small neighboring communities.

The South-Verona Community Psychiatric Service (CPS)

The South-Verona CPS comprises the following facilities:

The *Community Mental Health Centre (CMCH)*, open on all weekdays from 8 A.M. to 8 P.M., has been organized as a multiple-purpose facility where different activities take place, including morning report, planning of interventions, staff meetings, day care, and resocialization groups.

Domiciliary visits can be made in reply to emergency calls, to provide crisis intervention or, in the case of patients receiving long-term support, to avoid relapse and to minimize hospitalization. They are made by any member of the staff, including psychiatrists.

The *Psychiatric Unit* is an open ward of 15 beds located in the University general hospital.

The *Outpatient Department* provides psychiatric and psychological consultations, individual and family therapy.

The *Casualty Department* at the University general hospital is open 24 hours a day, seven days a week. During working hours the psychiatrist on duty is usually assisted in urgent intervention by a member of the team who is (or will be) responsible for the patient requiring the intervention. This is in order to extend to the emergency room the practice of therapeutic continuity (see below).

The *Psychiatric and Psychological Consultation Service* provides consultations for patients and doctors of other departments of the general hospital.

Finally, there are two *group homes* for patients discharged from the psychiatric hospital who can live on their own and one *supervised hostel* (8 beds) for difficult patients to be rehabilitated; they all belong to the CPS.

All these facilities are run by the same staff and constitute an integrated system of care. The CPS is staffed by nine psychiatrists, three psychologists, three social workers, and 28 psychiatric nurses. Besides running the service, the staff is also involved in research and in undergraduate and postgraduate teaching activities. There are also, at any given time, 8 to 10 residents in training (working full time, under supervision, for 12 months) and six to eight medical students (working part time, for four months). For maximal working efficiency the staff is divided into three teams, each being responsible for a defined sector of the area, with approximately 25,000 inhabitants.

Two or three members of the same team are always involved with each patient to ensure that a therapist is always available, despite turnover, shifts, vacations, and so forth. *Teamwork* is stressed and a *multidisciplinary approach* is emphasized, with doctors, nurses, psychologists, students, and social workers operating together as equal partners. *The same staff members remain involved with the same patient throughout the different settings of the CPS* and in different phases of the therapy, at the extramural as well as the intramural level. Thus, emphasis is placed on *longitudinal care* and on *therapeutic continuity.* In our CPS the emphasis on extramural activities is associated with an effort to change the whole concept of outpatient care, from mainly diagnosis or aftercare to being the pivot of both treatment and rehabilitation.

Other Services Available to the South-Verona Residents

The Provincial mental hospital of Verona now contains 350 long-stay patients, 18 of whom are from South-Verona (on December 31, 1986). Drug addicts as well as children and adolescents are treated by a specialized outpatient service, not belonging to the South-Verona CPS. In the Province of Verona (outside the South-Verona area) there are also two private psychiatric hospitals, with a total of 220 beds, but these beds are available also for patients from a much wider area. Moreover, a few neurological wards in general hospitals may admit patients with minor psychiatric disorders.

The South-Verona Psychiatric Case Register

All institutions mentioned above report data to the South-Verona Psychiatric Case Register, which began operating on December 31, 1978. Case-register data show that, despite the large availability of psychiatric beds and outpatient facilities by other agencies outside the South-Verona CPS, the majority of South-Verona residents requiring specialized psychiatric care are treated by our CPS (75). These data confirm that the South-Verona CPS is able to avoid a great deal of overlapping of care and of multiple service use.

The Style of Working in the South-Verona CPS

In South-Verona there is no split in responsibility between the local health authority and the local social service authority. Normalization, patient autonomy, and support to the families are the predominant goals of the South-Verona CPS.

The key operational elements of this service are extensive home support and home visiting, prompt crisis intervention, and integration and cooperation within the team, but the reduction of social distance and a sharing of skills must also be mentioned. Although each multidisciplinary district team (in charge of patients both at the community and at the hospital level) is coordinated by a psychiatrist, the doctors work with other staff (nurses, psychologists, social workers, and other therapists). An informal atmosphere encourages staff discussion and experimentation. Easy access of patients to the service and especially to the Mental Health Centre is ensured, and self-referrals are frequent (59).

Since the aim of the service is to integrate the patients into ordinary settings, they are encouraged to join activities available in the community, and the effort to integrate them within their natural network is given priority over establishment of separate, specialized settings.

Great attention is also paid to reviewing patients in community care at regular intervals in *ad hoc* meetings in which all the professionals of the district team take active part.

FROM LONG-STAY PATIENTS IN HOSPITAL TO LONG-TERM PATIENTS IN THE COMMUNITY

Our eight-year experience shows that in South-Verona while admissions to the mental hospital have been blocked, the total number of admissions to psychiatric beds has decreased (17) and the number of compulsory admissions has shown 90% decrease (61).

The number of long-stay patients (i.e., those in hospital for one year or more) has been decreasing over the years, and there is no evidence that new long-stay patients are accumulating (61). Instead patients in need of prolonged care are becoming long-term patients in the community, being assisted by the CPS, which provides inpatient care for short periods of time as well as day and outpatient/community care. These long-term patients are similar to those "chronic" patients who before the psychiatric reform were admitted to mental hospitals and became long-stay patients. These two groups of patients (long-stay and long-term), however, differ in their outcome in terms of subsequent patterns of care. In fact, a two-year follow-up study conducted using the South-Verona psychiatric case register showed that, while 88% of the long-stay patients remained long-stay in the following two years, only 45% of the long-term patients remained long-term in the same period (6).

These results, if confirmed for longer periods of time, would support the hypothesis that long-term community care may well replace long-term hospitalization in mental hospitals and lead to decreased dependence on the services and their chronic use.

Several case-register studies (17,61,75) showed that in South-Verona the majority of South-Verona residents requiring psychiatric care are treated outside the hospital only, confirming the community orientation of our service.

Comparing the South-Verona community-based psychiatric service with a Danish (Aarhus) institution-based service, it has been found that the incidence rates are similar in both areas. Admission rates as well as the one-year rate of persons in inpatient care are three times higher in Aarhus. Referrals to day and outpatient care (including home visits) are made 1.5 to 3.5 times as often in South-Verona, whereas the rates of persons in each of the three types of care are similar in the two centers. Compulsory admissions are higher in Aarhus (3.7/10,000 inhabitants) than in South-Verona (1.3/10,000 inhabitants) (46).

CONCLUSIONS

When psychiatric care is transferred from mental hospitals to the community, the characteristics and the standard of the new system of care need to be clearly defined, the steps that must be taken to develop these services need to be made explicit, and the ways in which the community care programs should be evaluated must be specified.

In the conclusions of the report on a WHO Working Group on *Changing Patterns in Mental Health Care* (73) the following general principles underlying the concept of comprehensive community mental health care are noted:

The services should be community-based, i.e. they should provide facilities for a defined area population small enough to permit most patients to be treated within easy travelling distance of their homes.

The services should be comprehensive, the sense that they provide a range of facilities, differentiated to meet the needs of persons suffering from any form of mental illness or handicap to be found in the area population.

The various agencies and services engaged in mental health care for each area population should be so effectively coordinated that each part of the system can contribute to the care of individual patients, according to needs, and that patients or their families do not suffer any disadvantage as a result of being transferred from one part of the system to another.

Services of equal quality and standard should be available to all persons in the service population who stand in need of mental health care, irrespective of financial or other considerations. (pp. 45–46)

The Italian psychiatric reform is based on all these principles, and they appear to have been put into practice wherever the reform has been properly implemented. But it should be made clear that "proper" implementation of any reform of this type requires adequate time; commitment from the individuals running the services as well as political and administrative commitment; new professional skills with a willingness on the part of the mental health professional to tolerate "more fluid roles and relationships" (39, p. 305) and to abandon "the protection of his medical status or his medical mystique" (p. 305); investment to be made in buildings, staff, and backup facilities; and a solid willingness to reach a *real* change.

All these elements are important, but the essential and most powerful one has probably been identified by Ramon (48): "For a real, non-cosmetic, change of the psychiatric system there is a need for *a changed professional and political attitude*, a fact that the Italians, for one, have understood perfectly" (p. 209).

ACKNOWLEDGMENTS

This study was supported by the Consiglio Nazionale delle Ricerche (CNR, Roma), Progetto Finalizzato Medicina Preventiva e Riabilitativa 1982–1987, contract no. 85.00786.56, and by the Regione Veneto, Ricerca Sanitaria Finalizzata, 1986. The authors are grateful to Mr. R. Fianco (Cattedra di Psicologia Medica, Universitá di Verona) for his assistance in the preparation of the manuscript.

REFERENCES

1. BACHRACH, L. L. (1983). Planning services for chronically ill patients. *Bulletin of the Menninger Clinic, 47* (2), 163–188.
2. BACHRACH, L. L. (1984). Asylum and chronically ill psychiatric patients. *American Journal of Psychiatry, 141,* 975–978.
3. BACHRACH, L. L. (1985). *The functions of semantics in mental health and mental retardation care.* Austin, TX: The University of Texas.
4. BACHRACH, L. L. (1985). Principles of planning for chronic psychiatric patients: A synthesis. In J. A. Talbott (Ed.), *The chronic mental patient.* New York: Grune & Stratton.
5. BACHRACH, L. L. (1986). The future of the state mental hospital. *Hospital and Community Psychiatry, 7,* 467–474.

6. BALESTRIERI, M., MICCIOLO, R., & TANSELLA, M. (1987). Long-stay and long-term patients in an area with a community-based system of care: A register follow-up study. *International Journal of Social Psychiatry*, in press.
7. BASAGLIA, F. (Ed.) (1968). *L'istituzione negata*. Torino: Einaudi.
8. BASAGLIA, F. (1981). Breaking the circuit of control. In D. Ingleby (Ed.), *Critical Psychiatry*. Harmondsworth: Penguin.
9. BASAGLIA, F., & ONGARO-BASAGLIA, F. (1971). *Noi matti: Dizionario sociale della psichiatria* (p. 12). Roma: L'Espresso-Colore.
10. BASAGLIA, F., & TRANCHINA, P. (1979). *Autobiografia di un movimento. 1961–1979. Dal manicomio alla riforma sanitaria*. Firenze: Unione Provincie Italiane, Regione Toscana, Amm.ne Prov.le di Arezzo.
11. BECKER, T. (1985). Psychiatric reform in Italy. How does it work in Piedmont? *British Journal of Psychiatry, 147*, 254–260.
12. BENNETT, D. H. (1978). Community psychiatry. *British Journal of Psychiatry, 132*, 209–220.
13. BENNETT, D. (1978). The Camberwell district services 1964–1974. The provision of alternatives to mental hospital care. In L. I. Stein, & M. A. Test (Eds.), *Alternatives to mental hospital treatment*. New York: Plenum Press.
14. BENNETT, D. H. (1978). *The changing pattern in mental health care in Trieste*. WHO Assignment Report. Copenhagen: WHO.
15. BOLLINI, P., MUSCETTOLA, G., PIAZZA, A., PUCA, M., & TOGNONI, G. (1986). Mental health care in Southern Italy: Application of case-control methodology for the evaluation of the impact of the 1978 psychiatric reform. *Psychological Medicine, 16*, 701–707.
16. BROWN, P. (1985). *The transfer of care: Psychiatric deinstituzionalization and its aftermath*. Henley-on-Thames: Routledge and Kegan Paul.
17. BURTI, L., GARZOTTO, N., SICILIANI, O., ZIMMERMANN-TANSELLA, CH., & TANSELLA, M. (1986). The South-Verona psychiatric service: An integrated system of community care. *Hospital and Community Psychiatry, 37*, 809–813.
18. CAPLAN, G. (1964). *Principles of preventive psychiatry*. London: Tavistock Publications.
19. CLARE, A. (1977). *Psychiatry in dissent*. London: Tavistock Publications.
20. CREER, C., & WING, J. K. (1974). *Schizophrenia at home*. Surbiton Surrey: National Schizophrenia Fellowship.
21. CREER, C. E., STURT, E., & WYKES, T. (1982). The role of relatives. In J. K. Wing (Ed.), *Long-term community care. Psychological Medicine* (Monograph Suppl. 2), 29–39.
22. DE SALVIA, D. (1977). *Per una psichiatria alternativa*. Milan: Feltrinelli.
23. DUPONT, A. (1980). A study concerning the time-related and other burdens when severely handicapped children are reared at home. *Acta Psychiatrica Scandinavica, 62* (Suppl. 285), 249–257.
24. FOWLER, N. (1982). Opening speech: "Working together." MIND Annual Conference, p. 5.
25. FRYERS, T., & WOLFF, K. (1985). Il controllo dei servizi di salute mentale in una città inglese. In M. Tansella (Ed.), *L'Approccio epidemiologico in psichiatria*. Torino: Boringhieri.
26. GIEL, R. (1980). The truth about psychiatric morbidity. *Acta Psychiatrica Scandinavica, 285* (Suppl.), 30–40.
27. GIEL, R. (1986). Care of chronic mental patients in the Netherlands. *Social Psychiatry, 21*, 25–32.
28. GOFFMAN, E. (1961). *Asylums*. New York: Doubleday.
29. HÄFNER, H. (1985). Changing patterns of mental health care. *Acta Psychiatrica Scandinavica, 71* (Supp. 319), 151–164.
30. HOGARTH, J. (1975). *Glossary of health care terminology*. Copenhagen: WHO Regional Office for Europe.

31. HORN TEN, G. H. M. M. (1984). Aftercare and readmission. A Dutch psychiatric case register study. *Social Psychiatrist, 19*, 111–116.
32. HORN TEN, G. H. M. M., & GIEL, R. (1978). Patronen in het network van de geestelijke gezondheidszorg. *Maandbl. Geestel Volksgez, 33*, 23–24 (cited by Giel, 1986).
33. JABLENSKY, A., & HENDERSON, J. (1983). *Report on a visit to the South-Verona community psychiatric service.* WHO Assignment Report. Geneva and Copenhagen: WHO.
34. JONES, K. (1979). Integration or disintegration of the Mental Health Service: Some reflections and developments in Britain since the 1950's. In M. Meacher (Ed.), *New methods of mental health care.* Oxford: Pergamon.
35. LANGSLEY, D. G. (1980). The community mental health center: Does it treat patients? *Hospital and Community Psychiatry, 31*, 815–819.
36. LANGSLEY, D. G., & YARVIS, R. M. (1978). Alternatives to hospitalization. The Sacramento story. In L. I. Skin & M. A. Test (Eds.), *Alternatives to mental hospital treatment.* New York: Plenum Press.
37. MAY, A. R. (1976). *Mental health services in Europe.* WHO Offset publication no. 23. Geneva: WHO.
38. MCCARTHY, M. (1985). Psychiatric care in Italy: Evidence and assertion. *Hospital Health Service Review, Nov.*, 278–280.
39. MECHANIC, D. (1978). Alternatives to mental hospital treatment: A sociological perspective. In L. I. Stein & M. A. Test (Eds.), *Alternatives to mental hospital treatment.* New York: Plenum Press.
40. MENDEL, W. M., & ALLEN, R. E. (1978). Rescue and rehabilitation. In L. I. Stein & M. A. Test (Eds.), *Alternatives to mental hospital treatment.* New York: Plenum Press.
41. MOLLICA, R. F. (1983). From asylum to community. The threatened disintegration of public psychiatry. *New England Journal of Medicine, 308*, 367–373.
42. MOROSINI, P., REPETTO, F., DE SALVIA, D., & CECERE, F. (1985). Psychiatric hospitalization in Italy before and after 1978. *Acta Psychiatrica Scandinavica, 71* (Suppl. 316), 27–43.
43. MOSHER, L. R. (1982). Italy's revolutionary mental health law: An assessment. *American Journal of Psychiatry, 139*, 199–203.
44. MOSHER, L. R. (1983). Recent developments in the care, treatment, and rehabilitation of the chronic mentally ill in Italy. *Hospital and Community Psychiatry, 34*, 947–950.
45. MOSHER, L. R. (1983). Alternatives to psychiatric hospitalization: why has research failed to be translated into practice? *New England Journal of Medicine, 309*, 1579–1580.
46. MUNK-JORGENSEN, P., & TANSELLA, M. (1986). Hospital and community-based psychiatry: A comparative study between a Danish and an Italian psychiatric service. *International Journal of Social Psychiatry, 32*(2), 6–15.
47. PAUL, G. L. (1969). Chronic mental patient. Current status — Future directions. *Psychological Bulletin, 71*, 81–94.
48. RAMON, S. (1985). Understanding the Italian experience. *British Journal of Psychiatry, 146*, 208–209.
49. REHIN, G. F., AND MARTIN, F. M. (1963), quoted by Freeman, H. L. (1983). District psychiatric services: psychiatry for defined populations. In P. Bean (Ed.), *Mental illness: Changes and trends.* New York: Wiley.
50. ROBB, J. H. (1986). The Italian health services: Slow revolution or permanent crisis? *Social Science Medicine, 22*, 619–627.
51. ROLLIN, H. R. (1977). De-institutionalization and the community: Fact and theory. *Psychological Medicine, 7*, 181–184.
52. Royal College of Psychiatrists (1974). *Memorandum on psychiatric manpower as it affects the psychiatric services.* London: Royal College of Psychiatrists.
53. SABSHIN, M. (1966). Theoretical models in community and social psychiatry. In L. M. Roberts, S. L. Halleck, & M. B. Loeb (Eds.), *Community psychiatry.* Madison: University of Wisconsin Press.

54. SEGAL, S. P., & AVIRAM, U. (1978). *The mentally ill in community based sheltered care: A study of community care and social integration.* New York: Wiley.
55. SERBAN, G. (1977). *New trends of psychiatry in the community.* Cambridge, MA: Ballinger.
56. STEIN, L., & TEST, M. A. (Eds.) (1978). *Alternatives to mental hospital treatment.* New York: Plenum Press.
57. STEIN, L. I., & TEST, M. A. (1978). An alternative to mental hospital treatment. In L. I. Stein & M. A. Test (Eds.), *Alternatives to mental hospital treatment.* New York: Plenum Press.
58. TANSELLA, M. (1986). Community psychiatry without mental hospitals — The Italian experience: A review. *Journal of the Royal Society of Medicine, 79,* 664–669.
59. TANSELLA, M., & BELLANTUONO, C. (1986). The view from abroad — Italy. In M. Shepherd, G. Wilkinson, & P. Williams (Eds.), *Mental illness in primary care settings.* London: Tavistock.
60. TANSELLA, M., & WILLIAMS, P. (1987). The Italian experience and its implications. *Psychological Medicine, 17,* 283–289.
61. TANSELLA, M., DE SALVIA, D., & WILLIAMS, P. (1987). The Italian psychiatric reform. Some quantitative evidence. *Social Psychiatry, 22,* 37–48.
62. TANTAM, D. (1985). Alternatives to psychiatric hospitalization. *British Journal of Psychiatry, 146,* 1–4.
63. TEST, M. A., & STEIN, L. I. (1978). The clinical rationale for community treatment: A review of the literature. In L. Stein & M. A. Test (Eds.), *Alternatives to mental hospital treatment.* New York: Plenum Press.
64. TEST, M. A., & STEIN, L. I. (1978). Training in community living: Research designs and results. In L. Stein & M. A. Test (Eds.), *Alternatives to mental hospital treatment.* New York: Plenum Press.
65. TORRE, E., MARINONI, A., ALLEGRI, G., BOSSO, A., EBBLI, D., & GORRINI, M. (1982). Trends in admissions before and after an act abolishing mental hospitals: a survey in three areas of northern Italy. *Comprehensive Psychiatry, 3,* 227–232.
66. WILLIAMS, P., DE SALVIA, D., & TANSELLA, M. (1986). Suicide, psychiatric reform and the provision of psychiatric services in Italy. *Social Psychiatry, 21,* 89–95.
67. WING, J. K. (1963). Mental health. The adult psychiatric patient in the community. *Public Health, 77,* 204–209.
68. WING, L. (1978). Planning and evaluation services for chronically handicapped psychiatric patients in the United Kingdom. In L. I. Stein and M. A. Test (Eds.), *Alternatives to mental hospital treatment.* New York: Plenum Press.
69. WING, J. K., & BROWN, G. W. (1970). *Institutionalism and schizophrenia.* London: Cambridge University Press.
70. WING, J. K., & OLSEN, P. (1979). *Community care for the mentally disabled.* Oxford: Oxford University Press.
71. World Health Organization (1971). *Trends in psychiatric care: Day hospitals and units in general hospitals.* Report on a symposium. Copenhagen: WHO Regional Office for Europe.
72. World Health Organization (1978). *The future of mental hospitals.* Report on a Working Group. Copenhagen: WHO Regional Office for Europe.
73. World Health Organization (1980). *Changing patterns in mental health care.* Report on a WHO Working Group. Copenhagen: WHO Regional Office for Europe.
74. WYKES, T., CREER, L., & STURT, E. (1982). Needs and the deployment of services. In J. K. Wing (Ed.), *Long-term community care. Psychological Medicine,* (Monograph Suppl. 2), 41–55.
75. ZIMMERMANN-TANSELLA, CH., BURTI, L., FACCINCANI, C., GARZOTTO, N., SICILIANI, O., & TANSELLA, M. (1985). Bringing into action the psychiatric reform in South-Verona. A five year experience. *Acta Psychiatrica Scandinavica, 71* (Suppl. 316), 71–86.

8

ATTENTION DEFICIT HYPERACTIVITY DISORDER

PAUL H. WENDER, M.D.

Professor of Psychiatry, Director of Psychiatric Research,
University of Utah School of Medicine,
Salt Lake City, Utah

INTRODUCTION

Attention deficit hyperactivity disorder (ADHD) is probably the most common diagnosis in child psychiatric outpatient clinics in the United States. ADHD has received multiple designations in the past: the hyperactive child syndrome; hyperkinesis; minimal brain dysfunction. Since motoric hyperactivity is neither diagnostically necessary nor pathognomonic, those designations are inappropriate. "Minimal brain damage" suggests an etiology that is rarely true and "minimal brain dysfunction," though having the virtue of nonspecificity, involves circular reasoning (behavior is disordered because the brain is dysfunctional and we know that the brain is dysfunctional because the behavior is disordered).

Before proceeding, we should address the question of why ADHD is diagnosed infrequently in England and appears to be an American disorder. The author presumes that there are a number of reasons, the first of which is that in England these children acquire a different label, probably conduct disorder. Academic child psychiatrists in North America would acknowledge that attention deficit hyperactivity disorder frequently occurs together with conduct disorder, but would state that "pure" forms of ADHD are, in fact, very common. The second reason that attention deficit hyperactivity disorder has apparently been neglected in Britain seems to be that psychopharmacological treatment, particularly stimulant drug treatment, is not commonly used for children. This is reflected by the paucity of

149

British scientific literature dealing with the effect of stimulant drugs on psychiatric disorders of childhood. When used with responsive ADHD children, stimulant medications may produce one of the most striking therapeutic effects we see in psychiatry. As practitioners we usually consider our patients lucky if we can return them to the *status quo ante*. Treatment with stimulants will often enable an ADHD child to function at a better level than he has ever functioned before. It is probable that the magnitude of this response has generated much of the current interest in — and literature about — ADHD in the United States.

In this chapter, assertions not referenced specifically will be found in the references of the monographs cited in the reference list.

SYMPTOMS

The *Diagnostic and Statistical Manual* of the American Psychiatric Association (Revised) (DSM-III-R) has changed the name of the syndrome formerly called Attention Deficit Disorder (ADD) to Attention Deficit Hyperactivity Disorder (ADHD) and changed the operational criteria for diagnosis. Diagnosing ADHD depends on the presence of a total number of symptoms characteristic of attentional problems, motor hyperactivity, and impulsivity. The major diagnostic change is that attentional deficits and impulsivity are no longer pathognomonic: A child could receive the diagnosis of ADHD with or without inattentiveness, with or without impulsivity, and with or without hyperactivity, so long as he manifested eight of 14 signs and symptoms reflecting such deficits. Nonetheless, it may be useful to describe the manifestations in these three areas.

Inattentiveness

Inattentiveness is usually a prominent feature of the syndrome. In toddlers and young children with severe ADHD, it may be present in most situations. In older and less severely affected children, inattentiveness may be situational and appears to be related to interest. The ADHD child may daydream when fractions are being taught but may pay complete attention to areas he finds of greater interest, such as tornados, earthquakes, dinosaurs, and wars. Most ADHD children are disorganized — a frailty that is most conspicuous at school. Disorganization appears to be partly the consequence of attentional lapses together with indifference to social (academic) demands. It is listed here for convenience.

Impulsivity

Impulsivity, another formerly pathognomonic attribute, is one whose manifestations change as a function of age. A school-age child may talk when silence is requested, may push ahead in lines, and may act without thinking. The nature of the impulsive behaviors obviously changes with age. This acting without thinking, together with a low tolerance for frustration, produces much difficulty for the ADHD individual in whom it persists through adolescence and into adult life. Impulsive symptoms which are seen in these older age groups and which are easily recognizable by the clinician are frequently indicators of persisting ADHD.

MOTOR SIGNS

Hyperactivity

"Hyperactivity" may be situational or cross-situational. It is very visible, easily measurable, and of no great pathological importance. "Hyperactive" children are no more active than their peers on the playground, but they are in the classroom, where it is disturbing to their teacher and classmates. The hyperactive ADHD child fidgets, squirms, and leaves his seat. Nonstop talking—"motor mouth"—*may* be an additional sign of hyperactivity.

Coordination Problems

ADHD appears to have an increased association with impaired coordination. ADHD children are often referred to as awkward or clumsy. Coordination difficulties manifest themselves in three areas: (1) balance—e.g., difficulty skating and riding a bicycle; (2) fine motor impairment—e.g., in kindergarten, failing to color within or cut along lines; difficulty tying shoelaces; messy handwriting (which may persist indefinitely, and which is, interestingly, often responsive to stimulant medication); and (3) hand-eye coordination—which renders the ADHD boy inept in baseball, basketball, and so forth and therefore not valued by his peers (who are excellent judges of athletic skill).

Altered Response to Social Reinforcement

ADHD children often do that which they should not and fail to do that which they should. They are at best forgetful and at worst obstinate and negativistic; forgetfulness characterizes the ADHD child; active resistance is more typical of the child with conduct disorder.

Altered Interpersonal Relations

ADHD children appear to begin their social lives by being outgoing but may — on the basis of repeated rejection — mix less and less with other children. They tend to be bossy, bullying, and domineering, all of which may alienate their peers and cause their exclusion from their peer group.

Altered Emotionality

For want of a better heading, I am listing a number of attributes under this excessively vague phrase. ADHD children have increased affective lability, with a tendency to get depressed or overexcited very easily. They are overreactive — ADHD children are readily upset and are often described as hot-tempered or "short-fused." Probably better classified as both a cognitive and affective attribute is low self-esteem. Whether this is a fundamental attribute, a learned attitude, or a combination of the two is uncertain. It is easy to see how ADHD children might acquire low self-esteem: they are rejected by other children, criticized by teachers, and experience chronic friction with their parents. They are poor athletes, poor students, and unfavorably compared to their siblings and peers. Under these circumstances, high self-esteem would be a manifestation of impaired reality testing. There may be a biological component to this. Many ADHD children and adults who respond favorably to stimulant medication experience an increase in their self-esteem long before their improved behavior has had time to produce positive feedback from others.

Associated Features

Two specific disorders and certain physical abnormalities seem to be associated with ADHD with an increased frequency: (1) specific developmental disorders (specific retardation in reading, spelling, and mathematics; and impaired coordination); (2) conduct disorders; (3) specific congenital anatomical stigmata. Children with ADHD have an increased number of stigmata, and children with an increased number of stigmata are more likely to have ADHD.

Changing Symptoms in Adolescence and Adulthood

As will be discussed in the section on prognosis, symptoms of ADHD frequently persist through adolescence and far into adult life. These will be discussed briefly at the end of this chapter.

PROGNOSIS

Until recently the accepted child psychiatric gospel was that "hyperactivity" diminished in late childhood and disappeared during adolescence. It was also believed that the "paradoxical response" to stimulants altered at this time and that "ex-hyperactive" patients developed the "normal" response to stimulant medication. Nonetheless, a few clinicians who treated many patients with "minimal brain dysfunction" or "hyperactivity" maintained that many of the children continued to have problems well into adult life and that they continued to manifest the same — beneficial — response to stimulant medication. None of these experienced clinicians published systematic accounts of their observations, and thus their findings were neglected by academic child psychiatrists.

In the past several years a number of systematic studies have investigated the postchildhood fate of children with ADHD. These studies have found that about 25 to 75 percent continue to have the behavioral and psychological abnormalities of ADHD (Cantwell) (2). This group of children is at increased risk for academic and vocational failure, legal transgressions, and alcohol and substance abuse. *Which* children are at *which* particular risk is uncertain. This is, among other reasons, because the samples studied did not discriminate clearly between children with ADHD alone and ADHD mixed with conduct disorder.

Studies are beginning to be done of adults with ADHD. The symptoms and signs they manifest are similar to those seen in the ADHD child, but the reasons they seek therapy are different: the child is *brought* for unacceptable *behavior* whereas the adult with ADHD usually comes voluntarily because of ego-dystonic *psychological symptoms*.

EPIDEMIOLOGY

Determining the prevalence of ADHD and associated disorders is subject to the same logical difficulties that exist in medicine when dealing with quantitative — rather than qualitative — differences. It is unclear where a cutting point between health and disease should be made for quantitative variables such as weight and blood pressure (it is obviously not true that a blood pressure of 141/91 is hypertension and 139/89 is not). The problem of defining disorders on the basis of quantitative differences is illustrated in studies of ADHD in which prevalence has often been determined on the basis of rating scales and on the decision that any child who is two (it should be 1.67) standard deviations above the mean has ADHD. This method produces the expectable result that about 3 or 4 percent of school-age children have ADHD. However defined, ADHD is, like other psychiatric conditions of childhood, much more common in males, with a probable sex ratio of 5 : 1 to 3 : 1. Women with symptoms of ADHD seem to "crop up" in later life, but what their behavior and psychological functioning were as children is unclear.

Prevalence estimates by experienced clinicians and based on categorical diagnosis yield rates that are much higher: of the order of 10 percent (e.g., Huessy and Gendron) (6). The prevalence of ADHD is thought to be appreciably increased in lower socioeconomic groups. Good data are not available.

ETIOLOGY

Until the past 10 or 15 years, the "hyperactive child syndrome" was believed to be the product of brain damage—hence the earlier designation "minimal brain damage." The origins of this notion are relevant. It appears that an ADHD-like syndrome—which had been described in the 19th century—was first observed on a large scale following the epidemic of von Economo's encephalitis that occurred after World War I. Following recovery from the acute encephalitis, many adults developed Parkinson's syndrome (some immediately, others much later) and many children developed a "postencephalitic behavior disorder." Contemporaneous descriptions of the latter sound very much like a mixture of ADHD and conduct disorder. In succeeding years, clinicians reported ADHD-like behavior as a sequel to lead poisoning, head injury, and pre- and perinatal difficulties. The correlations between the disorder and the putative insults were not high, and in some instances—such as head injury—the neurological insult was probably a manifestation of, rather than a cause of, the disorder. (Impulsive children run out in front of cars. One study found that ADHD children appeared in emergency rooms at five times the expected rate.)

In the 1960s and 1970s clinicians began to report an association between ADHD in children and other forms of psychopathology in their parents.

The relationships observed were an increased frequency of alcoholism and antisocial personality disorder in the fathers and a history of hyperactivity in childhood in the fathers and close male relatives. Of interest in this particular observation is the association between alcoholism and antisocial personality, which form two of the triad of associated disorders studied by the Washington University group (the third being Briquet's syndrome or somatization disorder [DSM-III-R]).

Association of a disorder in children and their parents may be a manifestation of either genetic or psychosocial transmission. The most powerful way of separating these effects is to employ the adoption strategy. There are three relevant studies. Safer (10) studied the siblings and half-siblings of "hyperactive" children in foster care. Approximately half the full siblings and one-quarter of the half-siblings manifested "hyperactivity" (which suggests dominant genetic transmission). The difficulties in interpretation of this study are due to the imprecision in diagnosis (to which I shall refer later) and the fact that all the children had been subjected to an abnormal environment for two or three years (which was the reason they were placed in foster care). Goodwin et al. (5) conducted a study in Denmark of the adopted-away adult sons of alcoholic and nonalcoholic fathers. The alcoholics' sons were at four times the risk for "hyperactive" behavior in childhood. Finally, Cantwell (3) and Morrison and Stewart (8) examined the parents of hyperactive children using the adoptive parents' technique. With this technique these investigators compared the nature and prevalence of psychopathology in the biological parents (who brought their own "hyperactive" children to clinic), the adoptive parents of "hyperactive" children (biological parents unknown), and the biological parents of a nonpsychiatric medical sample of children. They found an increased incidence of alcoholism, antisocial personality, and "hysteria" in the biological parents of the "hyperactive" children.

These studies clearly show genetic transmission — but of what? A major question in interpreting these studies has been raised by Stewart et al. (13). They have claimed that the increased frequency of psychopathology observed in the biological parents of "hyperactive children" may be limited to children with mixed ADHD and conduct disorder. Since most of the earlier studies did not subdivide their samples into ADHD children with and without conduct disorder, these studies will have to be replicated, paying careful attention to the diagnosis of the probands.

If ADHD is genetically transmitted, the next question is what the mediating biological mechanism(s) might be. On the basis of the data to be reviewed, it seems probable that many of the symptoms are produced by decreased activity in dopaminergic systems. The data consonant with this hypothesis are as follows. The von Economo's virus damaged dopaminergic neurons in adults. Patients dying of the disorder had destruction of dopaminergic neurons, particularly in the substantia nigra. Idiopathic Parkinson's syndrome is associated with decreased homovanillic acid (HVA is the principal metabolite of dopamine) in the cerebrospinal fluid (CSF). Furthermore, both postencephalitic and idiopathic Parkinson's syndrome respond to L-dopa, the immediate precursor of dopamine, as well as to direct dopamine agonists such as bromocryptine. One may *cautiously* extrapolate and hypothesize that similar neurons were damaged in children who developed postencephalitic behavior disorder—*but there are no supporting neuropathological data.*

The second group of data suggesting decreased dopaminergic activity in ADHD comes from the pattern of psychopharmacological responsiveness seen in ADHD children. ADHD responds best to drugs whose actions are dopaminergic. Methylphenidate is an indirect dopamine agonist (releasing dopamine from presynaptic stores); amphetamine is (among other things) an indirect dopamine agonist; and pemoline is likewise an indirect dopamine agonist. Tricyclic antidepressants (TCA) have been used to treat both ADHD children and adults. Their response is different both temporally and qualitatively from that seen in major depression. The TCAs are usually sedating and appear to decrease hyperactivity and improve mood, but appear not to increase concentration. The temporal response is characteristic: the TCAs work immediately but most ADHD patients become tolerant to them in about six weeks. This contrasts with major depressives, who usually do not respond to TCAs until four to six weeks and who usually do not develop tolerance. Since the action of the tricyclic antidepressants is presumed to be mediated by increased noradrenergic or serotonergic activity, it seems that these monoamines do not play a critical role in the pathogenesis of ADHD.

On the other hand, the monoamine oxidase inhibitors *do* improve the signs and symptoms of both ADHD children (19) and adults. The author and his colleagues have treated more than 30 ADHD adults (in open trial) with pargyline (16) and deprenyl (18), both—in low doses—specific MAO-B inhibitors. As with the TCAs, hyperactivity was reduced and mood improved. In addition, in responsive cases, hot temper, disorganization, and impulsivity diminished or disappeared, and concentration improved. There were two other differences between these MAOIs and the TCAs: when benefit occurred, it did so after four or more weeks, and when it did occur, tolerance did not develop. Physiologically, MAO-B is responsible for the oxidation of phenethylamine and dopamine. The effectiveness of a MAO-B inhibitor implies that ADHD symptoms are diminished by drug-induced increased phenethylaminergic and/or dopaminergic activity. However, the MAOI's action may well not have been specific. In the larger doses employed, l-deprenyl and pargyline may also inhibit MAO-A — which is responsible for the breakdown of norepinephrine, dopamine, and serotonin. The major clinical observation remains: that MAOIs were therapeutically efficacious and that the tricyclic antidepressants were not.

The last body of data compatible with the dopaminergic hypothesis comes from CSF studies of "hyperactive children" and adults with attention deficit hyperactivity disorder. Shaywitz et al. (11) found that hyperactive children had decreased CSF homovanillic acid compared to nonhyperactive controls (but only on the basis of some reasonable, but unproved metabolic assumptions). Shetty and Chase (12) found normal HVA in a group of hyperactive children but found an exceedingly high correlation between *de*creases in CSF HVA and the degree of improvement when treated with amphetamine. They explained their findings by hypothesizing that the degree of improvement was proportional to the degree of induced dopaminergic activity and that the greater this activity, the greater the feedback inhibition of endogenous dopamine production. Reimherr et al. (9) found a significantly decreased HVA concentration in a group of adult women (versus matched controls) with ADHD and a near-significant decrease in HVA in a group of men with ADHD. Of interest was the finding that the male subjects who were not benefited by treatment with stimulants — who in fact became worse — had significantly higher CSF HVA than did the controls.

Animal models for psychiatric disorders are always suspect. They are somewhat more acceptable in the case of ADHD because the behaviors that are relevant, inattentiveness, impulsivity, and noncompliance, can be studied in animals. Bareggi et al. (1) investigated CSF metabolites and brain slices in a hybrid strain of dogs which was difficult to discipline and found that some responded to amphetamine with increased compliance. These responsive animals had decreased norepinephrine, dopamine, and HVA in brain slices and decreased CSF HVA — a finding consistent with the dopamine hypothesis.

The dopaminergic hypothesis, even if correct, fails to answer several questions. Chief among them is the increased association of ADHD with conduct disorder and specific developmental disorders. Neither syndrome responds to stimulant medications, and an explanation of their pathophysiology must lie elsewhere.

Evaluation

The full evaluation of the child with suspected ADHD involves: (1) a past and current behavioral and psychological history from the child's parents and teachers; (2) an educational evaluation of the child; (3) a clinical examination of the child.

With few exceptions, the most important diagnostic information is obtained from the child's caretakers and teachers. A number of structured psychiatric interviews for parents and the child have been developed in the United States. They were keyed to DSM-III diagnostic categories and were useful in obtaining standardized data, particularly for trainees. (Slight modification will be necessary to key them to DSM-III-R.) It is useful to interview both the mother and father, since parents often disagree. In addition to often having (implicitly) different criteria, it must be remembered that the child's mother spends more time with the child and is likely to see him in a larger number of social situations than is the father.

Teachers are in a particularly advantageous position to evaluate a child's functioning. To begin with, they have usually seen many children of the child's age and are therefore very aware of behavioral norms. In addition, they see him engaged in the two most important developmental tasks of childhood: learning in the classroom, and forming relationships with peers. Teachers are also in an excellent position to assess particular ADHD problems: inattentiveness; motor restlessness when quiet is demanded; impulsivity; disorganization; tolerance to academic frustration; and the difficulties with peers that cause much trouble to ADHD children—stubbornness and bossiness.

A number of teacher and parent questionnaires have been used to evaluate psychopathology. The most widely used one in the United States is the Conners' Abbreviated Teacher's Rating Scale. This is a 10-item questionnaire which is filled out by the child's teacher. It has been administered to tens of thousands of children. In the United States it has been usual to employ a particular cutoff score as diagnostic of ADHD and to use the scale to monitor behavioral changes in drug trials. A number of psychologists have expressed dissatisfaction with it recently, feeling that the usual cutoffs overdiagnose and that it fails to distinguish between ADHD and conduct disorder. There are a number of suggested alternatives. The most thoroughly researched of the new tests, devised by Ullmann et al. (14), rates a child's classroom functioning in four areas: hyperactivity, inattentiveness, social maturity, and conduct disorder. It is new and its practical usefulness remains to be documented.

The next area that must always be evaluated is the child's intelligence and level of academic performance. Academic underachievement is almost a hallmark of ADHD. For a particular child it is important to determine to what extent it is the result of ADHD alone or of the specific developmental disorders with which ADHD is frequently associated. The DSM-III-R definition of developmental disorders in reading and arithmetic is that there is a significant impairment in the development of these skills not accounted for by mental retardation, hearing or visual defects, or inadequate schooling. The operational definition of impairment is the difference between time (in months) of predicted reading age (on the basis of chronological age and IQ) and actual reading age. The magnitude that qualifies as "significant" is arbitrary—in the United States it is about 24 months. This evaluation is relatively straightforward. It requires administration of a standardized intelligence test and a standardized test of achievement in reading, spelling, and arithmetic. The intelligence test must be individually administered, since group tests depend on the child's reading, which is one of the areas to be tested. There are no widely accepted tests for motor competence. This can be crudely evaluated on the basis of age-specific motor tasks: coloring within lines; cutting with scissors along lines; writing; tying shoelaces, and so forth. Hand-eye coordination can be crudely evaluated by skill in throwing, catching, and batting a ball.

The interview with a child is likely, in most instances, to be less informative than the history and educational evaluation. It has been repeatedly observed that, at least for short periods of time, most ADHD children can be relatively quiet and attentive within the examiner's office, and thus failure to observe "hyperactivity" in these circumstances is not diagnostically significant. The presence or absence of anatomical stigmata and/or motor problems is also not diagnostic. The child's own account of his history is usually not helpful. The individual examination of the child is most useful in detecting other psychiatric symptomatology, for example affective disorder and psychosis. An appreciable number of parents are unaware of anhedonia and/or suicidal preoccupations associated with the former, or of bizarre fantasies (which may sometimes be elicited by drawings and projective storytelling techniques) associated with the latter.

TREATMENT

There are four major components to the management of a child with ADHD: (1) education of the parent and child about the problem; (2) drug therapy; (3) psychological and behavioral therapies; (4) specific educational procedures.

Explanation of the Problem to Parents

The physician must educate the parents about the nature of ADHD. The notion that psychological problems in children may have specific biological bases is not well known. Psychological dogma — at least in the United States — asserts that the child's personality, both his assets and his liabilities, are the product of upbringing. If the child has problems, it is usually assumed that they are parental in origin. The first point to make in the explanation is that ADHD is a psychiatric disorder — frequently genetically transmitted — which produces certain specific behavioral problems. Next, the physician should explain what these problems are: attentional difficulties; impulsivity; decreased sensitivity to social reinforcement; affective liability; quick temper; and so forth. He should explain that if the child responds to medication, the parents should see a marked improvement in *these* symptoms. However, the symptoms have existed for years, have affected the child's environment, and may have produced psychological changes that remain even if the biological disorder is brought under control by medication.

If specific developmental disorders are present, a full explanation of them is necessary. The parents need to understand that their child can have normal or superior intelligence despite being unable to master certain rote skills.

A major goal in educating the parents is to communicate to them that to the best of our current knowledge their child's problems are not their fault. The physician must avoid both explicit and implicit guilt provocation. However, the physician must also be aware that often at least one parent has ADHD and that family disruption and physical abuse are very common. What the parents must learn, with the physician's help, is how to deal with the child's current difficulties.

Finally, the physician should explain the therapeutic plan.

Explanation of the Problem to the Child

This phase of treatment will be greatly facilitated if the initial diagnostic sessions have been held with the child present. Most children see the whole evaluative and therapeutic procedure as punitive and many will feign ignorance if they can. If the child has participated in the initial meetings and knows the physician knows what the problems are, the latter can occupy the role of an ally rather than that of a prosecuting attorney. The physician should offer an age-appropriate explanation of ADHD. One therapeutic goal in working with the child is to help him perceive the behavioral difficulties he has had and to help him to learn how they are diminished by medication. In addition, the physician wants to communicate to the child that the latter has a certain degree of "free will" and responsibility for his own behavior. The rationale is that the physician does not want the child to say: "I couldn't help it — I've got a chemical difference." One's goal is to have the child try, without blaming him — even tacitly — for failing. The objective is to motivate the child, letting him take credit for his successes without making him feel guilty for his failures — easier said than done.

PHARMACOLOGICAL MANAGEMENT

In the United States stimulant drugs play the preeminent role in the treatment of the ADHD child. Between 60 and 80 percent of ADHD children respond favorably to these agents. In perhaps one-half this number, the effects are dramatic. Responding children function at a higher level than they ever have before. Hyperactivity diminishes or disappears; attention span is lengthened and academic performance may improve dramatically; motor abnormalities may be modified — sloppy handwriting becomes neat. Far more important are the changes in impulsivity and response to social expectations. The child begins to think before he acts and starts to behave in accordance with the shoulds and should nots he has heard for years. Frustration tolerance increases and temper outbursts diminish. Affective lability smooths out and excitements as well as depressions disappear. Social behavior which had been antipathetic to others changes subtly and the child develops friendships. These changes often produce a "virtuous cycle" — positive feedback with gradually improving behavior.

In the United States four stimulant drugs are employed: d-amphetamine (DA); methamphetamine (MA); methylphenidate (MP); pemoline (P). The percentage of children who have a favorable response is approximately equal for the first three — pemoline is considerably less effective on a percentage basis. However, considerable individual variation exists, and any child may do better on any one of the four. Idiosyncratic and allergic reactions are virtually unknown with DM, MA, and MP, and chemical monitoring is unnecessary. Two to three percent of individuals receiving P develop abnormalities in liver function tests, so that periodic monitoring is necessary. The drugs differ in potency and duration of action. DA and MA are equally potent; MP has one-half their potency, while P has one-quarter the potency of DA and MA. Individual doses of DA and MA last approximately four hours. MP lasts two to three hours and P may last as long as 12 hours. DA and MA are usually given two or three times a day, MP three (occasionally four) times a day, and P, once or (occasionally) twice a day. The usual doses are: D and M, 10–40 mg/day; MP 20–80 mg/day; P 18.75–112.5 mg/day.

The most common side effects are those one would expect from a sympathomimetic drug: appetite loss, insomnia (if the dose is given too late in the day), tics, and headaches. These can readily be controlled by a reduction in dose. Insomnia can usually be controlled by diminishing the last dose of the day or administering it earlier. If insomnia persists, modest doses of thioridazine at bedtime (10–50 mg) will usually control the problem. Tolerance does not generally develop to the stimulants; when it occurs, it is gradual and appears over a year or two. There is not complete cross-tolerance among the stimulants, so that rotation of stimulants (e.g., MP for DA or MA) is usually satisfactory. (Some recent clinical experience suggests that children with apparent ADHD who develop rapid tolerance may actually be suffering from a major ("vital," "endogenous") depression and that they respond dramatically to treatment with tricyclic antidepressants). One concern with the stimulants has been that they were found to slow growth velocity. This seems to be so, but the degree is slight and long-term follow-up studies show no diminution in expected height. Because of concerns with growth and other possible effects of chronic administration, many clinicians give children "drug holidays" during vacations and weekends. This is an acceptable procedure if the child's only difficulties are in school. If, however, the disorder causes problems with his family and peers, it is doing the child and his family no favor to withhold medications during such periods. Several other drugs have been employed in the treatment of ADHD. Neuroleptics are rarely useful. Tricyclic antidepressants (TCAs) are effective only briefly, as discussed earlier. Lithium — tried because of the ADHD child's affective lability — is also ineffective. MAO inhibitors have been found to be effective in very small trials with ADHD children and larger trials with ADHD adults.

Short-term drug therapy is clearly of benefit. The appropriate question is whether continuing treatment — as long as signs and symptoms are disabling — continues to suppress these signs and symptoms. There are no studies of long-term drug treatment and there never will be: random assignment to placebo treatment for 10 years is neither ethically nor clinically feasible. The experience of older clinicians who have followed ADHD children through adolescence and young adulthood is that medication continues to control symptoms and helps in academic, vocational, and social adaptation. The major treatment problem is not tolerance to medication. Motivating the patient to take medication is often the problem. The child-adolescent-adult must come to appreciate the nature and extent of his problems, accept the need for medication, and then be prepared to accept and use psychological and educational help. The therapeutic problem with the ADHD child who has remained untreated until adolescence is that by this time he has a long history of failure in school, difficulties with his parents and peers, low self-esteem, and possibly substance abuse and delinquency.

Simple psychological management can be summarized as being characterized best by firm, mutually agreed upon rules. Many authors report that behavioral modification techniques are useful with younger (below age 10 or 11) ADHD children. Reports of the effectiveness of various behavioral strategies may be found in Ross and Ross and Barkley. Most of the studies that have been conducted do not compare response to behavioral therapies with that of a group receiving stimulant medication, nor have they employed large numbers or evaluated long-term outcome. The results reported so far are disappointing. One well-controlled study compared the effects of behavior modification plus stimulant drug and stimulant drug alone and behavior modification alone. It found that behavior modification was considerably less effective than medication alone and that the combination was only minimally more effective than medication alone. Furthermore, the effects of behavior modification disappeared fairly rapidly when reinforcement was discontinued (Gittelman-Klein et al.) (4). Obviously, psychological techniques must form the mainstay of treatment for children unresponsive to medication. Quite a few useful techniques have been discovered by parents and teachers and conveyed to child psychiatrists. These, plus other suggestions, may be found (I report somewhat immodestly) in a book I have written for parents (20).

Effect of Stimulant Medication in Mixed ADHD

ADHD frequently occurs in conjunction with specific developmental disorders in reading, spelling, and mathematics. In children who have both syndromes, the best that can be expected from medication is that it reduces or eliminates the behavioral characteristics that interfere with learning and "leaves" the specific learning problems. One study has found that methylphenidate was ineffective for purely "learning disabled" children while special teaching techniques were more effective than an equivalent period of attention control (i.e., giving the child contact with an adult who uses no specific teaching techniques). The issue of treatment of specific developmental disorders is a separate topic. From a practical standpoint, it is uncertain which kinds of techniques can be expected to help which kinds of children and to how great a degree. From the standpoint of the child and his family, the meaning of these learning problems must be carefully explained. Most children and their parents perceive the specific developmental disorder in reading as evidence of mental retardation. They should be disabused of this notion. Affected children are usually delighted to learn that they are not "dumb" — they are "dyslexic." In children who have ADHD without SDDs, medication may facilitate learning but it cannot compensate for past failures to master school subjects. For such children, remedial education is necessary.

In children with mixed ADHD/conduct disorder, stimulants may diminish not only the "pure" ADHD symptoms, but some of the manifestations of conduct disorder as well. The drug responsiveness of this important group requires further study.

The overall approach the author employs with regard to therapeutic trials is based on the "payoff matrix." This is formal, perhaps pedantic terminology for the simple procedure of calculating the benefits and costs of the four logical possibilities. They are based on whether or not the child has ADHD and the consequences of a trial of stimulant medication being given or not given. If ADHD is present and medication is given, the chances are approximately 60 to 80 percent the child will achieve a significant clinical benefit; if the child does not have ADHD, the only loss will be very mild discomfort (irritability, anxiety) for several hours; if the child does have ADHD and is an "undiscovered" good responder and is not given stimulant medication, the loss is considerable — continuing impaired functioning which is minimally responsive to psychosocial intervention; (finally, of course, if the child does not have ADHD and medication is not given, there are no benefits and no costs of a drug trial).

ADHD in Adolescents and Adults

As mentioned, it is being increasingly observed that ADHD persists into adolescence and adulthood. We are just beginning to explore ADHD in adults: its symptomatology, differential diagnosis, biological and psychological test correlates, and therapeutic responsiveness to medication and psychological interventions. DSM-III recognized that ADHD persists into adult life and suggested that hyperactivity disappears while inattentiveness and impulsivity remain. That was probably incorrect. Hyperactivity usually persists, but in a more muted form. The ADHD adult will report that he is uncomfortable sitting still and that he prefers to be up and on the go, and he may be observed to be ceaselessly fidgeting. The only group of investigators who have proposed tentative operational criteria has been that of this author and his colleagues, Reimherr and Wood. The "Utah criteria" require that the individual qualified as a child for a diagnosis of ADHD with hyperactivity, that he continues to have both hyperactivity and attentional problems, and that he has two of the following problems: impulsivity, labile affect, hot temper, extreme overreactivity to stress, and disorganization. (A fuller description of these characteristics is provided in Table 1.)

Three random-assignment placebo-controlled trials of stimulant medication in adults with ADHD have been conducted. We found pemoline (15) (chosen because of its low abuse potential) and methylphenidate (17) to be demonstrably more effective than placebo in putative adult ADHD patients. Approximately 60 to 70 percent of these patients had a moderate to marked therapeutic response — one that was not only statistically, but also clinically significant — with both behavioral and symptomatic improvement. As mentioned earlier, our group has also conducted *open* trials of two MAO inhibitors, pargyline and *l*-deprenyl. These also produced moderate-to-marked therapeutic benefit in approximately two-thirds of the patients treated. (Obviously these findings will have to be replicated in a placebo-controlled design.) A third placebo-controlled study, by Mattes et al. (7), failed to document the efficacy of methylphenidate. We believe his and our studies to be noncomparable because he included diagnostic categories that we exclude (such as borderline personality disorder) and he failed to obtain ratings by a spouse or "other" person living with the patient. We have found it mandatory to obtain observations from someone in the patient's immediate environment. ADHD adults, like ADHD children, are often grossly unaware of their behavioral differences before treatment or the responses of their behavioral differences to treatment.

Now it is necessary for other investigators to apply the tentative "Utah criteria" for adult ADHD and determine their usefulness. In addition, of course, other investigators must attempt to replicate our drug studies to make sure that our results are not the product of biased perception.

SUMMARY

ADHD is a common psychiatric diagnosis in North America, frequently associated with specific developmental disorders and conduct disorder, and has probably been hiding itself elsewhere for some time, concealed

Table 1
Utah Criteria for the Diagnosis of ADHD

I. Childhood history consistent with ADHD of childhood
II. Broad Criteria
    A. Both characteristics #1 and #2, and one characteristic of #3 through #6
        1. More active than other children, unable to sit still, fidgitiness, restlessness, always on the go, talking excessively
        2. Attention deficits, sometimes described as "short attention span," characterized by inattentiveness, distractibility, inability to finish school work
        3. Behavior problems in school
        4. Impulsivity
        5. Overexcitability
        6. Temper outbursts
    B. Presence in adulthood of both characteristics #1 and #2 — which the patient observes or says others observe about him — together with two of characteristics #3 through #7
        1. Persistent motor hyperactivity as manifested by restlessness, inability to relax, "nervousness" (meaning inability to settle down — not anticipatory anxiety), inability to persist in sedentary activities (e.g., watching movies, TV, reading newspaper), being always on the go, dysphoria when inactive.
        2. Attention deficits as manifested by: Inability to keep mind on conversation, distractability (being aware of other stimuli when attempts are made to filter them out); inability to keep mind on reading materials; difficulty keeping mind on job; frequent "forgetfulness" — often losing or misplacing things, forgetting plans, etc.; "mind frequently somewhere else."
        3. Affective lability: Usually described as antedating adolescence and in some instances as far back as the patient can remember. Manifested by definite shifts from a normal mood to depression or mild euphoria or excitement; depression described as "down," "bored," or "discontented"; mood shifts usually last hours to at most a few days and are present without significant physiological concomitants; mood shifts may occur spontaneously or be reactive.
        4. Inability to complete tasks: The subject reports lack of organization in job, running household, or performing schoolwork; tasks frequently not completed; subject switches from one task to another in haphazard fashion; disorganization in activities, problem solving, organizing time.
        5. Hot temper, explosive short-lived outbursts. Subject reports he may have transient loss of control and be frightened by his own behavior. Easily provoked or constant irritability. Temper problems interfere with personal relationships.

(continued)

Table 1
(*Continued*)

6. Impulsivity: Subject makes decisions quickly and easily without reflection, often on the basis of insufficient information to his own disadvantage. Inability to delay acting without experiencing discomfort. Manifestations include: poor occupational performance; abrupt initiation or termination of relationships (e.g., multiple marriages, separations, divorces); antisocial behavior such as joy-riding, shop-lifting; excessive involvement in pleasurable activities without recognizing risks of painful consequences, e.g., buying sprees, foolish business investments, reckless driving.
7. Stress intolerance: Subject cannot take ordinary stresses in stride and reacts excessively or inappropriately with depression, confusion, uncertainty, anxiety, or anger. Emotional responses interfere with appropriate problem solving. Subject experiences repeated crises in dealing with routine life stresses.

C. Absence of the following disorders
   1. Antisocial personality disorder
   2. Major affective disorder
D. Absence of signs and symptoms of the following disorders
   1. Schizophrenia
   2. Schizoaffective disorder
E. Absence of the following characteristics of schizotypal or borderline personality disorders
   1. Magical thinking
   2. Ideas of reference
   3. Recurrent delusions
   4. Odd communications
   5. Inadequate rapport in face-to-face interactions
   6. Suspiciousness or paranoid ideation
   7. Prolonged anger
   8. Identity disturbances (in borderline sense)
   9. Inability to tolerate being alone
   10. Physically self-damaging acts
   Associated features: Marital instability; academic and vocational success less than expected on the basis of intelligence and education; alcohol or drug abuse; atypical responses to psychoactive medications; familial history of similar chacteristics; family histories of ADHD in childhood, alcoholism, drug abuse, antisocial personality, and Briquet's syndrome.
F. Child temperament questionnaire (Connor's abbreviated rating scale): Although not necessary for diagnosis, a score of 12 or greater as rated by the patient's mother is helpful for diagnostic purposes and may be predictive of treatment response.

among the group of children diagnosed as having "conduct disorder." ADHD appears to be genetically transmitted, and many of its features are probably linked to underactivity of dopaminergic systems. Its short-term response to stimulant medication is striking. Medication frequently enables the child to function more effectively and happily than he has ever done before. ADHD frequently persists into adult life, where current evidence suggests that it continues to respond to medication. The pharmacological response may be as valuable theoretically as it is clinically. The simultaneous chemical alteration of restlessness, inattentiveness, frustration tolerance, disorganization, inability to control anger, and social noncompliance is clearly of great interest and may provide a powerful clue to an understanding of the biological underpinnings of these symptoms.

REFERENCES

Monographs

BARKLEY, R. A. (1981). *A handbook for diagnosis and treatment.* New York: Guilford Press.
CANTWELL, D. P. (Ed.). (1975). *The hyperactive child.* New York: Spectrum.
ROSS, D. M., & ROSS, S. A. (1982). *Hyperactivity. Current issues, research, and theory* (2nd ed.). New York: Wiley.
WEISS, G. (1986). *Hyperactive children grown up.* New York: Guilford Press.
WENDER, P. H. (1971). *Minimal brain dysfunction in children.* New York: Wiley.
WENDER, P. H. (1987). *The hyperactive child, adolescent and adult. Attention deficit disorder through the lifespan.* New York: Oxford University Press.

Articles

1. BAREGGI, S. R., BECKER, R. E., GINSBURG, B. E., & GENOVESE, E. (1979). Neurochemical investigation of an endogenous model of the "hyperkinetic syndrome" in a hybrid dog. *Life Sciences, 24,* 481.
2. CANTWELL, D. P. (1985). Pharmacotherapy of ADHD in Adolescents: What do we know, where should we go, how should we do it? *Psychopharmacology Bulletin, 21,* 251.
3. CANTWELL, D. P. (1975). Genetic studies of hyperactive children. In R. R. Fieve, D. Rosenthal, & H. Brill (Eds.), *Genetic research in psychiatry.* Baltimore: Johns Hopkins University Press.
4. GITTELMAN-KLEIN, R., ABIKOFF, H., POLLACK, E., KLEIN, D. F., KATZ, S., & MATTES, J. (1980). A controlled trial of behavioral modification and methylphenidate in hyperactive children. In C. K. Whalen & B. Henker (Eds.), *Hyperactive children: The social ecology of identification and treatment.* New York: Academic Press.
5. GOODWIN, D. W., SCHULSINGER, F., HERMANSEN, L., GUZE, S. B., & WINOKUR, G. (1973). Alcohol problems in adoptees raised apart from alcoholic biological parents. *Archives of General Psychiatry, 28,* 238.
6. HUESSY, H. R., & GENDRON, R. (1970). Prevalence of the so-called hyperkinetic syndrome in public school children of Vermont. *Acta Paedopsychiatrica, 37,* 243.
7. MATTES, J. A., BOSWELL, L., & OLIVER, H. (1984). Methylphenidate effects on symptoms of attention deficit disorder in adults. *Archives of General Psychiatry, 41,* 1059.

8. MORRISON, J. R., & STEWART, M. A. (1973). The psychiatric status of the legal families of adopted hyperactive children. *Archives of General Psychiatry, 28*, 888.
9. REIMHERR, F. W., WENDER, P. H., EBERT, M. H., & WOOD, D. R. (1984). Cerebrospinal fluid homovanillic acid and 5-hydroxyindoleacetic acid in adults with attention deficit disorder, residual type. *Psychiatry Research, 11*, 71.
10. SAFER, D. J. (1973). A familial factor in minimal brain dysfunction. *Behavior Genetics, 3*, 175.
11. SHAYWITZ, B. A., YAGER, R. D., & KLOPPER, J. H. (1976). Selective brain dopamine depletion in developing rats: An experimental model of minimal brain dysfunction. *Science, 191*, 305.
12. SHETTY, T., & CHASE, T. N. (1976). Central monoamines and hyperkinesis of childhood. *Neurology, 26*, 1000.
13. STEWART, M. A., DeBLOIS, C. S., & CUMMINGS, C. (1979). Psychiatric disorder in the parents of hyperactive boys and those with conduct disorder. *Journal of Child Psychology and Psychiatry, 21*, 283.
14. ULLMANN, R. K., SLEATOR, E. K., & SPRAGUE, R. L. (1984). A new rating scale for diagnosis and monitoring of ADHD children. *Psychopharmacology Bulletin, 20*, 160.
15. WENDER, P. H., REIMHERR, F. W., & WOOD, D. R. (1981). Attention deficit disorder ("minimal brain dysfunction") in adults: A replication study of diagnosis and drug treatment. *Archives of General Psychiatry, 38*, 449.
16. WENDER, P. H., WOOD, D. R., REIMHERR, F. W., & WARD, M. (1983). An open trial of pargyline in the treatment of attention deficit disorder, residual type. *Psychiatry Research, 9*, 329.
17. WENDER, P. H., REIMHERR, F. W., WOOD, D., & WARD, M. (1985). A controlled study of methylphenidate in the treatment of attention deficit disorder, residual type, in adults. *American Journal of Psychiatry, 142*, 547.
18. WOOD, D. R., REIMHERR, F. W., & WENDER, P. H. (1983). The use of *l*-deprenyl in the treatment of attention deficit disorder, residual type (ADD,RT). *Psychopharmacology Bulletin, 19*, 627.
19. ZAMETKIN, A., RAPOPORT, J. L., MURPHY, D. L., LINNOILA, M., KAROUM, F., POTTER, W. Z., & ISMOND, D. (1985). Treatment of hyperactive children with monoamine oxidase inhibitors. *Archives of General Psychiatry, 42*, 969.
20. WENDER, P. H. (1987). *The hyperactive child, adolescent and adult: Attention Deficit Disorder through the lifespan*. New York, Oxford: Oxford University Press.

9

THE PREMENSTRUAL
SYNDROMES

BERNARD L. FRANKEL, M.D.

Departments of Psychiatry and Medicine,
George Washington University Medical Center,
Washington, DC

and

DAVID R. RUBINOW, M.D.

Alcohol, Drug Abuse, and Mental Health Administration, NIMH,
Intramural Research Program, Bethesda, Maryland

INTRODUCTION

The exact nature of the relationship between mood and behavioral disturbances and menses has been a source of controversy among researchers and clinicians for more than 50 years despite the fact that descriptions of this relationship are centuries old. The Biblical Ezekiel, for example, warned against coming "near a woman in her impurity" (26) and Hippocrates attributed a host of behavioral and cognitive symptoms to "retained menstrual blood" (84). In more recent times, a number of cases of menstrually related mood disturbances (mostly mania) were reported (67,88). For example, in 1890 Icard compiled an extensive list of behavioral and mood disturbances that he associated with menstruation. These included melancholia, hallucinations, illusions, lying, morbid jealousy, delirious and impulsive insanity, nymphomania, erotomania, homicidal and suicidal mania, dipsomania, kleptomania, and pyromania (42). These early

---

This chapter summarizes material that has been published elsewhere (22,72–77).

efforts to describe menstrually related mood and behavioral disorders reflected uncertainty about whether they were discrete disorders or exaggerations of normal experience.

The era of modern research in the area of menstrually related mood disorders was ushered in by Robert Frank's description in 1931 of 15 women who developed seizures, bronchial asthma, and "indescribable tension" in the 7 to 10 days preceding the start of menstruation (29). Since his report, over 150 different symptoms have been purported to vary with the menstrual cycle (19,57). In general, the subsequent articles about the nature of the "premenstrual tension syndrome" or "premenstrual syndrome(s)" suffer from significant conceptual and methodological imprecision resulting from the failure to use a clear, testable definition of menstrually related syndromes that might allow for consistency and generalizability across studies. Further, in addition to problems with definition, little attention has been directed toward the capacity of the menstrual cycle to act as a modulator of preexisting psychiatric disorders or vulnerabilities.

METHODOLOGICAL ISSUES

The remarkable progress and discoveries in medicine over the last 50 years have led to a proliferation of etiological hypotheses about premenstrual syndromes. These generally have been based on the purported fluctuation during the menstrual cycle of some newly discovered factor, its regulation by reproductive endocrine hormones, or its potential mediation of the central nervous system (CNS) effects of reproductive endocrine hormones. Table 1 lists some of the proposed etiologies for premenstrual syndromes.

Attempts to precisely define an etiology and identify effective treatments for the premenstrual syndromes have been unsuccessful mainly as a result of a variety of study design flaws. The most common and serious error has been the use of inaccurate diagnostic methods to select the samples of women studied. Since the syndrome was tied to a physiological occurrence (menstruation), was characterized by somatic and behavioral symptoms, and was treated with medication, it is understandable that efforts to diagnose premenstrual syndrome reflected the traditional symptom-oriented methods and techniques of medical diagnosis. While helpful with regard to other disorders, these methods may not be reliable in diagnosing the premenstrual syndrome for a number of reasons.

First, multitudinous symptoms representing virtually every organ sys-

Table 1
Proposed Etiologies for Premenstrual Syndromes*

Ovarian hormonal
  Estrogen
  Progesterone
Fluid and electrolyte hormonal
  Prolactin
  Aldosterone
  Renin/angiotensin
  Vasopressin
Other hormonal
  Endorphins/enkephalins — Melanocyte-Stimulating Hormone
  Glucocorticoid
  Androgen
  Insulin
  Melatonin
Neurotransmitter
  Monoamine (5-hydroxytryptamine, norepinephrine, dopamine)
  Acetylcholine
Other
  Vitamin B_6/magnesium
  Psychological factors
  Prostaglandins

---

*From *The American Journal of Psychiatry, 141*, 63–172, 1984. Copyright 1984, the American Psychiatric Association. Reprinted by permission.

tem have been implicated as key diagnostic features of the premenstrual syndrome. Even the commonly reported symptoms (e.g., irritability, mood changes, and peripheral edema) are neither necessary nor sufficient for diagnostic purposes. This great diversity of reported symptoms has generated efforts to define premenstrual syndrome subtypes (1,33). However, these subsyndromes are not mutually exclusive and must be viewed as descriptors rather than diagnoses. At present, therefore, it appears that the type of symptom has little value in diagnosing premenstrual syndrome.

Second, evaluation of the *severity* of the symptoms of the premenstrual syndrome has been problematic. Measures of severity that are categorical rather than dimensional have been utilized in many studies; such measures are insufficiently sensitive to differences in severity and overly sensitive to the influence of reporter bias. The variance in a subject's threshold for rating a symptom as "severe," for example, may depend on her belief about where she is in her menstrual cycle at the time of the rating (79). Moreover, because many of the symptoms are subjectively experienced, there are few objective correlates for an observer to detect and assess. Furthermore, the recollection and perception of these symptoms may be quite inaccurate, as Faratian et al. (27) demonstrated in a group of women whose perceptions of their premenstrual weight gain and abdominal bloating significantly exceeded the objective measurements of these changes.

A third important source of methodological error in diagnosis has been the insufficient appreciation of the critical importance of the *timing* of the appearance of symptoms in relation to menses in contrast to the *type* of symptom experienced. Despite the diagnostic importance of symptom timing, several investigators have suggested that recalling *when* symptoms appear may be even more inaccurate than remembering *what* the symptoms are (78). Supporting this hypothesis is the finding that, when assessed *prospectively* with daily ratings over several cycles, 40 to 50 percent of patients presenting with a typical history of premenstrual syndrome will not show any evidence of a relationship between symptomatic variation and menstrual cycle phase (24,75,80). In addition to this issue of recall of timing, there is disagreement among investigators about the specific time interval around menstruation that should be examined (19,48,53,58, 89,92).

A fourth unresolved methodological issue involves the nature of the baseline in reference to which menstrually related symptoms should be measured. The important distinctions among the premenstrual *appearance* of symptoms, the premenstrual *exacerbation* of preexisting symptoms, and the premenstrual *continuation* of symptoms rarely are addressed. Furthermore, few authors have attempted to define the acceptable amount of variance in a symptom over the course of the menstrual cycle (65), despite numerous reports that women with premenstrual syndrome may be symptomatic at other times in their cycles (16,81). The degree of symptom *change* in relation to baseline is of greater relevance than the nature and severity of the premenstrual symptom examined without reference to the rest of the menstrual cycle.

Finally, the rating instruments used in many studies to assess menstrually related symptomatology may introduce another source of error. If a rating scale for measuring symptom severity does not provide a sufficiently broad range of dimensional options, then the process of recording symptoms prospectively may be compromised. A bias in information processing has been described which consists of a change in a patient's threshold for rating a symptom as present as a function of where in the menstrual cycle she believes herself to be (79). The use of dichotomous scales only aggravates this problem of alteration in the threshold for response, as demonstrated by the discrepancy between ratings of symptoms simultaneously performed with visual analog and dichotomous rating scales (J. Steege, personal communication).

The diagnosis of premenstrual syndrome, therefore, should be accomplished by means of prospective symptom assessment on a daily basis over several cycles utilizing rating scales such as visual analog scales that allow sufficient dimensional options. The importance of this requirement is emphasized by the observation that the baseline descriptions of premenstrual symptom type and severity could not distinguish those women who subsequently provided confirmatory evidence of a menstrually related mood disorder from those in whom such a disorder was prospectively disconfirmed (72). The selection of samples on the basis of a subject's history of premenstrual syndrome without prospective confirmation of the accuracy of that history is, unfortunately, characteristic of the premenstrual syndrome literature. Given the consequent heterogeneity in samples and the ungeneralizability of the data obtained, it is not surprising that convincing evidence is lacking for specific biological correlates of this syndrome as well as for the superiority of any of the many proposed treatment regimens.

DIAGNOSTIC CRITERIA

As noted above, the diagnosis of premenstrual syndrome cannot be established on the basis of history alone. Rather, there are two key requirements: (1) symptoms must appear or be significantly exacerbated during the premenstrual phase of the menstrual cycle; and (2) this premenstrual phase specificity of symptoms must be confirmed prospectively over the course of several cycles. Two formal sets of diagnostic criteria have incorporated these diagnostic prerequisites. The criteria of the NIMH Premenstrual Syndrome Workshop (62) specified that in the five days prior to menses as compared with the five days following cessation of menses there must be at least a 30 percent increase in symptom severity in at least two out of three cycles. Similar prospective confirmation is required as a criterion for the diagnosis of the APA defined "periluteal phase dysphoric disorder" (4).

ETIOLOGIES/BIOLOGICAL STRATEGIES

Most etiological hypotheses since Frank's report have implicated endocrine abnormalities (Table 1). (See Refs. 70 and 71 for reviews of the numerous etiologies and their rationales.) The most frequently cited etiological theory attributes premenstrual symptoms to altered gonadal steroid activity in the form of the following: (a) decreased estrogen secondary to decreased renal clearance (29), decreased hepatic clearance (14), or increased gonadotropin secretion (7); (b) unopposed estrogen due to inadequate luteal phase activity with progesterone deficiency (43); or (c) an altered estrogen-progesterone ratio (32). Roles for prolactin or aldosterone in premenstrual syndrome also have been suggested, although less frequently than for the gonadal steroids (5,6,8,12,34,44,49,60,61,63,64,66). Other factors implicated include vitamin B[6] (14), glucose metabolism abnormalities (59), melanocyte-stimulating hormone (71), peptide hormones such as endorphins and vasopressin (13), prostaglandins (96), glucocorticoids (70), and central monoamines (70,71). Finally, several psychological theories of the pathogenesis of menstrually related mood disorders also have been proposed and reviewed elsewhere (30). Absence of methodological comparability and rigor across studies has diminished the likelihood of demonstrating any systematic syndrome-related changes in endocrine activity. Although menstrually related mood disorders are, by definition, linked to a biological event (i.e., menstruation), it still remains to be determined whether the symptoms are *entrained to* or *caused by* menstrual cycle-related biological events. It is similarly unclear whether menstrually related symptoms represent a normal response to abnormal endocrine activity or an abnormal response to normal endocrine events (56).

As part of an attempt to explore the biology of premenstrual syndrome, Rubinow et al. (unpublished data) studied baseline hormonal function in patients diagnosed with premenstrual syndrome and normal controls. Patients and control subjects completed visual analog scale ratings of mood (depression and anxiety) twice daily for three months (75). Patients selected for this study had at least a 30 percent increase in mean negative mood symptomatology in the week prior to menses compared with the week following menses. (See Figure 1 for sample analog scale-derived graphs.)

Analysis of variance with repeated measures did not yield any significant effects for diagnosis or for the interaction of diagnosis and time for any of the hormones studied. Thus, patients with premenstrual syndrome could not be differentiated from controls on the basis of abnormal or different levels or rhythms of circulating reproductive hormones or related

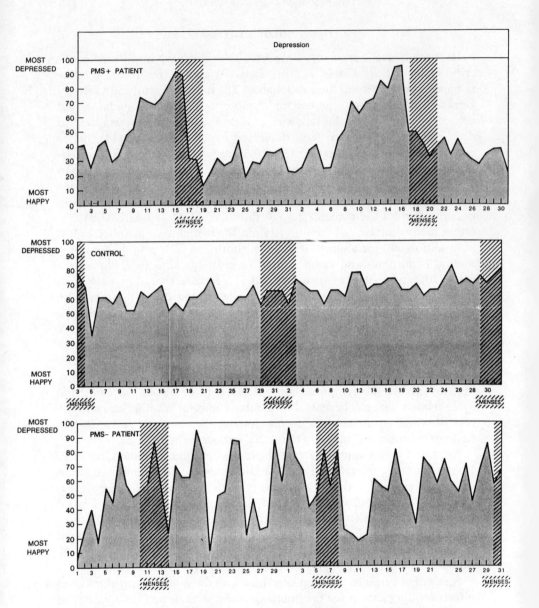

Figure 1. Daily A.M. depression self-ratings in relation to menses in three women: PMS+patient, control, PMS−patient. (Reprinted with permission from Rubinow et al. [77], p. 87.)

factors. These results are in accord with those of Backstrom et al. (9), who, in contrast to their earlier reports (7,10), found no differences in plasma estradiol, progesterone, testosterone, or androstenedione in women with large and small amounts of cyclical mood changes as determined by ratings on visual analog scales. It seems improbable that additional studies will demonstrate a baseline "hormonal lesion" in patients with carefully diagnosed premenstrual syndrome. However, there may exist a dynamic endocrine abnormality that is demonstrable only when the system is challenged rather than sampled under baseline conditions.

The thyrotropin-releasing hormone (TRH) stimulation test is an endocrine challenge strategy employed by Roy-Byrne et al. in a study of 14 women with prospectively confirmed premenstrual syndrome and nine controls (73). No follicular-luteal phase differences in basal or maximal values of TSH or prolactin were found within either of the two groups of women or between groups. In addition to replicating previous observations of the absence of menstrual cycle phase-related differences in basal prolactin levels in women with premenstrual symptoms (87), these results extend earlier findings by demonstrating that stimulated prolactin levels of such women do not differ from those of controls. A similar lack of effect of menstrual cycle phase on a neuroendocrine test reported to display state-dependent abnormalities in depression, the dexamethasone suppression test, was also observed by Haskett et al. (38) and Roy-Byrne et al. (74).

Patients symptomatic during the month of testing (10 of the 14) had significantly greater variance in the maximal change in TSH following TRH infusion in both phases of their cycles. In 9 of 19 TRH tests performed by Roy-Byrne et al. in patients who were symptomatic during the month of testing, the maximal stimulated TSH was beyond the established normal range (73,82). Stimulated change in TSH levels of greater than 32 μIU/ml in 4 of the 10 symptomatic patients suggested the presence of subclinical hypothyroidism. Three other patients had blunted responses (less than 7 μIU/ml) to TRH stimulation. These abnormal responses to TRH stimulation were found in the luteal *and* follicular phases in some patients and in only *one* of these phases in other patients. Because of the high prevalence of a history of affective or anxiety disorder in this patient sample compared with the controls, the abnormal response to TRH stimulation observed in the patients may have been an epiphenomenon of a preexisting psychiatric disorder rather than a characteristic of premenstrual syndrome. (Abnormal responses of TSH to TRH stimulation have been described as trait, as well as state, markers for major affective disorders [18,51].)

Nevertheless, the finding of abnormal TSH responses in four patients without a history of affective disorder and the equal prevalence of a significant psychiatric history in the patients with abnormal ($n = 7$) or normal ($n = 7$) TSH responses suggest that abnormal responses to TRH stimulation may define a group of premenstrual syndrome patients with particular phenomenological, biological, and/or treatment-response characteristics. This and other neuroendocrine challenge strategies should be pursued in larger cohorts of patients with precisely characterized premenstrual syndrome.

TREATMENT

Studies of proposed treatment regimens for premenstrual syndrome (Table 2) generally have suffered from the same methodological shortcomings as have the investigations of its possible etiologies. In 1983, Rubinow and Roy-Byrne critically reviewed a number of treatment studies (76) and concluded that despite anecdotal reports of the successful use of many therapeutic agents, none had clearly demonstrated superiority to placebo. De-

Table 2

Proposed Treatments for Premenstrual Syndromes*

Hormonal
  Progesterone
  Progestins/oral contraceptives
  Antihormonal, danazol
  Androgens
Psychotropics
  Lithium
  Monoamine oxidase inhibitors
  Sedative-hypnotics
Other
  Bromocriptine
  Pyridoxine
  Dietary restriction
  Diuretics
  Prostaglandin precursors/inhibitors

*From *The American Journal of Psychiatry, 141,* 163–172, 1984. Copyright 1984, the American Psychiatric Association. Reprinted by permission.

spite a continual accumulation of treatment trials and the addition of new agents to the therapeutic armamentarium (e.g., alprazolam, GnRH), this conclusion has not changed.

Diagnostic Overlap

Because affective symptoms have frequently been reported in most descriptions of premenstrual syndrome, the existence of a special relationship between premenstrual symptoms and specific psychiatric disorders has been hypothesized (17,20,45,54). In patients with major affective disorder, about a 60 percent prevalence of "premenstrual affective syndrome" has been observed. This is higher than the prevalence reported in some controls (25,40,47), similar to that reported in other controls (23), and similar to that found in schizophrenics (40). Studies also have been performed of the prevalence of affective disorder in women reporting premenstrual mood changes. A lifetime diagnosis of major depressive disorder was observed in 57 to 100 percent of women in five different cohorts meeting the criteria for "premenstrual full depressive syndrome"; of the women in these five groups only 0 to 20 percent were found to have no history of mental illness (35). Several investigators have reported an increased lifetime history of depression and an increased frequency of subsequent presentation with affective disorder in college women complaining of premenstrual syndrome (83,95). Except for a subsample of women in one study (35), none of the patients in these studies had their premenstrual mood changes documented with prospective confirmation; i.e., premenstrual syndrome was diagnosed solely on the basis of history.

Therefore, using the Schedule for Affective Disorders and Schizophrenia-Lifetime (SADS) interview (86), DeJong et al. studied the prevalence of psychiatric history in 57 women whose presenting symptoms of a menstrually related mood disorder were subsequently confirmed (PMS +) or disconfirmed (PMS −) by the prospective methodology described above. Twenty-one of the twenty-four PMS − patients (88 percent) had a significant past psychiatric history, while of the 33 PMS + patients only 15 (45 percent) had such a history (chi square, 10.57; df = 3; $p < .05$) (22). Thus, the excess of psychiatric (and especially affective) disorders that has been found in previous studies of women with premenstrual syndrome may reflect a disproportionate contribution of positive psychiatric history from those women who would not have provided prospective confirmation of their presenting menstrually related mood changes (i.e., PMS − women). In order to clarify the prevalence of premenstrual syndrome and its association with affective disorder, further epidemiological studies utilizing prospective diagnostic methods are necessary.

Modulation of Preexisting Psychiatric Disorders

Reports of menstrually related exacerbation or linkage/recurrence of psychiatric disorders suggest the ability of the menstrual cycle to modulate psychiatric disorders (15,21,28,31,50,85,90). Both the "atypical psychoses" (39,98) and the "periodic psychoses of puberty" (3) are characterized by the recurrence or exacerbation of symptoms during the late luteal and menstruation phase of the menstrual cycle. The disproportionate incidence of psychiatric admissions and suicide attempts during the perimenstruum (20,46,52,93), as well as the recrudescence of symptoms only during the premenstruum in some clearly diagnosed psychiatrically ill patients (28,97,98), also underscores the potential importance of the influence of menstrual cycle phase on the course of psychiatric illness.

The capacity of the menstrual cycle to act as a powerful entrainer of a variety of episodic disorders has been noted (55). Despite anecdotal observations of the apparent premenstrual clustering of episodic disorders such as panic attacks and bulimic episodes, documentation of these observations currently is lacking. There is great need for detailed evaluations of the family history, course, and treatment-response characteristics of patients with menstrually influenced psychiatric disorders.

MODELS AND CONCLUSIONS

Two major conceptual shortcomings have marred efforts to elucidate the basic mechanisms and biobehavioral implications of menstrually related mood syndromes. One is the use of constricted, mutually exclusive biological or psychological models as explanatory paradigms; the other is the conceptualization of premenstrual syndrome as a unitary, isolated disorder with attendant lack of consideration of the menstrual cycle as a modulator or entrainer of other disorders. Menstrually related mood syndromes are biopsychosocial complexities whose understanding necessitates newer models that integrate and organize the clinical data more effectively.

In the *sensitization or "kindling" model*, the repeated administration of a stimulus over time produces increasingly stronger effects and profound, long-term changes in behavior and brain activity (68). Accordingly, the repetitive experience of a dysphoric state in the setting of the premenstruum might influence the development or course of an affective illness in a genetically predisposed individual. In addition, the clinically observed propensity for premenstrual symptoms to increase in duration and severity with time might be explained on the basis of premenstrual sensitization. Finally, the marked influence of environment on symptomatic expression seen in menstrually related mood disorders may be the analog of the context dependency observed in amygdala kindling (69).

The *learned helplessness model* has been used to explain the behavioral and biological changes that occur (e.g., immunological dysfunction and depletion of forebrain norepinephrine) in a rat subjected to uncontrollable shock; such changes are not found in the rat that controls the shock delivered to both rats under otherwise identical conditions (91,94). Therefore, it appears to be the former rat's "perception" of being unable to control the shock administered (rather than the characteristics of the shock itself) that leads to the development of both the behavioral and biological dysfunction. In view of the bidirectionality of the relationship between biological and perceptual-cognitive-behavioral processes, it can be hypothesized that early experiences of "loss of control" may influence not only subsequent psychological, but related biological functioning as well.

Finally, the *state model* of psychological functioning may help us understand much of the diversity of symptoms and treatment responses described in patients with premenstrual syndrome. This model proposes that the normal human psyche is made up of a number of discrete experiential or behavioral states, each characterized by specific ideas, perceptions, memories, emotions, attitudes toward self and others, and so forth. It has been suggested that psychotherapy may effect behavioral changes by delineating these states, identifying the state-to-state transition patterns, and providing strategies that patients may use to interrupt a maladaptive, stereotyped state transition and substitute a more adaptive state for the dysfunctional one (41). In accordance with this model, the menstrual cycle may biologically choreograph or facilitate state changes instead of causing specific symptoms. Premenstrual syndrome, therefore, would not be conceptualized as a symptom-specific disturbance, but rather as a disorder characterized by a menstrual cycle-linked transition into a specific experiential state, usually, but not exclusively, with dysphoria and/or irritability as its predominant features. Biological and psychological characterization of the point of premenstrual state transition (the "switch") is likely to foster understanding of the key processes involved in the transition between other experiential states that occur in normal as well as maladaptive human functioning.

Premenstrual syndrome research may increase our knowledge about the predisposition, onset, and course of psychiatric disorders. Properly conducted, it must draw on many areas, including endocrinology, chronobiology, neurobiology, behavioral psychology, and social psychology. In so doing, it promises to extend the limits of our knowledge of each of these areas as well as the interactions among them. For this promise to be realized, it is necessary to complement, not replace, careful history taking and psychosocial assessment with modern neurobiological techniques, all within the context of carefully defined methodologies.

REFERENCES

1. ABRAHAM, G. E. (1980). The premenstrual tension syndromes. In I. K. McNall (Ed.), *Contemporary obstetric and gynecologic nursing, Vol. 3.* St. Louis: Mosby.
2. ABRAHAM, S. (1984). Premenstrual or postmenstrual syndrome. *Medical Journal of Australia,* Sept. 15, p. 327.
3. ALTSCHULE, M. D., & BREM, J. (1963). Periodic psychosis of puberty. *American Journal of Psychiatry, 119,* 1176.
4. American Psychiatric Association—Workgroup to Revise DSM-III (1985). *Draft: DSM-III-R in development.* Washington, DC: American Psychiatric Association Press.
5. ANDERSCH, B., ABRAHAMSSON, L., WENDESTAM, C., OHMAN, R., & HAHN, L. (1979). Hormone profile in premenstrual tension: Effects of bromocriptine and diuretics. *Clinical Endocrinology (Oxford), 11,* 657.
6. ANDERSEN, A. N., LARSEN, J. F., STEENSTRUP, O. R., SVENDSTRUP, B., & NIELSEN, J. (1977). Effect of bromocriptine on the premenstrual syndrome: A double-bind clinical trial. *British Journal of Obstetrics and Gynaecology, 84,* 370.
7. BACKSTROM, T., WIDE, L., SODERGA, R., & CARSTENSEN, H. (1976). FSH, LH TeBG-capacity, estrogen and progesterone in women with premenstrual tension during the luteal phase. *Journal of Steroid Biochemistry, 7,* 473.
8. BACKSTROM, T., & AAKVAAG, A. (1981). Plasma prolactin and testosterone during the luteal phase in women with premenstrual tension syndrome. *Psychoneuroendocrinology, 6,* 245.
9. BACKSTROM, T., SANDERS, D., LEASK, R., DAVIDSON, D., WARNER, P., & BANCROFT, J. (1983). Mood, sexuality, hormones, and the menstrual cycle. II. Hormone levels and their relationship to the premenstrual syndrome. *Psychosomatic Medicine, 45,* 503.
10. BACKSTROM, T., & CARSTENSEN, H. (1974). Estrogen and progesterone in plasma in relation to premenstrual tension. *Journal of Steroid Biochemistry, 5,* 257.
11. BALDESSARINI, R. J. (1984). Risk rates for depression. *Archives of General Psychiatry, 41,* 103.
12. BENEDEK-JASZMANN, L. F., & HEARN-STURTEVANT, M. D. (1976). Premenstrual tension and functional infertility: Aetiology and treatment. *Lancet, 1,* 1095.
13. BICKERS, W., & WOODS, M. (1951). Premenstrual tension—Rational treatment. *Texas Report on Biological Medicine, 9,* 406.
14. BISKIND, M. S. (1943). Nutritional deficiency in the etiology of menorrhagia, metrorrha-

gia, cystic mastitis and premenstrual tension: Treatment with vitamin B complex. *Journal of Clinical Endocrinology and Metabolism, 3*, 227.

15. COOKSON, B. A., QUARRINGTON, B., & HUSZKA, L. (1967). Longitudinal study of periodic catatonia: Long-term clinical and biochemical study of a woman with periodic catatonia. *Journal of Psychiatric Research, 5*, 15.

16. COPPEN, A., & KESSEL, N. (1963). Menstruation and personality. *British Journal of Psychiatry, 109*, 711.

17. COPPEN, A. (1965). The prevalence of menstrual disorders in psychiatric patients. *British Journal of Psychiatry, 111*, 155.

18. COWDRY, R. W., WEHR, T. A., ZIS, A. P., & GOODWIN, F. K. (1983). Thyroid abnormalities associated with rapid cycling bipolar illness. *Archives of General Psychiatry, 40*, 414.

19. DALTON, K. (1964). *The premenstrual syndrome*. Springfield, IL: Charles C Thomas.

20. DALTON, K. (1959). Menstruation and acute psychiatric illness. *British Medical Journal, 1*, 148.

21. DANZIGER, L., KINDWALL, J. A., & LEWIS, H. R. (1948). Periodic relapsing cataonia: A simplified diagnosis and treatment. *Diseases of the Nervous System, 9*, 330.

22. DEJONG, R., RUBINOW, D. R., ROY-BYRNE, P. P., HOBAN, M. C., GROVER, G. N., & POST, R. M. (1985). Premenstrual mood disorder and psychiatric illness. *American Journal of Psychiatry, 142*, 1359.

23. DIAMOND, S. B., RUBINSTEIN, A. A., DUNNER, D. L., & FIEVE, R. R. (1976). Menstrual problems in women with primary affective illness. *Comprehensive Psychiatry, 17*, 541.

24. ENDICOTT, J., & HALBREICH, U. (1982). Psychobiology of premenstrual change. *Psychopharmacology Bulletin, 18*, 109.

25. ENDICOTT, J., HALBREICH, U., SCHACHT, S., & NEE, J. (1981). Premenstrual changes and affective disorders. *Psychosomatic Medicine, 43*, 519.

26. EZEKIEL (18.6) (1954). *The holy scriptures*. Philadelphia: The Jewish Publication Society of America.

27. FARATIAN, B., GASPAR, A., O'BRIEN, P. M., JOHNSON, I. R., FILSHIE, G. M., & PRESCOTT, P. (1984). Premenstrual syndrome: Weight, abdominal swelling and perceived body image. *American Journal of Obstetrics and Gynecology, 150*, 200.

28. FELTHOUS, A. R., ROBINSON, D. B., & CONROY, R. W. (1980). Prevention of recurrent menstrual psychosis by an oral contraceptive. *American Journal of Psychiatry, 137*, 245.

29. FRANK, R. T. (1931). The hormonal causes of premenstrual tension. *Archives of Neurological Psychiatry, 7*, 1053.

30. GANNON, L. (1981). Evidence for a psychological etiology of menstrual disorders: A critical review. *Psychological Report, 48*, 287.

31. GLICK, I. D., & STEWARD, D. (1980). A new drug treatment for premenstrual exacerbation of schizophrenia. *Comprehensive Psychiatry, 21*, 281.

32. GREENE, R., & DALTON, K. (1953). The premenstrual syndrome. *Britith Medical Journal, 1*, 1007.

33. HALBREICH, U., ENDICOTT, J., SCHACHT, S., & NEE, J. (1982). The diversity of premenstrual changes as reflected in the Premenstrual Assessment Form. *Acta Psychiatrica Scandinavica, 65*, 46.

34. HALBREICH, U., BEN-DAVID, M., ASSAEL, M., & BORNSTEIN, R. (1976). Serum-prolactin in women with premenstrual syndrome. *Lancet, 2*, 654.

35. HALBREICH, U., & ENDICOTT, J. (1985). Relationship of dysphoric premenstrual changes to depressive disorders. *Acta Psychiatrica Scandinavica, 71*, 331.

36. HALBREICH, U., ENDICOTT, J., & NEE, J. (1982). Premenstrual depressive changes: Values of differentiation. *Archives of General Psychiatry, 40*, 535.

37. HASKETT, R. F., STEINER, M., OSMUN, J. N., & CARROLL, B. J. (1980). Severe premenstrual tension: Delineation of the syndrome. *Biological Psychiatry, 15,* 121.
38. HASKETT, R. F., STEINER, M., & CARROLL, B. J. (1984). A psychoendocrine study of premenstrual tension syndrome. *Journal of Affective Disorders, 6,* 191.
39. HATOTANI, N., ISHIDA, C., YURA, R., MAEDA, M., KATO, Y., & NOMURA, J. (1962). Psycho-psychological studies of atypical psychoses — Endocrinological aspect of periodic psychoses. *Folia Psychiatrica et Neurologica Japonica, 16,* 248.
40. HURT, S. W., FREIDMAN, R. C., CLARKIN, J., CORN, R., & ARONOFF, M. S. (1982). Psycho-pathology in the menstrual cycle. In R. C. Freidman (Ed.), *Behavior and the menstrual cycle.* New York: Marcel Dekker.
41. HOROWITZ, M. (1979). *States of mind.* New York: Plenum Press.
42. ICARD, S. (1890). *La femme pendant la periode menstruelle.* Paris: Felix Alan.
43. ISRAEL, R. S. (1938). Premenstrual tension. *Journal of the American Medical Association, 110,* 1721.
44. JANOWSKY, D. S., BERENS, S. C., & DAVIS, J. M. (1973). Correlations between mood, weight, and electrolytes during the menstrual cycle: A renin-angiotension aldosterone hypothesis of premenstrual tension. *Journal of Psychosomatic Medicine, 35,* 143.
45. JANOWSKY, D. S., GORNEY, R., & KELEY, B. (1966). "The curse": Vicissitudes and variations of the female fertility cycle. *Psychosomatics, 7,* 242.
46. JANOWSKY, D. S., GORNEY, R., CASTELNUOVO-TEDESCO, P., & STONE, C. B. (1969). Premenstrual-menstrual increasings in psychiatric admission rates. *American Journal of Obstetrics and Gynecology, 103,* 189.
47. KASHIWAGI, T., MCCLURE, J. M., JR., & WETZEL, R. D. (1976). Premenstrual affective syndrome and psychiatric disorder. *Diseases of the Nervous System, 37,* 116.
48. KRAMP, J. L. (1968). Studies of the premenstrual syndrome in relation to psychiatry. *Acta Psychiatrica Scandinavica, 203 (Suppl.),* 261.
49. KULLANDER, S., & SVANBERG, L. (1979). Bromocriptine treatment of the premenstrual syndrome. *Acta Obstetrica Gynecologica Scandinavica, 58,* 375.
50. LINGJAERDE, P., & BREDLAND, R. (1954). Hyperestrogenic cyclic psychosis. *Acta Psychiatrica Neurologica Scandinavica, 29,* 335.
51. LOOSEN, P. T. (1985). The TRH induced TSH response in psychiatric patients: A possible neuroendocrine marker. *Psychoneuroendocrinology, 10,* 237.
52. MANDELL, A. J., & MANDELL, M. P. (1967). Suicide and the menstrual cycle. *Journal of the American Medical Association, 200,* 792.
53. MAY, R. R. (1976). Mood shifts and the menstrual cycle. *Journal of Psychosomatic Research, 20,* 125.
54. MCCLURE, J. N., JR., REICH, T., & WETZEL, R. D. (1971). Premenstrual symptoms as an indicator of bipolar affective disorder. *British Journal of Psychiatry, 119,* 527.
55. MENNINGER-LERCHENTHAL, F. (1960). *Periodizitat in der psychopathologie (neuro- und allgemeinpathologie).* Wein: Wilhelm Maudrich Verlag.
56. MERRIAM, G. R., BRODY, S. A., & ALMEIDA, O. F. X. (1983). Endocrinology of the menstrual cycle: Implications for premenstrual syndrome. Presented at the NIMH Premenstrual Syndrome Workshop, Bethesda, MD, April 14–15.
57. MOOS, R. H. (1968). Typology of menstrual cycle symptoms. *Gynecology, 103,* 390.
58. MOOS, R. H. (1968). The development of a menstrual distress questionnaire. *Psychosomatic Medicine, 30,* 853.
59. MORTON, J. H. (1950). Premenstrual tension. *American Journal of Obstetrics and Gynecology, 60,* 343.
60. MUNDAY, M. R., BRUSH, M. G., & TAYLOR, R. W. (1981). Correlations between progesterone, oestradiol and aldosterone levels in the premenstrual syndrome. *Clinical Endocrinology (Oxford), 14,* 1.

61. MUNDAY, M. (1977). Hormone levels in severe premenstrual tension. *Current Medical Research Opinion, 4(Suppl. 4)*, 16.
62. NIMH Workshop on Premenstrual Syndrome (1983). Rockville, MD, April 14.
63. O'BRIEN, P. M. S., CRAVEN, D., SELBY, C., & SYMONDS, E. M. (1979). Treatment of premenstrual syndrome by spironolactone. *British Journal of Obstetrics and Gynaecology, 86*, 142.
64. O'BRIEN, P. M. S., & SYMONDS, E. M. (1982). Prolactin levels in the premenstrual syndrome. *British Journal of Obstetrics and Gynaecology, 89*, 306.
65. PARLEE, M. B. (1973). The premenstrual syndrome. *Psychological Bulletin, 80*, 454.
66. PERRINI, M., & PILIEGO, N. (1959). L'aumento dell'aldosterone nella sindrome premenstruale. *Minerva Medicine, 50*, 2897.
67. PINEL, P. (1799). *Nosographie philosophique on la methode de l'analyse applique a la medicine.* Paris: Maraden.
68. POST, R. M., & BALLENGER, J. C. (1981). Kindling models for the progression development of behavioral psychopathology: Sensitization to electrical, pharmacological and psychological stimuli. In H. M. Van Praag, M. H. Lader, O. J. Rafaelse, E. J. Sachar (Eds.), *Handbook of biological psychiatry*, Part IV. New York: Marcel Dekker.
69. POST, R. M., WEISS, S. R. B., PERT, A., & UHDE, T. W. (1986). Chronic cocaine administration, sensitization and kindling effects. In S. Fisher, A. Raskin, & E. H. Uhlenhuth (Eds.), *Cocaine: Clinical and biobehavioral aspects.* New York: Oxford University Press.
70. RAUSCH, J. L., & JANOWSKY, D. S. (1982). Premenstrual tension: Etiology. In R. C. Friedman (Ed.), *Behavior and the menstrual cycle.* New York: Marcel Dekker.
71. REID, R. L., & YEN, S. S. C. (1981). Premenstrual syndrome. *American Journal of Obstetrics and Gynecology, 139*, 85.
72. ROY-BYRNE, P. P., RUBINOW, D. R., HOBAN, M. C., PARRY, B. L., ROSENTHAL, N. E., NURNBERGER, J. I., & BYRNES, S. (1986). Premenstrual changes: A comparison of five populations. *Psychiatric Research, 17*, 77.
73. ROY-BYRNE, P. P., RUBINOW, D. R., HOBAN, M. C., GROVER, G. N., & BLANK, D. (1987). TSH and prolactin response to TRH in patients with premenstrual syndrome. *American Journal of Psychiatry, 144*, 480–484.
74. ROY-BRYNE, P. P., RUBINOW, D. R., GWIRTSMAN, H., HOBAN, M. C., & GROVER, G. N. (1986). Cortisol response to dexamethasone in women with premenstrual syndrome. *Neuropsychobiology, 16*, 61–63.
75. RUBINOW, D. R., ROY-BYRNE, P. P., HOBAN, M. C., GOLD, P. W., & POST, R. M. (1984). Prospective assessment of menstrually related mood disorders. *American Journal of Psychiatry, 141*, 684.
76. RUBINOW, D. R., & ROY-BYRNE, P. P. (1984). Premenstrual syndrome: Overview from a methodologic perspective. *American Journal of Psychiatry, 141*, 163.
77. RUBINOW, D. R., ROY-BYRNE, P. P., HOBAN, M. C., GROVER, G. N., STAMBLER, N., & POST, R. M. (1986). Premenstrual mood changes: Characteristic patterns in women with and without premenstrual syndrome. *Journal of Affective Disorders, 10*, 85.
78. RUBLE, D. R., & BROOKS-GUNN, J. (1979). Menstrual symptoms: A social cognition analysis. *Journal of Behavioral Medicine, 2*, 171.
79. RUBLE, D. N. (1977). Premenstrual symptoms: A reinterpretation. *Science, 197*, 291.
80. SAMPSON, J. A., & PRESCOTT, P. (1981). The assessment of the symptoms of premenstrual syndrome and their response to therapy. *British Journal of Psychiatry, 138*, 399.
81. SAMPSON, G. A., & JENNER, F. A. (1977). Studies of daily recordings from Moos menstrual distress questionnaire. *British Journal of Psychiatry, 130*, 265.
82. SAWIN, C. T., HERSHMAN, J. M., BOYD, A. E., LANGCOPE, C., & BACHARACH, P. (1978). The relationship of changes in serum estradiol and progesterone during the menstrual

cycle to the thyrotropin and prolactin responses to TRH. *Journal of Clinical Endocrinology and Metabolism, 47*, 1296.

83. SCHUCKIT, M. A., DALY, V., HERRMAN, G., & HIARMAN, S. (1975). Premenstrual symptoms and depression in a university population. *Diseases of the Nervous System, 36*, 516.

84. SIMON, H. (1978). *Mind and madness in ancient Greece.* Ithaca, NY: Cornell University Press.

85. SIMPSON, G. M., RADINGER, N., ROCHLIN, D., & KLINE, N. S. (1962). Enovid in the treatment of psychic disturbances associated with menstruation. *Diseases of the Nervous System, 23*, 589.

86. SPITZER, R. L., & ENDICOTT, J. (1975). *Schedule for affective disorders and schizophrenia — Lifetime version.* New York: New York State Psychiatric Institute, Biometrics Research.

87. STEINER, M., HASKETT, R. F., CARROLL, B. J., HAYS, S. E., & RUBIN, R. T. (1984). Plasma prolactin and severe premenstrual tension. *Psychoneuroendocrinology, 9*, 29.

88. SUTHERLAND, H. (1892). Menstruation and insanity. In D. H. Tuke (Ed.), *A dictionary of psychological medicine.* Philadelphia: P. Blakistone.

89. SUTHERLAND, H., & STEWART, I. (1965). A critical analysis of premenstrual syndrome. *Lancet, 1*, 1180.

90. SWANSON, D. W., BARRON, A., FLOREN, A., & SMITH, J. A. (1964). The use of norethynodrel in psychotic females. *American Journal of Psychiatry, 120*, 1101.

91. SWENSON, R. M., & VOGEL, W. H. (1983). Plasma catecholamine and corticosterone as well as brain catecholamine changes during coping in rats exposed to stressful footshock. *Pharmacological and Biochemical Behavior, 18*, 689.

92. TAYLOR, J. W. (1979). The timing of menstruation-related symptoms assessed by a daily symptom rating scale. *Acta Psychiatrica Scandinavica, 60*, 87.

93. TONKS, C. M., RACK, P. H., & ROSE, M. J. (1968). Attempted suicide in the menstrual cycle. *Journal of Psychosomatic Research, 11*, 319.

94. VISINTAINER, M. A., VOLPICELLI, J. R., & SELIGMAN, N. E. P. (1982). Tumor rejection in rats after inescapable or escapable shock. *Science, 216*, 437.

95. WETZEL, R. D., REICH, T., McCLURE, J. N., JR., & WALD, I. (1975). Premenstrual affective syndrome and affective disorder. *British Journal of Psychiatry, 127*, 219.

96. WOOD, C., & JAKUBOWICZ, D. (1980). The treatment of premenstrual symptoms with mefenamic acid. *British Journal of Obstetrics and Gynaecology, 87*, 627.

97. WILLIAMS, E. Y., & WEEKES, L. R. (1952). Premenstrual tension associated with psychotic episodes. *Journal of Nervous and Mental Disorders, 116*, 321.

98. YAMASHITA, I., SHINOHARA, S., NAKAZAWA, A., YOSHIMURA, Y., ITO, K., & TAKASUGI, K. (1962). Endocrinological study of atypical psychosis. *Folia Psychiatrica et Neurologica Japonica, 16*, 293.

10

AIDS AND PSYCHIATRY

SAMUEL W. PERRY, M.D.

Professor of Clinical Psychiatry, Cornell University Medical College,
New York City

PAUL JACOBSEN, PH.D.

Instructor of Psychology, Cornell University Medical College,
New York City

and

JOHN MARKOWITZ, M.D.

Instructor in Psychiatry, Cornell University Medical College,
New York City

INTRODUCTION

Since first recognized in 1981, acquired immunodeficiency syndrome (AIDS) has become a serious public-health emergency that challenges many fields of medicine, including psychiatry. Human immunodeficiency virus (HIV), the cause of AIDS, now infects more than one million people in the United States and millions more in other countries. As of October 1987, more than 42,350 cases of AIDS have been reported in the United States. The number of cases reported thus far is only the beginning of the expected toll, since at least two-thirds of those who are currently infected will in the coming years develop the disease. Furthermore, the epidemic is growing every day as persons who are infected spread the virus. HIV is transmitted in only a few ways: by anal or vaginal intercourse; by mother

Supported in part by NIH research grant #MH 42277-01.

187

to fetus or newborn infant; and by exchange of contaminated blood, such as from transfusions or intravenous drug use.

This chapter describes the psychiatric issues raised by the disease in five overlapping adult populations: (1) medically hospitalized patients with AIDS; (2) outpatients with AIDS and AIDS-related complex (ARC); (3) patients with AIDS-related dementia (ARD); (4) asymptomatic individuals who have been infected by the HIV virus; and (5) psychiatrically hospitalized patients with AIDS-related disorders. Psychiatric interventions are suggested for each group based on the relevant literature and on the authors' clinical and research experiences. The chapter concludes with comments regarding noninfected populations who seek psychiatric consultation because of emotional problems related to the epidemic. Additional readings are then provided.

MEDICALLY HOSPITALIZED PATIENTS WITH AIDS

Available medical evidence suggests that infection with HIV, a retrovirus that damages the body's immune system, is the first step in the development of AIDS (i.e., opportunistic infections and/or malignancies, such as an aggressive form of Kaposi's sarcoma or a non-Hodgkin's lymphoma). Although some drug treatments may prolong survival, AIDS is ultimately fatal. Over 80 percent of patients with AIDS die within two years, although approximately 15 percent have been known to survive for three years or more. Of all those infected by the HIV virus, hospitalized AIDS patients pose the least perplexing problems in terms of psychiatric management. The reasons for consultation are familiar to psychiatrists who regularly see patients in the general hospital: depression, delirium, and denial.

The "depression" in many hospitalized patients with AIDS does not represent a pathological process, but instead is a normal grief response about having a fatal illness. The psychiatrist can help such patients by indicating that the sadness is an appropriate reaction and by conveying an empathic understanding. In some cases, however, a more pathological process may be present, which is characterized by alienation, irrational guilt, diminished self-esteem, and suicidal ideation. These depressive symptoms are dynamically related to conscious and unconscious conflicts regarding what the disease means to the particular patient and how it was acquired, such as homosexual encounters, intravenous drug abuse, or heterosexual promiscuity. Psychiatric interventions are then indicated. For milder depressions, an effective intervention is the psychodynamic life narrative: the psychiatrist places the patient's illness in the context of his life course and his specific character style and concerns, thereby enhancing the comfort of a positive transference and providing an intellectual mastery over the conflicts related to having AIDS. This personally tailored intervention is preferable to more global, less specific reassurance.

For more severe depressions, psychopharmacotherapy is indicated. Nothing about AIDS in itself precludes the use of antidepressant medication. The choice of drugs will be influenced by the patient's psychiatric and medical condition. More activating drugs, such as imipramine or desipramine, are preferred for lethargic patients with pulmonary infections because they can increase alertness and respiratory movements. These drugs have the additional advantage of enabling the psychiatrist to regulate the dosage by making sure that blood levels have reached the therapeutic range. An antidepressant with more anticholinergic action, such as amitriptyline, may beneficially increase sedation and diminish diarrhea in agitated depressed patients with gastroenteritis.

The suicide potential among depressed patients with AIDS is a major consideration. Although no prospective data are available to document the incidence of suicide in this population, recent reports indicate that fatal suicide attempts are increasingly common and higher than in patients with other illnesses. Depressed patients with AIDS often view their suicidal ideation and intent as reasonable, considering the social stigma of the disease and its malignant and ultimately fatal course; however, in the presence of a depression, the psychiatrist must not accept this explanation. Instead, the patient can be told that suicidal ideation is a common symptom accompanying depression and that "rational" suicide cannot be evaluated until the patient's mood lifts. In the meantime, 24-hour companions or psychiatric hospitalization may be required to prevent the patient from acting on his feelings of guilt, worthlessness, and social ostracism.

Delirium occurs in more than 50 percent of medically hospitalized patients with AIDS. The delirium can be caused by systemic illness (for example, septicemia or electrolyte imbalance), by direct central nervous system diseases that have arisen secondarily as a result of the immune deficiency (such as lymphoma, toxoplasmosis, or meningoencephalitis), and by direct HIV infection of the central nervous system (see below). The delirium can be treated with the usual psychotherapeutic and pharmacological strategies familiar to a consultation-liaison psychiatrist, including frequent orientation, titration of external stimuli, and small doses of neuroleptics for sedation and frightening misperceptions or hallucinations. Because a delirious patient with AIDS can arouse intense anxiety in the staff and other patients if he wanders the halls or becomes uncooperative, there is a tendency to rely too heavily on continuous restraints. A preferable alternative is to arrange for hospital personnel or family and friends to stay with the patient and guide him toward appropriate behavior.

In addition to depression and delirium, denial is the third major reason why psychiatrists are asked to see hospitalized patients with AIDS. The consultation is prompted by the staff's concern that the patient is remaining unreasonably hopeful despite the presence of a fatal illness. When the denial has become so extreme that it interferes with the patient's receiving palliative medical care or when it jeopardizes others because the patient refuses to practice risk-reducing behaviors, then the psychiatric consultant must confront the patient and, with medication and psychotherapy, reduce the underlying panic that is responsible for the rigid denial. More often, however, the consultant must take a liaison role and remind the staff that denial of a fatal illness can be an adaptive defense if it does not prevent the patient from getting supportive medical care and does not jeopardize others. Staff's insistence that the patient come to terms with his fate derives in part from an unconscious need to perceive the patient as sick and therefore categorically different from the healthy caretaker; therefore, when the patient with AIDS admits he is ill, the staff member feels relieved: "The patient is different than me; he is ill and I am fine."

Although the therapeutic interventions for depression, delirium, and denial in medically hospitalized patients with AIDS are basically the same as for others with severe illnesses, the countertransference problems are different in both degree and kind. Most pervasive is the fear of contagion, even though well-documented studies have shown that casual contact poses no risk. The staff's fear of contagion will be reduced when they are informed of specific precautions to be taken when caring for AIDS patients (see Table 1).

An educational approach may not be sufficient to overcome the staff's fear of contagion. An exaggerated concern is often fueled by irrational, unconscious forces. For example, the patient with AIDS may represent illicit impulses in the caregiver: by avoiding the patient with AIDS, the staff member may unconsciously be avoiding his or her own concerns about homosexuality, sexual activity, or substance abuse. An appreciation of these dynamics will help the psychiatrist not to become disheartened when a "rational" discussion does not produce the desired result. It may be necessary to serve as a role model and accompany the staff member into the phobic situation. On an encouraging note, the initial fear of contagion

Table 1
Recommended Precautions for Prevention of
Human Immunodeficiency Virus (HIV) Infection in the Clinical Setting*

- Routine HIV antibody screening for staff is not recommended. The risk of contracting this bloodborne virus is very low, and it is not spread by casual contact. While the risk of contracting hepatitis B virus from an infected needle is 6 to 30 percent, an AIDS-infected needlestick carries a less than 1 percent risk. Precautions are the same as for other bloodborne infections.
- Handle potentially infective needles, scalpel blades, and other sharp instruments with extraordinary care.
- Put disposable sharp instruments in puncture-resistant containers as close as possible to the area of use. Do not recap, remove, or otherwise manipulate used needles.
- Gloves alone may suffice for exposure to blood or body fluids. For more extensive contact and invasive procedures, use gowns, masks, and eye coverings.
- Wash hands thoroughly and immediately if accidentally exposed to blood.
- To obviate the need for mouth-to-mouth resuscitation, keep mouthpieces and ventilatory equipment near patients who might require resuscitation.
- Pregnancy does not increase the risk of infection. But because infants may contact HIV infection perinatally, pregnant health care workers should be especially aware of these precautions.
- Wear gloves to clean spilled blood or body fluids. Clean the area with soap and water or household detergent, followed by household bleach.
- Consult a physician if exposed to HIV by a cut, a needlestick, or a splash in the eye or mouth.
- Routine HIV antibody screening of all patients is not recommended.

*Adapted from Centers for Disease Control: *Morbidity and mortality weekly report, 34*, 681–695, 1985.

diminishes as staff members acquire more experience in treating patients with AIDS.

A second common countertransference reaction is a tendency to stereotype the patient on the basis of his being a member of a high-risk group. Prejudices against homosexuals, substance abusers, and sexually active women may predispose the staff to assume that the patient with AIDS was highly promiscuous or socially irresponsible. The psychiatrist can reduce these prejudices and resultant stereotyping by reminding the staff of the heterogeneity within the designated high-risk groups and by pointing out those aspects of a patient that make him or her a unique individual.

A third common countertransference problem is the failure to find the appropriate empathic distance with these relatively young patients infected with a fatal disease. On the one hand is the problem of being too close—of sympathetically identifying with the patient to the point that the caregiver is overwhelmed by what he presumes the patient must be experiencing. On the other hand is the problem of being too distant—of emotionally detaching oneself and viewing the patient as an AIDS "victim." Both sympathetic identification and detached pity prevent the caregiver from relating to the patient as a unique individual, and both extremes can contribute to staff "burnout" as more and more young patients with AIDS are admitted to the medical services and die. Assuming a liaison role, the psychiatrist can decrease these problems by providing a forum to ventilate staff reactions, by identifying the frustration and guilt generated by unrealistic expectations, and by indicating that a given patient's reaction to his illness may be quite different than the staff assumes.

OUTPATIENTS WITH AIDS AND AIDS-RELATED COMPLEX

Although one thinks of AIDS as being an acute fatal illness, most patients with the disease are outpatients, many of whom remain highly functional between exacerbations of the disease. In addition, there are approximately 20 times as many patients who have milder physical symptoms caused by HIV infection but who do not have AIDS. These patients with milder symptoms are said to have an "AIDS-related complex" (ARC). It is not known to what extent ARC may predict the eventual development of frank AIDS, but current estimates are that about one-half will go on to develop the fatal disease within three years. ARC constitutes a broadly defined category and includes persistent generalized lymphadenopathy, fatigue, fever, weight loss, diarrhea, and widely varying neurological signs and symptoms (described below).

Standardized longitudinal studies have documented that the psychological morbidity in outpatients with AIDS and ARC is extraordinarily high. At least one-third have an affective disorder or a severe adjustment disorder with anxiety and/or depression. These patients live under the sword of Damocles. Physical symptoms that previously would have been ignored—a dry mouth, a mild cough, a slight rash—could for them be an early sign of thrush, an opportunistic pneumonia, Kaposi's sarcoma, and eventual death.

Given the heterogeneity of outpatients with AIDS and ARC, no single therapeutic strategy is likely to be widely applicable, but four general principles can be kept in mind. First, the psychiatrist should appreciate that although the patient may appear to have no current severe physical problems, the patient has concluded that he is sick and accordingly may have assumed the sick role—that is, regressed to a more dependent state and delegated normal responsibilities to an idealized caregiver. This understandable regression is a "state" phenomenon and should not be confused with "trait" characterological problems. Under other circumstances, many of these patients would not appear helpless, dependent, obsessional, hypochondriacal, or self-absorbed. A premorbid personality disorder should not be presumed without adequate documentation.

Second, given the patient's heightened awareness of physical symptoms, the psychiatrist should not prematurely deflect the patient from somatic to psychological issues. Many patients with AIDS and ARC (for example, homosexual and bisexual men, substance abusers, and prostitutes) are wary about how they will be judged, if not prejudged, by the psychiatrist. By at first focusing on the physical symptoms, by accepting the patient's somatic concerns, and by conveying medical knowledge about AIDS and ARC, psychiatrists can tighten the therapeutic alliance. This initial, more physicianly role will make the psychiatrist's later questions about the psychological aspects of the patient's life appear more acceptable and accepting—such as "How has the chronic fatigue affected your work, your mood, and the relationship with your lover?"

A third general principle is that the psychiatrist should recognize the value of clarification, abreaction, suggestion, and supportive techniques. Because of the intense distress and desperation these patients express, the psychiatrist may mistakenly conclude that standard psychotherapeutic interventions will not be helpful enough. On the contrary, many of these patients are confronted with a double-barreled situation: they are constantly exposed through the media or illness in friends to AIDS-related issues, yet they may have no one with whom they can openly share their most intimate concerns. Providing an empathic holding environment, correcting cognitive and somatic distortions about AIDS (for instance, "I'm contaminated" or "I'm worthless"), discouraging unreasonable experimental treatments that will deplete financial resources, and facilitating last-chance reconciliations with rejecting family members can all be helpful.

A fourth principle is that major affective disorder should not be overdiagnosed in this population. Somatic symptoms associated with AIDS and ARC are similar to vegetative symptoms of depression (fatigue, sleep disturbance, anorexia, and weight loss). These symptoms do not in themselves warrant the prescription of antidepressant medication, especially in the absence of psychological symptoms (irrational guilt, suicidal ideation, and a profound loss of self-esteem). Responding to his own feelings of helplessness, the psychiatrist may be inclined to resort to pharmacotherapy without clear indications. This response can "medicalize" problems that more appropriately require interpersonal support.

Outpatient psychotherapy for patients with AIDS and ARC can catalyze other countertransference reactions that are more pronounced than those invoked in the protected environment of a general hospital. Most prominent is the unwarranted fear of contagion when these "contaminated" patients read the psychiatrist's magazines in the waiting room, sit in his office, or use his bathroom. Concerns about what can be considered an invasion of the psychiatrist's physical space can be a displacement of fears about invasion of the psychiatrist's internal world, unconscious fears that are heightened as these patients form an intimate, sustained relationship.

Another countertransference reaction can be an irrational need to assume the stance of an omnipotent expert about AIDS, mastering the medical literature and intellectually expanding on the immunological intricacies of the disease. This posture of omnipotence is partly a response to the psychiatrist's own feelings of helplessness and partly a response to the idealization delegated by the regressed patient in his search for certainty and authority. The danger of this fragile omnipotent stance is that it leads to eventual disillusionment and it impedes a more genuine human exchange with the frightened patient.

Finally, for countertransferential reasons the psychiatrist may prematurely refer patients to self-help groups, such as substance abuse programs or those provided by gay-men's health organizations for persons with AIDS or ARC. Although a homogeneous group format can reduce the alienation experienced by many patients, some individuals are simply too overwhelmed or too concerned about confidentiality to accept such a referral. In addition, some are too distressed by egodystonic homosexuality to participate in a group process with those who are more open about and comfortable with being gay. A premature referral may induce feelings of rejection, the same feelings that brought the patient to psychotherapy.

PATIENTS WITH AIDS-RELATED DEMENTIA (ARD)

During the first three years after AIDS was identified, clinicians were puzzled not only by the high frequency of organic mental disorders among hospitalized patients with AIDS, but also by the severity of these disorders.

The profound dementias seemed disproportionate to the clinical condition, laboratory values, and gross neuropathological findings. Furthermore, the history of many of the patients revealed that cognitive deficits and psychological problems predated signs of immune deficiency. We now know that these puzzling clinical features can be explained by the mounting evidence that HIV directly infects the central nervous system and causes a subacute encephalopathy with diffuse gliosis.

Even with this knowledge, the diagnosis of AIDS-related dementia (ARD) may be difficult to make because: (1) the cognitive deficits are often subtle, delayed, and not detected by standard questions asked during a mental status examination; (2) the insidiously developing cognitive problems may mimic many functional disorders; and (3) initially the neurological examination, laboratory values, and electroencephalograms, cerebral spinal fluid, and computed axial tomography of the brain may all be normal. This difficulty is compounded because many of these high-risk individuals have psychosocial stressors that can explain their emotional problems. Nevertheless, there are clues to making the diagnosis of ARD: HIV seropositivity on the ELISA and Western blot tests; the absence of a premorbid personal or family history of psychiatric illness; neuropsychological testing; and soft signs of organicity, such as imbalance, tremor, avoidance of complex tasks, forgetfulness, personality change, irritability, impulsivity, and sensitivity to alcohol and other drugs.

Although AIDS-related dementias are typically atypical, they do tend to cluster into two broad categories: an insidious depression characterized by apathy, withdrawal, fatigue, hypersomnia, weight loss, anorexia, psychomotor retardation, and subtle cognitive deficits; and an acute psychotic presentation with delusions, hallucinations, psychomotor agitation, mania with grandiosity, and more profound cognitive impairment.

The psychiatric interventions for ARD are similar to the general management of organic mental disorders. The psychiatrist can help the patient establish structure in daily living, set limits appropriate to the patient's current capacities, decrease hypochondriacal preoccupations with reasonable reassurance, reduce self-destructive or impulsive acts, and help the patient with financial matters, including preparation of a will.

Neuroleptics can be helpful for psychotic disorganization and agitation, and antidepressants or psychostimulants may be helpful for fatigue, weakness, and diminished affectivity. If family members are available, they should be counseled about providing the patient with maintenance care and arranging for eventual institutionalization. These services will be increasingly difficult to acquire, so early arrangements are necessary.

INDIVIDUALS WITH HIV ANTIBODIES

Because HIV harbors itself within the cells, the presence of antibodies does not mean that one is now immune to the virus. On the contrary, most individuals who have antibodies also have the virus in their systems. They are potentially contagious, and after a prolonged incubation period of months or years, an unknown percentage will go on to develop an AIDS-related disorder. This percentage was initially believed to be about 10 percent, but it appears to be rising as seropositive individuals are followed for longer periods. The percentage may be at least as high as 60 percent.

As more and more individuals are tested for HIV antibodies, psychiatrists can anticipate frequent consultations for seropositive individuals. Their concerns will not only be about possibly developing a fatal disease, but also about infecting others or about never being able again to have normal sex or children. They may also have guilt about how they acquired the virus and want advice about whom they should tell and how.

Although psychiatrists cannot magically eradicate these concerns and the existing uncertainty, they can provide several positive interventions. First, the psychiatrist can help the seropositive subject effectively appraise his situation. We know that severe stress can lead to misperceptions and distortions that can make a situation seem more malignant than it actually is. By applying a psychoeducational approach, the psychiatrist considers not only the facts, but also the psychological determinants that lead to the distortions.

Second, the psychiatrist can use well-documented techniques of stress inoculation, including palliative relaxation techniques, cognitive appraisal, and cognitive reframing. Benzodiazepines may be indicated for the intense panic that may occur immediately after the individual is notified of seropositivity, but nonpharmacological methods of reducing anxiety should be taught. The stress of seropositivity will be chronic, perhaps lifelong, and continuous use of anxiolytics may lead to physical and psychological dependency. Third, the psychiatrist can help the seropositive individual in daily problem solving. Although this approach seems no more than common sense, it can be a valuable resource that may be unavailable elsewhere for someone alienated from potential support systems. For example, the patient may not know the potentially hazardous consequences of telling an employer about his seropositivity, and he may not know how to tell a spouse, lover, or family member about what the antibody test means and what risk-reducing behaviors must now be practiced.

Fourth, an important role for the psychiatrist is to help the infected patient prevent the spread of the epidemic. Table 2 lists the basic high-risk behaviors that must be changed. These behaviors are easy to describe but not so easy to practice. One of the most difficult aspects of treating seropositive patients is that the psychiatrist's alliance must be with the distressed patient, yet the psychiatrist must also ally himself with the public to reduce the spread of the disease. This dual role can pose a strain. For example, when a seropositive patient admits that he is practicing unsafe anonymous sex, or is not telling his wife that he is infected, or is sharing needles in a "shooting gallery," the psychiatrist may fear that confronting the patient about such behavior will threaten the therapeutic alliance and prevent the patient from receiving necessary support.

Our experience has not confirmed this fear. On the contrary, by allying with the patient's healthier ego functions and by stating directly from the start that one goal of treatment will be to help the patient act responsibly, we have found that the therapeutic bond has been strengthened. In addition, the patient's guilt about having acquired the infection is countered by the pride that comes from now protecting others; the patient's uncertainty about his medical condition is countered by his sense of mastery over his current behavior. To reinforce the statement that a high priority is to reduce the spread of the epidemic, the psychiatrist can inquire about the patient's risk-reducing behaviors even if the patient does not volunteer such information, can ask how the patient has informed past and present

Table 2
Risk-Reducing Behaviors for Persons with HIV Antibodies*

Abstinence is the only certain method of preventing sexual transmission of HIV virus.

Sexual practices with a partner at any risk for or known to have HIV infection should not allow exchange of blood or bodily secretions.

A condom should be worn for all sexual activity.

Anal intercourse is strongly discouraged.

Avoid mucous membrane contact with blood, semen, preejaculate secretions, vaginal secretions, saliva, urine, and feces.

Intravenous drug use is discouraged. If use persists, needles and other injection equipment should not be shared or reused.

---

*Adapted from Centers for Disease Control: *Morbidity and mortality weekly report, 34* (Suppl.), 75S–76S, 1985.

partners at risk, can role-play with the patient about how future partners will be informed, and can invite partners and spouses to attend a session at which appropriate precautions are discussed. No legal precedent has yet been set regarding whether the psychiatrist is obligated to warn and protect an individual known to be at imminent risk of being infected by a seropositive patient, but moral and ethical reasons dictate that the psychiatrist should make every effort to have the patient prevent the spread of the disease.

PSYCHIATRICALLY HOSPITALIZED PATIENTS WITH AIDS-RELATED DISORDERS

The two most common AIDS-related reasons for psychiatric hospitalization are depression with suicidal ideation and acute psychotic disorganization precipitated by either ARD or the psychosocial stress of an HIV infection. The psychotherapy and pharmacotherapy provided for these patients does not differ substantially from therapy of other patients with these diagnoses. On the contrary, problems in management are more likely to arise if the staff insists on treating patients with AIDS-related disorders in a special manner beyond the precautions itemized in Table 1. Some patients may be too physically ill, disorganized, or demented to participate either in ward activities or in physical and occupational therapies, but most patients with HIV seropositivity or ARC can attend all ward activities and eat with other patients. Like the general public, the staff and other patients may be concerned about casual contact with an HIV-infected individual; the chief of service will need to take a direct educational and positive modeling role in allaying these unrealistic fears. Other patients frequently learn about a patient's HIV infection, but the staff is under no obligation to disclose this information, which, like other illnesses in other patients, is confidential. If the hospital has a policy of listing hepatitislike precautions on the patient's door, these can be posted without revealing the diagnosis of AIDS.

In addition to the problem of treating HIV-infected patients as special and of inappropriately isolating them from ward activities, another problem that commonly occurs in psychiatric hospitals is that the diagnosis of ARD is missed. As discussed above, AIDS-related organic mental disorders can mimic many functional conditions, including mania, major depression, and schizophreniform disorders; however, these organic problems may be more refractory to treatment and may be associated with more impulsivity, violence, and suicidal potential. Given the increasing prevalence of the AIDS epidemic through heterosexual spread, ARD must be considered in the differential diagnosis of every patient and not be restricted to certain higher-risk groups.

NONINFECTED PATIENTS WITH HIV-RELATED DISORDERS

The anxiety generated by the AIDS epidemic affects many individuals who are not infected by HIV. These populations include: (1) individuals at increased risk for infection, who require counseling to maintain their seronegativity, such as by entering substance abuse programs or by changing their sexual practices; (2) family members and friends of HIV-infected patients, who require a confidential forum to discuss their profound grief, their ambivalence toward the sick loved one, and their rationale and exaggerated concerns about becoming infected themselves and ostracized by others; (3) AIDS caretakers, who experience disillusionment, social withdrawal, and substance abuse as a result of the stress posed by the epidemic; and (4) individuals with prior anxiety and somatization disorders, who now focus their avoidance and hypochondriacal complaints on issues related to AIDS.

The psychiatrist can be enormously helpful to these groups if interventions combine a specific understanding of the individual patient with a general knowledge of HIV infections. To obtain this knowledge, the psychiatrist has a responsibility to stay abreast of the rapid advances in the field by reviewing the relevant medical and psychiatric literature. In this regard, the references listed are suggested for background information, with the realization that reviewing more recent publications will also be necessary.

ADDITIONAL READINGS

1. *Confronting AIDS: Directions for public health, health care and research.* Washington, DC: National Academy Press, 1986.
2. HOLLAND, J. C., & TROSS, S. (1985). The psychosocial and neuropsychiatric sequelae of acquired immunodeficiency syndrome. *Annals of Internal Medicine, 103,* 760–764.
3. MILLER, D., WEBER, J., & GREEN, J. (Eds.) (1986). *The management of AIDS patients.* London: Macmillan.
4. NAVIA, B. A., JORDAN, B. D., & PRICE, R. W. (1986). The AIDS dementia complex. I. Clinical features. *Annals of Neurology, 19,* 517–524.
5. PERRY, S. W., & JACOBSEN, P. (1986). Neuropsychiatric manifestations of AIDS spectrum disorders. *Hospital and Community Psychiatry, 37,* 135–142.
6. PETITO, C. K., NAVIA, B. A., CHO, E. S., et al. (1985). Vacuolar myelopathy pathologically resembling subacute combined degeneration in patients with acquired immunodeficiency syndrome. *New England Journal of Medicine, 312,* 874–879.

11

THE BORDERLINE DOMAIN: THE "INNER SCRIPT" AND OTHER COMMON PSYCHODYNAMICS

MICHAEL H. STONE, M.D.

*Professor of Clinical Psychiatry, Cornell University Medical College;
Director, Psychotherapy Service, Extended Treatment Division,
New York Hospital–Westchester Division, White Plains, New York*

INTRODUCTION

Borderline, as a diagnostic label, has become increasingly popular in the United States and on the European continent, particularly since the term was "legitimized" in 1980 through its inclusion in the third revision of the *Diagnostic and Statistical Manual* (DSM-III). In the 1930s and 1940s "borderline" was used chiefly within the American psychoanalytic community to denote cases that were not clearly psychotic yet somehow not amenable to classical psychoanalytic treatment (26): these cases were "borderline" with respect to analyzability. Most American analysts regarded their borderline patients as incipient or attenuated instances of schizophrenia (5,34), i.e., as "borderline" with respect to schizophrenia, as well. These early definitions were vague and imprecise. Efforts were made to develop more stringent criteria, most notably by Knight (13), who drew attention to the borderline patient's fragility of defenses despite an outward display, often, of healthier coping mechanisms, and by Kernberg (11), who established the "boundaries" of the borderline: the presence of ego diffusion (which demarcated the borderline from the neurotic level) and the presence of adequate reality-testing capacity (demarcating the borderline from the psychotic level of psychic function). Kernberg also underlined, as inhering to this psychostructural definition of "borderline," a number of other qualities: primitivity of defenses, impulsivity, impairment in sublimatory capacities, and a tendency toward disorganizing anxiety in situations regarded as only moderately stressful by better-integrated persons.

In recent years, the Kernberg definition has itself been criticized as imprecise, particularly from the standpoint of *etiology*. The similarity of symptoms and defenses did not harken back to any homogeneity of primary causative factors, although certain factors that came rather late in development (problems in separation/individuation) were emphasized as important contributors to the genesis of borderline conditions. It was recognized in the 1970s that relatively few borderline patients could be regarded as incipient schizophrenics, especially by the more rigorous diagnostic criteria that were (finally) being introduced into the United States from Britain and the Continent, where such criteria had long been standard. One could in fact speak of a borderline "domain" that, however uniform in defense mechanisms and ego fragility, was bewilderingly heterogeneous etiologically: a good many cases seemed, if attenuated examples of anything, to be attenuated forms of affective, not schizophrenic, psychosis (1,27). In Britain, until very recently, "borderline" was not considered a useful term: patients who would be so designated in the United States might be called, in Britain, narcissistic (24) or be seen as exhibiting a "false self" (32). More biologically oriented British psychiatrists subsumed some of these cases under headings more closely related to well-defined and more widely accepted nosological entities (cf. Paykel's "atypical depression" [20]).

In the last decade, several syndromal definitions of *borderline* have been elaborated. The criteria of Gunderson and Singer (10) were more empirically based, stressing observational and anamnestic data (manipulative suicide gestures, disturbances in close relationships) rather than intuitive and inferential conclusions about defensive patterns or about the solidity of one's identity. Still more "computer-friendly" were the eight items of the DSM-III definition (extracted mainly from the Kernberg and Gunderson criteria), where inference is kept to a minimum. The simplicity of the DSM definition, coupled with America's powerful position within the international psychiatric community, has led to (a) widespread adoption of the term "borderline" throughout the world, (b) increasing popularity of the DSM definition at the expense of the broader and more intuitive definitions, (c) increasing spread of the borderline label into the larger, nonpsychoanalytical segment of the psychiatric community, despite the analytical origins of the concept, and (d) a *re*definition of borderline in the direction of an *affective/irritable* constellation, whereas "borderlines" as defined by broad criteria generally show a *mixture* of affective and "schizotypal" traits. The DSM description is not without its usefulness. It is rather similar to the 19th-century concepts of the melancholicocholeric and sanguineocholeric temperaments and happens also to single out the suicide-prone from the non-suicide-prone Kernberg borderlines (29). But the DSM version of borderline represents, in my opinion, too sharp a break with tradition, too simplistic an approach, and too skewed a definition to perform well all the functions this label was invented to subserve.

The DSM definition of borderline has also (by dwelling only on symptoms) become decoupled from its origins as a signifier of attenuated forms of the classical psychoses. This tends to discourage the clinician from looking deeper, in his "borderline" cases, for signs of such vulnerability. In some samples, this vulnerability will be present in half or more of the "borderline" cases. There is really no reason to jettison broad definitions of borderline, nor is there any rationale for claiming that one or another borderline construct is the "right" one. The Kernberg definition, or the less sharply bounded concepts of the basic fault (2) or the false self (32), continue to have considerable usefulness. They provide handy descriptive labels, providing "coverage" for many otherwise undiagnosible cases (especially in young people, where later definable conditions are seen *in statu nascendi*). In addition, the broad definitions serve as an index of "in-between" function, namely, the fragile, disaster-prone function of certain persons who for the most part are unable to keep their problems hidden like ordinary ("neurotic-level") folk, yet who are clearly not continuously psychotic, either. Borderline can be used, in other words, as a coarse lens for viewing certain patterns of thought and behavior — later to be examined under oil immersion for finer details as to specifics and subtype. The sentiments expressed here I find echoed in Gallwey's excellent chapter on borderline psychodynamics (8).

In relation to the broader definitions of borderline, I have recently formed the impression that there is rather a close fit between these definitions and the area on a bell curve of mental health, applicable to a whole community or country, and situated between the 1st and the 2nd standard deviation (SD) from the norm.

Figure 1 represents such a whole population, whose members would be distributed, presumably, in good Gaussian fashion, where about 5 percent of persons enjoy clearly superior levels of mental health, integrity of per-

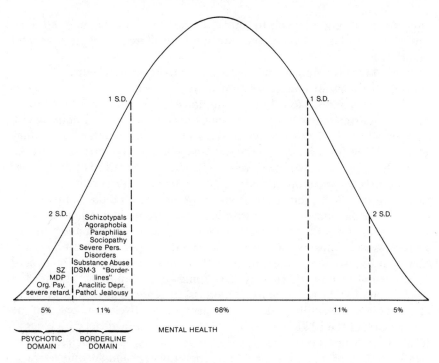

Figure 1. Bell curve of a whole population.

sonality, leadership ability, and so forth, placing them at 2 SD from the average. Somewhat less exuberant, but still recognizably better-than-average health is enjoyed by the 11 percent of the population situated between the 1st and 2nd SD. On the other pole, one would find a twentieth of the population in a psychotic condition, its ranks made up of chronic schizophrenics (usually about 1 percent in any population), bipolar manics (.5 percent), unipolar depressives, "organic" psychoses, and severely retarded persons. Between this extreme and the large "average" segment one would find a collection of fairly ill but nonpsychotic persons: severe agoraphobes, schizotypal ("borderline schizophrenic") persons, sociopaths, those who abuse alcohol and drugs to any significant degree, severe anorexia/bulimia cases, paraphiliacs, persons exhibiting marked personality disorders of other types or else exhibiting one of the Kraepelinian temperaments associated with manic-depression (including the cyclothymics), and the more narrowly defined borderlines of Gunderson or the DSM-III. It is likely that all these people would make up a tenth (or just over) of the population—in what might be said to constitute the borderline domain: all those between 1 and 2 SD from the norm in the direction of poor mental health.

Viewed in this manner, the borderline domain would occupy about the same dimensions in one generation as in the next, since many factors conspire to keep the shape of the population curve similar over long periods of time. (Distortions would come about only in unusual circumstances, such as when the British convicts and their guards debarked at Sydney Cove in 1788: for a few years the not very populous country of Australia would have had a curve skewed to the left.) The proportions of the various diagnostic subtypes *within* this domain would, and apparently *do*, change from one decade to the next. There has been an absolute increase, for example, in the number of anorexia/bulimia cases in Switzerland over the past 20 years (30); this is probably true throughout America and Western Europe as well. Meanwhile the ranks of the severe phobias, hysteria cases, obsessive handwashers, and so forth that filled the pages of Janet and Freud at the turn of the century have somewhat dwindled. Whether the proportion of DSM-III borderlines is on the increase or has remained rather constant is difficult to guess: the concept is a relatively new one and the case reports of the 1920s and earlier do not always provide us with clues as to whether or not the various items were present. Epidemiological surveys relative to this question did not exist a generation ago and are only currently getting underway (viz., in Sweden, cf. Kullgren [14]).

The borderline domain as sketched in Figure 1 would overlap considerably both with the realm of type A (concealed ego deficiencies resulting from early prolonged infantile deprivation) plus type B (schizoid encapsulation of destructive impulses) patients outlined by Gallwey (7, p. 133) and with the realm of Kernberg's borderline level ("borderline personality organization") patients. There would be small areas of dysjunction: some schizotypal patients, for example, or patients with pathological jealousy might show a poor enough reality-testing capacity in the interpersonal sphere to qualify in Kernberg's psychostructural model as "psychotic" in structure.

THE INNER SCRIPT

Intensive psychotherapy with patients of any diagnostic category has as one of its goals the elucidation of the patient's inner script. By this phrase I refer to the fundamental wishes, coupled with one's fundamental self-image, as these evolve during early development. The script constitutes the basic plan around which one's life is organized; it becomes the embodi-ment of one's hopes, which thus animates one and gives a sense of purpose and direction to one's life. This idea of an inner script is related to the psychoanalytic concept of the repetition compulsion; only here, the focus is on the nature of the hidden drama mobilizing the repetitive behavior — not on the repetitive acts, *per se.*

There is a relationship between the inner script and Winnicott's notion of the "true," in contradistinction to the "false," self (33). The differences between true and false self are easier to appreciate in emotionally ill than in healthy persons. In health, for example, the false self "is represented by the whole organization of the polite and mannered social attitude" (33, p. 143) in order to fit into society more smoothly (less abrasively, less shock-ingly, etc.) than would be the case were the true self to preside over day-to-day behavior. In lesser degrees of health, the degree of compliance (viz., with the parents' demands) may be so great and so at variance with the underlying true self as to yield an individual lacking in spontaneity.

At the other extreme (of emotional ill health) Winnicott mentions (33, p. 142) that the false self "sets itself up as real . . . but, in living relation-ships, the False Self begins to fail": the (presumably more acceptable) facade breaks down, and unacceptable or exaggerated tendencies (often in the direction of possessive control) assert themselves.

Applying these general remarks of Winnicott to patients in the border-line domain, Gallwey offers a number of theoretical refinements (8). In his type A personality, formed primarily in relation to early deprivation, one finds (1) a "deformed sense of identity" prone to collapse under stress, with ensuing loss of psychological containment; (2) a poverty of defenses against emotional turbulence; (3) a reduced capacity to manage separations, giv-ing rise to clinging, ambivalence, and violent jealousy; and (4) a continual sense of sensual starvation, along with a general depressive affect and primitive feelings of revenge (pp. 133–134). Some of the extreme measures that borderline persons of this sort resort to, by way of coping with these intolerable feelings, include possessiveness, "acting out" (including promis-cuity, sexual perversions), sensation seeking (including substance abuse), exploitativeness, and oscillations (within intimate relationships) between masochism and cruelty (p. 135). The false self in borderline patients of this type can, in Gallwey's experience, give rise either to an "openly disturbed personality or, when the deprivation is not too great and the defensive reaction well balanced, to a very convincing pseudo-normality" (p. 135). In the latter situation there might be too little in the way of overt symp-toms to trigger a DSM diagnosis of "borderline personality."

Gallwey's type B personalities consist of persons who "do have a coherent area of ego functioning in their own right" (and who therefore do not exhibit a false self in quite the way Winnicott spoke of it), but "who maintain it by operating a functional independence from more actively disturbed areas of their personality" (p. 140). Some of these type B persons maintain the split organization with a fair degree of success and personal fulfillment. But they are vulnerable to breakdown, in the form of either social collapse or social offending. Certain grandiose, secretive schizoid individuals can be understood as borderlines of this type, likewise certain schizoid criminals, especially those who present an innocuous face to the world, hold steady jobs and positions of respect in the community, but who become dominated episodically by the ordinarily disowned, dystonic secret self. These persons function as "dual personalities" of the Jekyll and Hyde type, and would be exemplified by a number of celebrated murderers, such as the Boston Strangler (7) and Dennis Nilsen, the serial killer/necrophile in England (16). Patients of this sort often appear better motivated for psychotherapy than they really are and, as Gallwey mentions (8, p. 143), often seduce their therapists into a sense of reassurance about how "well" the treatment is progressing. In the background of these type B "dual personalities" one is more likely to find childhood abuse rather than mere deprivation. The disowned, hidden self is walled in by shame — usually about incest, parental brutality, or shattering verbal humiliation. Cases of "multiple personality," though rare, are among the more flamboyant examples of this type of splitting; recently, we have become aware that a history of incest or brutalization is a universal feature of this condition (12).

What I mean by the inner script consists of the mental program elaborated over the years by which the individual hopes to realize the aims of the true self. These cherished hopes and recurrent fantasies help establish the patterns of discourse and behavior by which the person is known, but may also include fantasies whose implementation would be socially repugnant and which are (except during periods of breakdown) kept well under wraps. Someone who grew up poor, but with nurturing parents, may develop an inner script characterized by a relentless ambition to accumulate wealth, with the hope of making his own, and perhaps his parents', old age more comfortable. This is a rather adaptive, often realizable, and relatively unembarrassing script not requiring much concealment from one's fellows. The inner script of many of our borderline patients, in contrast, is dominated by motifs of revenge, total control of others, murder of rivals, and so forth. The more unrealistic the script, the more — once it becomes teased out and recognized during the course of therapy — it will need to be modified, and toned down or kept in check. An important goal of therapy will be to help the patient make compromises, acceptable to both self and society. The more malignant the script, the more difficult (sometimes impossible) the task. In this chapter, however, the focus is not so much on therapeutic considerations as on elucidation of some of the more typical "scripts" discernible in the lives of borderline patients. The following are some illustrative clinical vignettes.

Case A

Once I treated a graduate student in his midtwenties who came from a lower-middle-class family, of which he was the only member to attain this level of education. A borderline man with depressive symptoms and a rather impulsive life-style, he had grown up apart from his father (who was in the armed forces) until he was three. His mother resented being "stuck" with a baby whom she had to care for without the father's help; she often expressed the wish, in her not infrequent moments of anger, that he had never been born. By the time the father returned, the pattern of interaction changed, to the extent that the father humiliated the boy verbally — against which abuse the mother now protected him, to the point of becoming hovering and openly seductive. The patient had been consistently homosexual since his early teens.

Out of all this, and coupled with the growing realization that he was brighter than most of the people around him, an inner script took shape. According to this script, he was nearly as great as Christ, and he was destined to make great discoveries and work wonders that would rescue the fallen and restore the lame. There was little in his script of a typically Oedipal nature: he hoped to "cure" his mother (of her depression) and his sister (of her recklessness and drug abuse), but these aims were not sexualized. His inner script was primarily that of a savior — who, among other things, rescues women in distress, but does not marry one of them. Much of this grandiosity still burned within him, as he entered treatment in the midst of an unhappy love affair and in the midst of difficulty maintaining his academic standards. During the course of psychotherapy (which spanned some four years) his script became clear to both of us. Fortunately he had the motivation and personal wherewithal to achieve an acceptable compromise with his script: his "savior complex" (not a grotesque fantasy to begin with) served as the impetus to enter one of the "helping" professions, where he now works effectively, earning the respect of his colleagues.

Some borderlines, in contrast to the preceding, base their lives (unwittingly) on an absurd and pathetic inner script, or else one whose actualization would bring distress and injury to others. By the time we as therapists see certain patients of this type, they have often been enmeshed in this script for years on end and are powerless to get out of it. Worse still, the endless energy they expend in trying to realize what is, unbeknown to them, a self-defeating plan for life has robbed them of the skills necessary to become an effective person in the real world. Misdirected single-mindedness is not easily reversed; there may be plenty of zeal, but none for tasks that would promote genuine growth and individuation. A borderline patient whose life has been quite literally a waste, up until the time his condition comes under the scrutiny of a therapist, can hardly acknowledge this sorry fact with any equanimity. Such acknowledgment would of course be devastating — until such time, later in treatment, when enough skills had been acquired and developed, at some vocation or hobby or social grace, to permit the patient, now looking back from a position of some accomplishment, to admit the barrenness that had once characterized his life.

Case B

A young woman had been hospitalized for a breakdown during her sophomore year at college. She had become increasingly depressed, promiscuous, and impulsive and had developed a number of somatic complaints, including globus hystericus. The depression itself followed on the heels of progressive difficulty making friends. She was snobbish, disdainful toward her classmates, and indifferent to the social conventions governing the keeping of appointments. A suicide gesture following a social rebuff had precipitated the hospital admission. Once in the hospital, her "script" became discernible rather quickly.

The only child of a wealthy couple who divorced when she was four, she had been raised by her mother. She had never seen her father again in the 16 years between his leaving and her hospitalization. He had remarried and had several children by his second wife. The patient grew up with the belief that her father was timid and had been frightened off by his imperious and unforgiving ex-wife, avoiding all contact not only with the latter but, regrettably for the patient, with his daughter as well — since he would have had to confront her mother in order to regain any contact with her. As she grew up, fantasies began to take shape and condense into a central script, whose main ingredients were (1) the wish to be reunited with her father and (2) an imaginary scene in which she, as a now famous ballerina, is greeted by her father, who rushes in backstage after her stunning performance and falls on his knees, begging her forgiveness for all the years of neglect. The script took on so consuming a character that it would be fair to say she was no longer guided by the script; the script had "become" her. There *was* no self apart from it, in the sense that she eschewed all activities and developed no abiding interests except those related to her fantasies.

This patient, who was intensely narcissistic and rejecting of help, frittered away precious years attempting to pursue a career for which she had no skill (her script "demanded" it), such that, at 22, she had to begin her life over — educating herself in subjects she detested in order to support herself by work for which she had no enthusiasm. I was never able to get this patient to go through the steps necessary to achieve an autonomous, if less glittering, life than the one to which she aspired. In comparison to the graduate student of the previous example, she was more grandiose and less disciplined. She broke off treatment after two years, moved to a different city, and found a temporary job helping with decorations in a department store.

Regarding that facet of her script that governed her romantic relationships, the theme of paternal rejection was played out repeatedly in her (1) choosing men who treated her shabbily and then "dumped" her and (2) rejecting out of hand any men from her own background, who were conventional, stable, and kind. This pattern continued until her late thirties, when her father's second wife died. He now sought out his daughter for solace and the two were reunited, after a lapse of 30 years. By now she had largely overcome her need to "punish" him for his neglect. She also was able to accept a compromise with respect to her grandiose "ballerina" fantasy: she was content to open a salon for interior decorating, became successful, and married a suitable partner.

Case C

A 20-year-old woman was readmitted to hospital because of repeated acts of superficial wrist cutting and a recent overdose of antidepressant medication. Her first breakdown occurred shortly before she was to leave home for the first time to enter college and was also precipitated by self-mutilation (with bits of broken glass). She was raised in an emotionally aloof family environment. There was no history of abusiveness or of molestation. Her father, mildly alcoholic, had a depressive episode during her adolescence. She felt particularly "abandoned" at this time because of his remoteness and preoccupation with his own worries. Since that time she herself had become preoccupied with wishes to "be a baby": " . . . if I had my way, I'd be totally self-indulgent," she told her therapist. These wishes evoked considerable self-condemnation ("if I allowed myself to have all these needs granted, they'd call me crazy and put me on a back ward. Yet they're just normal baby needs"). During an exercise in dance group (emphasizing "self-expression") while in hospital, instead of dancing she crawled on the floor and sucked her thumb to demonstrate her being a "baby."

This patient was consciously in touch with her inner script and had some awareness that, much as she condemned it as infantile, the craving for motherly attentiveness was in itself neither eccentric nor socially repugnant.

One's inner script, as can be seen from these examples, reflects one's central dynamics, and represents the child's dream for some magical resolution of the key conflicts preserved, in somewhat modified form, into adult life.

The scripts of these patients, however unrealistic and unrealizable in their original form, were relatively benign. They were impossible only in practical terms, but not impossible logically. It is possible, at least in the abstract, for someone to become a well-known dancer and to have a dramatic reconciliation with one's father. Scripts such as these need to be pared down in the course of treatment, but a therapist would not feel constrained to encourage the abandonment of the script altogether. Many borderline patients, in contrast, have inner scripts that are inherently contradictory, and therefore logically impossible. A patient who bends all his energies to the attainment of the logically impossible is, of course, licked before he starts. In this situation the therapist has the task not only of attenuation — of helping the patient move from the grandiose to the life-sized — but also of persuading the patient to sacrifice his most cherished self-image and dream for a quite different dream that is of no interest to him.

Case D. An "Impossible" Script

Some years ago I worked with a borderline, dysthymic woman in her late thirties who exemplified the situation of the impossible script. A lonely and rather eccentric woman born to a schizophrenic mother, she grew up on a mammoth estate, cut off from the society of ordinary people until well into her teens. Hers was a life of "splendid isolation," shared only with her three siblings (one of whom was schizophrenic) and the household servants. Her mother was often in the hospital for long stretches; her father left the family when the patient was 12. Having completed some college, she "bummed around the world" for about 10 years, finally settling into a bohemian neighborhood in a large city, where she worked at an uninspiring job, supplementing her income with family money. She longed, as it emerged in therapy, for a close, symbiotic relationship with a homosexual man. Homosexual men, in her opinion, were more tender, more artistic and sensitive than the usual run of heterosexual men. From analysis of her dreams, it became apparent, as might be anticipated, that such a man would represent the actualization of a deep wish for union with the primal mother—a wish rendered the more poignant by virtue of the emotional unavailability of her real mother, either during the patient's infancy or at any other time.

The patient actually fell in love with a homosexual man, of considerable artistic achievements, who lived a few doors away. Every day she wasted hours to catch a glimpse of him and felt "on air" if he said good morning or if he thanked her perfunctorily for the cookies she baked and deposited with a note by his door two or three times a week. The man had been living there with his homosexual partner for some 15 years and gave not the slightest evidence of interest in a neighborly friendship, let alone any romantic involvement, with my patient. In effect, her "script" was logically impossible. She "wanted" a sexual relationship with a man—but only with a man guaranteed not to reciprocate her feelings. It was very difficult to get her to look at the nature of her script and at its built-in inconsistency, since this put me in the position of treading on what was, for her, sacred soil. Either alternative—to live without male companionship or to grow comfortable with a conventional heterosexual relationship—would have spared her the continual immersion in a fantasy world, where she repeatedly suffered humiliation and rejection. Eventually she adopted the first of these solutions and departed from the hopeless script, but some five years of twice-weekly therapy were required to effect this change.

Case E. An Impossible Script, Incompatible with Life

A 27-year-old single man was admitted to hospital because of alcohol abuse and a serious suicide attempt. Once on the inpatient psychotherapy unit he "sealed over," exhibiting denial of underlying despair and emptiness. In personality he was noted to be narcissistic, with particularly strong feelings of grandiosity and entitlement. He had done little with his life after graduating from college, subsisting on a (generous) allowance from his wealthy parents. His father was a self-made millionaire; his mother was from "old wealth" and came from a prestigious family. The patient was chronically beset by feelings of inadequacy, specifically that he could never measure up to the achievements of his father or maternal grandfather. His father tended to soft-pedal these issues, whereas his mother made it clear she expected him to be "great." (At *what*, was never spelled out.) The patient developed a two-layered inner script: the superficial aspect compelled him to achieve preeminence at something, and to feel humiliated if he failed. The deeper aspect, in rebellion against this program, compelled him to seek revenge against those responsible for saddling him with this burden in the first place. Mother was the chief author of the superficial script and the chief target of the hidden layer.

While in hospital, shortly after one of his mother's infrequent visits, he made a near-fatal suicide attempt. He experienced the episode as reflecting his sense of failure and shame. Evidence soon surfaced that the more important dynamic element was revenge. His suicide, alone, could humble mother and her lofty aspirations; it constituted the perfect mechanism for "killing" the (as he saw her) giant who tried to crush him. A Sampson-like script of this sort might have succeeded in ruining his mother's life—but at the certain cost of his own life. The revenge motif figures in the inner script of many suicidal borderline patients. Such patients, of course, remain at risk until they are enabled, through psychotherapy (if the latter is successful), to give up this motif for a script (i.e., a life program) that does not demand the sacrifice of the patient.

The preceding scripts took shape in relation to family environments predisposing, via deprivation, primarily to type A personalities.

Still more self-defeating scripts are found among borderline patients, in cases where contradictory values—themselves stemming from persistent splits in good and bad images of key figures in their lives—determine an intense and exquisitely balanced ambivalence in object relations (especially, vis-à-vis the love partner). In this situation the ultimate destruction of all love relationships is guaranteed.

Many women who have been incest victims (and their number is strikingly high in samples of borderline patients) have extremely polarized love-hate attitudes toward men, particularly if the sexual abuse involved the father.

Case F

A 32-year-old woman was referred for psychotherapy following a suicide gesture that had occurred in the context of a deteriorating marriage. She had had sexual relations with her father for 10 years up through her late adolescence. She had become inordinately dependent on the love and attention of men and, at the same time, murderously vengeful toward them. Hers was what one might call the "Salome" script—since it called for seducing, via her unusual attractiveness, a man whom she would then set about destroying via provocations and public humiliation. Perhaps a more appropriate appellation for the governing motif of her life would be the "Carmen" script, inasmuch as the guilt she felt in connection with the incest was as keen as the vengefulness. The guilt, in turn, inclined her toward the kind of provocativeness (threatening to "screw the first guy I meet in a bar" as a "retaliation" for some minor "failing" on the part of a man who was deeply attached to her) that sometimes triggered physical assault and murderous threats from her lovers.

This patient was in effect programmed to pass sequentially from a positive "scene" to a negative "scene," and back again: lovemaking led to enjoyment but also (1) guilt and (2) fear of abandonment ("men are all unfaithful cads who manipulate and take advantage"); these, in turn, led to retaliation of a sort that would hurt both the man and herself; this constituted expiation and revenge at the same stroke, thus entitling her to another round of lovemaking and enjoyment. It goes without saying that a script of this sort—and it is a common one in borderlines—is *logically*— not merely *practically*—impossible: one can retain the affection perhaps, but not the devotion of a man one tries to ruin. Thus, the patient must either give up (the acting out of) vengefulness or give up men. As a further complication, such women tend not to choose stable men (who would tire, after a while, of the repetitive scenes) but, rather, choose men who are jealous and volatile (as these patients' fathers often were and as they themselves have become). In the unfolding of the life drama of these women, there is often a tragic final act: every Don José has his limit.

Case G. Encapsulation of Aggressive Impulses in a Borderline Schizoid Psychopath

An architect in his late twenties was referred for consultation because of having strangled his wife nearly to death the week before.

He had grown up in an affluent home, the younger of two children born to a successful merchant. The family was respected in the community and appeared outwardly harmonious. The marital relationship was stormy; the atmosphere within the four walls of the house was in striking contrast to the impressions of the neighbors. The father was irascible and often violent, arguing with his wife over trivia, badgering his son to "be a man," to excel at sports (at which he was graceless and inept), and to get better grades. Only the patient's older sister escaped the father's wrath — which engendered murderous envy on the part of the patient. Once when the father dressed him down for using illicit drugs, the patient (then 14) kicked the father in the groin and got beaten severely as a punishment. After this, he kept mostly to himself; he had no close friends.

At university, the patient was preoccupied with fantasies of strangling or shooting anyone who had "wronged" him. He purchased a gun with which to kill his roommate for having made an ethnic slur, but held himself back only because the opportunity never presented itself to "do it and get away with it." In romantic relationships he quickly became pathologically jealous, which eventually drove away any woman he courted. When he was 22 he became engaged, but six months later his fiancée left him for another man, whereupon he let himself in her apartment and strangled her cat. Engaged again four years later and apprenticed to an architect firm, he grew violently angry at his new fiancée during an argument about his sexual performance, whereupon he tried to drown *her* cat in the bathroom sink. A few months after their marriage he accused her of breaking an "oath" she had made to him on their wedding day: her only "offense," actually, was to have passed an examination that elevated her professionally to a status similar to his own. It was on this occasion that he choked her to the point of losing consciousness. Upon recovery, she complained to his family, who now urged psychiatric consultation.

He showed no remorse for, nor any insight into, any of his violent actions, which seemed inexplicable to him, as if "something came over me." To his co-workers he appeared bright and capable, but aloof, abrasive, and hypercritical.

Comment. This patient demonstrates the classic split or "dual" personality (Jekyll and Hyde), often mistakenly considered schizophrenic. The *schiz-* of the latter term refers, of course, only to the split between intellect and affect in schizophrenic persons, not to the compartmentalization of certain disowned affective states (rage or lust, usually) within separate, dissociated "personalities" that switch on and off in relation to internal or external pressures. The schizoid psychopath such as the patient in the vignette exemplifies Gallwey's type B borderline. The disowned and dystonic "beta-self" seems so foreign to the main (alpha) self in such borderlines that premature and overforceful interpretive efforts on the part of a therapist may have disruptive, even shattering, effects rather than an integrative effect. Where antisocial features are particularly prominent, as in the case above, treatment is usually futile. The well-documented case of the Chicago serial killer John Gacy, also considered a borderline schizoid psychopath, illustrates this phenomenon (4).

In the above vignette, the disowned feelings were mostly aggressive, though aggressive outbreaks could be triggered not only by external threats of bodily harm, but also by actions on the part of women that had the effect of calling into question the patient's manliness. He did not appear to struggle against unacceptable homosexual fantasies. In John Gacy, the latter were present and were kept under lock in the "beta-system": murderous aggression could be unleashed both by threats of harm and by young men who awakened the disowned homoerotic feelings. The splitting, projective identification and denial that characterize the defensive posture in borderlines of this type are mobilized usually by a simultaneous love and hatred for the same parent — who in many instances engenders far more hatred than the average parent. This was certainly true of the patient above and of John Gacy (both of whose fathers had been habitually cruel). One must keep in mind, however, that similar defenses and a similar type of borderline-level "dual personality" may occur for largely constitutional reasons (as in the case of Nancy Spungen [25]) or deprivational reasons (Dennis Nilsen: the death of his grandfather).

In admittedly oversimplified language, we may view Gallwey's type A and B borderlines as reactions to "sins of omission" versus "sins of commission." The balance between these factors affects amenability to psychotherapy. There is less shame attached to being deprived than to being a participant in secret and socially unacceptable sexual acts. Even if one were purely an unwilling participant, one may grow up feeling like a pariah, with envy and hatred toward the larger world of persons not victimized in this manner. In cases where an incestuous relationship has been prolonged over years and not merely episodic or a solitary occurrence, an evenly divided ambivalence is the more customary reaction. Righteous indignation is counterbalanced by excitement, adoration, and intense shame at having enjoyed what society regards as sinful. It is this kind of background that especially conduces to the formation of a compartmentalized secret self that makes little or no contact with the main, socially acceptable facade ("false") self. In dealing with borderlines of this sort, the clinician encounters a wall of denial or repudiation that may be insurmountable.

Parental brutalization will predispose even more powerfully to the formation of a split self into evil and good components: chronic and unprovoked violence stimulates revenge fantasies so strong as to lead, in some instances, to parenticide; in others, to murder of strangers who, in the eyes of the perpetrator, symbolize the offending parent. An example of chronic abuse (on the part of outwardly respectable parents) culminating in parenticide is to be found in the account of the Dresbach case by Mewshaw (18). Probably the majority of the type B schizoid-psychopathic borderlines have experienced brutalization or molestation at the hands of primary caretakers; the dystonic and socially unacceptable aspect of those "split" personalities are often mobilized into action through the use of alcohol. Borderline persons of this sort may resort to alcohol specifically because of its disinhibiting affects, in order to catalyze (and also to justify) the emergency of the disavowed self. By "justify" I refer, of course, to the tendency of such persons to disclaim ownership of the resulting behavior: "It wasn't really me that did that — I was under the influence . . . ," as though that somehow excuses the antisocial behavior. This dynamism brings up the subject of *willed dyscontrol*, which I feel is sufficiently important to the understanding of borderline "dynamics" to warrant discussion under a separate heading. From the standpoint of therapy, meantime, it is easier to deal with patients who have been short-changed than with those who have been egregiously misused or hurt, since in the latter the developing inner script will be constructed around *revenge*. The true self will strive not after a second helping (which does not hurt anyone), but rather murder. The borderline adult who has been beaten repeatedly as a child does not readily walk away from his preoccupation with revenge/murder even while aware of the unacceptability of acting out these motifs. Hence these dynamics tend to remain hidden, denied, and encapsulated within the "beta-system" (the set of unacknowledged splitoff parts of the total self, as Gallwey refers to it).

THE WILL TO BE OUT OF CONTROL

In a trenchant observation regarding criminal psychopaths, Wilson and Herrnstein (31) spoke of their demonstrating again and again the *will* to be out of control. There are many ways this can be demonstrated. The paranoid "macho man" who hangs out in bars, especially those located in whatever part of town his type of people are not accepted, has already elected to place himself in an environment where sharp disagreements and provocations are highly likely to occur. Add a few shots of whiskey into the mix, radically weakening impulse control, and it is no longer surprising that a few shots of a different kind may soon be exchanged.

This mechanism, quite obvious in the careers of many antisocial persons, operates with great frequency in the lives of many borderline patients as well — sometimes more subtly, sometimes not. One even has the impression that there is something about this *willed dyscontrol* that is of the very essence of what we wish to convey when we call someone borderline, absent which, we tend to apply other labels altogether. Perry and Klerman (21) in their comparative essay on different borderline diagnostic systems mentioned (accurately) that only the item *impulsivity* was included across the board in all systems. This points to the same phenomenon I have characterized as willed dyscontrol, though impulsivity is a more neutral word, lacking any reference to any conscious decision to let all hell break loose.

The motives for willed dyscontrol are not the same for all borderlines; rather, the mechanism appears as an "overdetermined" path, paved partly by constitutional factors (in some patients), partly by sociocultural factors, and partly as an outgrowth of adverse patterns of interactions with key persons (usually family members) in one's early environment.

A constitutional push in the direction of dyscontrol may come in the form of increased genetic vulnerability to manic-depression, specifically, to the bipolar II or bipolar I form. Or it may come in the form of organic impairment (including grand, and petit mal, and temporal lobe epilepsies), the latter contributing to a lowering of frustration tolerance.

A common sociocultural factor is substance abuse on the part of the parents: there tends to be more alcoholism in children of alcoholics (especially among the sons) than in children of parents who drink in moderation. Something similar may be so in connection with marijuana abuse.

Many borderline patients spend their whole lives consumed with vengeful fantasies, trying endlessly to "get even," with the result that they neither get even nor get anything out of the intimate relationships they disrupt in the process.

Some borderline patients deal with an intolerable past by getting into endless crises — the latter amounting to a running defense against the pain of dealing with the noxious interactions of the early environment. In therapy, one sees continual acting-out — as a way of sidestepping the task of exploring, and coming to terms with, the painful areas. Partly this is to avoid the pain; partly, to keep it perpetually "alive" (unconsciously) — since certain painful patterns may constitute all the borderline person knows and can adjust to. These patterns become precious in this paradoxical way and are not lightly sacrificed in favor of more adaptive, less stormy modes of interacting with others. This paradox is reflected in the popular epigram, "better the devils you know than the devils you don't know."

One borderline woman in her late twenties came from a background where the parents argued continually, their strife culminating in the father's killing the mother with a shotgun in full view of the daughter (then 13). The patient was never able to come to terms with this tragedy. Instead she led a chaotic life, abusing marijuana and other drugs, drinking to excess, taking up with violent men who treated her (at best) shabbily, coming to her sessions sporadically, and comporting herself at every job in such a way as to get fired with some regularity. Her nomadism and maltreatment of her body were painful enough, it is true, but considerably less so than it would have been (in her own psychic economy) to look squarely at what may have taken place between father and mother.

The "scenes" created by borderline patients often appear as the extensions into adult life of childhood tantrums, and it is no surprise that repetitive tantrums played a large role in the early lives of many borderline patients, according to their own report as well as the recollections of their parents. By no means is it their only function to serve as a resistance to exploration of conflict-laden areas; the "scene" often serves as a power maneuver for controlling the behavior of those who are important to the borderline person. In addition, and quite independent of these "important others," the scene may act as an escape valve for intolerable tension (especially in the Gallwey type B borderline). This function is particularly in evidence with borderline women premenstrually. Elsewhere I have expressed the view that, in comparison to women in general (some 4 to 7 percent of whom suffer severe premenstrual tension; cf. Ref. 19), borderline women have a much heightened incidence of the combined hostile and depressed feelings that make up this syndrome (28). Interrelated with these phenomena, the "scene," with its elements of provocativeness and willed dyscontrol, may reenact a highly important and ambivalently regarded event of childhood. Again, incestuous experiences often lead to this pattern, since a tabooed encounter of this sort, simultaneously exciting and infuriating, would tend to be acted out repeatedly later on — both as a way of reliving the intense pleasure and as a way of gaining mastery over a trauma: the child-victim turns aggressor and symbolically victimizes her original aggressor via a "scene" with spouse or lover.

The phenomenon under discussion here — willed dyscontrol — is related to another feature commonly present in persons eventually identified as borderline, namely intense *craving*. This craving is often discernible early in the lives of borderline patients and serves as a kind of prelude to the impulsivity, including the willed dyscontrol, that characterizes borderline conditions of any sort. We turn our attention to this craving in the following section.

CRAVING

Borderline patients whose symptoms lie mostly in an affective rather than in a cognitive direction are especially likely to exhibit intense craving; i.e., the phenomenon is more visible in the depressive or depressive/hypomanic than in the schizotypal subtypes. The further diagnostic distinctions that we make are themselves often a reflection of the favorite channel through which the craving is to be satisfied. A number of these are outlined in Figure 2. As suggested by this diagram, the factors contributing to this craving include constitution, deprivation, and abuse. In clinical practice every conceivable mixture and interaction between these factors are encountered. There is not a very close correspondence between the etiological factors and the eventual avenue of satisfaction. Hypersexuality and possessiveness, for example, can develop as sequelae either of the parental deprivation or of parental seduction/overstimulation. Revenge-dominated behavior, however, stems largely from abuse or molestation.

As a corollary to this theme of abnormal craving in borderlines, one may state that, in comparison to the normal/neurotic population, borderline persons almost invariably feel, and often genuinely were, *unloved* by at least one parent. Healthier persons, having received more consistent (and less conditional) love and having assimilated this fact, over time, into an internalized conviction of worthiness to receive another's love, are less frantic about finding a sexual partner. Once having found a suitable mate, the healthier person does not resort to drastic measures to bind that person's affection: there is no need for exerting the kind of total control one finds in the life story of the pathologically jealous person. Most persons who become "borderline," in contrast, have lived in a life-and-death atmosphere, worry incessantly about rejection and loss, and tend to choose partners not so much out of similarity of taste and values as out of a perception that the partner can be dominated. The goal is to ensure against abandonment. The more primitive aspects of intimacy are emphasized rather than the more mature aspects. Borderline persons, as a rule,

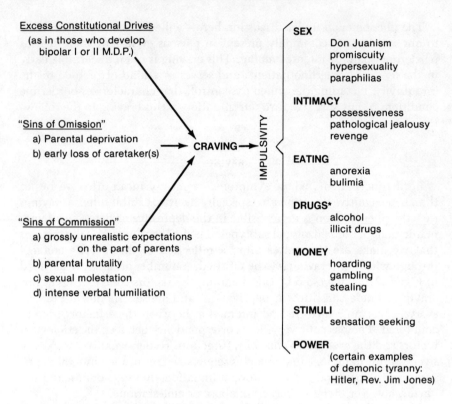

Figure 2. Factors contributing to craving.

will use sex more to "prove" being loved, to dominate, and to bind than to express tenderness and a joyful sense of connectedness to the beloved. Since no amount of affection can convince the borderline that he or she is genuinely lovable in a *permanent* (as opposed to transitory) way, the craving for demonstrations of "love" tends to be insatiable. Worse still, the borderline person often doubts the motives of a love partner, out of a conviction of unlovability. The love partner is forever regarded as suspect, along the lines of the famous quip of Groucho Marx: "Any club that'll have me can't be worth joining."

Borderlines are prone toward certain abnormalities in intimate relationships that are reminiscent of first love: it is normal, when a young person falls in love for the first time, to assume that no one else will do and that no other person in the whole world could replace the beloved. The language of everyday life with which we attempt to capture these emotions itself reflects the at times disturbing proximity of being-in-love to madness. Thus, lovers are "crazy" for one another (or "mad" about one another); they pine for one another, waste away with grief after a rejection or loss, and so forth. A possessive lover, if jilted, grows "insane" with jealousy and may be moved to murder the abandoning partner or (as in the situation exemplified by Eugene Onegin and Lensky) to fight to the death with the person who has "stolen" the heart of the unfaithful partner. There is not always a sharp line of demarcation between the normal/neurotic and the borderline in this realm, though in actual practice we make reasonable distinctions, based on the age of the participants, the intensity of the emotions, and the frequency with which someone becomes involved with the kind of hopeless passion I have been alluding to.

Many people have experienced a "hopeless infatuation" at least once. The story of La Traviata serves well as an archetype: Alfredo Germont falls hopelessly in love with the beautiful courtesan, Violetta — but the affair is crushed by the elder Germont, for whom such a match would be intolerable. Alfredo is not portrayed in pathological terms as though he were "borderline" (Verdi, in any case, does not provide us with a follow-up). But those who remain mired throughout most of their lives in a love relationship guaranteed not to flourish often exhibit the other attributes of borderline personality organization as well. The "hopelessness" of these relationships centers, psychodynamically, around the forbidden incestuous object; it is an absolute *precondition* (unknown to the lover) that the beloved be unavailable, for one reason or another, or else this person would not have awakened such passionate feelings to begin with. Alfredo laments that "if only" Violetta did not have a "past," everything would have worked out, whereas had Violetta been the girl next door, he would not have fallen in love with her. To be sure, one sees this mechanism in certain neurotic patients. But in borderline patients hopeless love of this sort is often a recurring feature; the accompanying emotions are so intense as to provoke all manner of inappropriate and impulsive behavior. Since this form of craving has been described with special verisimilitude and beauty by Cervantes, we might call it "quixotic love."

Though many forms of craving involve food, drink, and drugs, those mediated by sex or by "anal" dynamisms (hoarding, stealing) still subserve very primitive needs in borderline patients. It is thus simplistic and not altogether correct to characterize them as "oral," even in the case of bulimia. Craving relates to fundamental issues of security and survival. The persons or objects craved are symbolically connected to nurturing mother with her small infant (for whom she supplies the basic needs of being soothed and fed). The infatuation or adoration we note in the attitude of the borderline adult toward a love object is (usually) an amalgam of genuine Oedipal longings superimposed on more primitive longings related to the basic (and "pre-Oedipal") mother-child symbiosis. The latter is generally the predominant, if initially hidden, element in borderline love; the Oedipal aspects, merely a thin patina.

A DOUBLE DYNAMIC UNDERLYING STORMY RELATIONSHIPS IN BORDERLINE PERSONS

Having examined some of the common inner scripts that program the lives of borderline patients, and having highlighted their tendency toward willed dyscontrol and intense cravings, we are in a better position to understand some of the dynamics underlying the cyclical upheavals that characterize their intimate life. These upheavals are especially noticeable in the lives of mood-disordered borderlines; they are less visible among schizotypal (borderline schizophrenic) patients, many of whom avoid closeness altogether.

Borderline patients often find themselves trapped between the mutually contradictory feeling states of love and mistrust. Both are experienced in the exaggerated manner typical of their highly polarized emotions. The love is characterized by adoration and desperate clinging (so as to avoid loneliness). The mistrust may come in the form of pathological jealousy or intense fear of rejection. As a relationship progresses from first encounter to sexual intimacy, the borderline person is required to trust the partner (if the relationship is to flourish) — yet cannot. Burnham (3) spoke of similar situations as exemplifying a "need-fear" dilemma. Borderlines programmed to mistrust (i.e., those who have been victims of physical abuse or sexual molestation) often deal with this dilemma in a cyclical fashion. The key elements of the cycle are outlined in Figure 3. In this diagram *intimacy* and *mistrust* are represented as two orthogonal variables. In order to appreciate the applicability of the diagram to the borderline's "stormy" relationships, it will be useful for the reader to walk with me through one such cycle. The patient in clinical vignette F, above, provides a dramatic example:

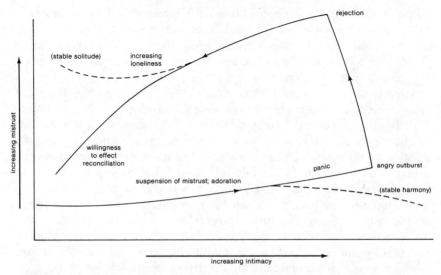

Figure 3. Cyclical on-again/off-again pattern of stormy relationships in certain borderline persons.

This woman (whom we shall call B) met a man (M) following the breakup of her marriage. Though predisposed to mistrust men (she had been an incest victim and saw her mother betrayed by her father; she expected all wives to be betrayed by their husbands; only lovers could— temporarily—be trusted), she nevertheless suspended this mistrust in the first flush of romantic infatuation. Here she was propelled by intense lone-liness and craving for attachment. The cycle begins, therefore, as at the lower left of the diagram, with consciously recognized mistrust at the minimum and intimacy minimal initially, but rapidly increasing. She soon reached a point of maximal dependency and intimacy. The conviction that her very survival depends on the trustworthiness of the lover activates the hitherto suppressed mistrust. High dependency coupled with high mistrust cannot coexist and form an explosive mixture. She becomes panicky, casti-gates M for some tiny fault (forgetting to buy the right brand of cigarettes) or for an imagined "wrong" (she "catches" M "looking at another woman," when actually he was not), and creates an angry "scene." The angry out-burst has the effect of rapidly decreasing the level of intimacy: the cycle moves up (toward maximal mistrust) and to the left. B rejects M through her accusations; M now leaves. At first B experiences feelings of "good riddance." A few days go by, however, and loneliness mounts. As loneliness, in its intensity, begins to surpass the level of mistrust, B enters a new region of *catastrophic* (as opposed to gradual) change: she is now, as loneliness awakens fears for her survival, eager for *reconciliation*. Mistrust is abrogated (suppressed, actually, and rendered temporarily unconscious). B pleads with M to come back. The two are reunited, each full of hope that "this time it will be different." The cycle begins anew.

A reconciliation that follows an argument, it should be mentioned, is greater proof of still being loved than mere steadfastness in a calm relationship. Borderline persons have a damaged self-image and have inordinate fear of rejection. To mistreat a lover and *still* be loved is a potent tonic for a flagging self-esteem — therefore, the paradoxical quality of the on-and-off nature of the borderline's intimate relations. What is destabilizing for an ordinary person is stabilizing (although imperfectly so) for the borderline: the periodic reconciliations provide the necessary reassurance to perpetuate the (admittedly fragile and stormy) relationship. Another term sometimes used to characterize this type of relationship is "sadomasochistic." The main point is that while the relationship may end abruptly at any moment, it may, if the emotions are titrated carefully, last for years.

In the case of the borderline patient in case F the cycle would last, at most, one month. Premenstrual tension was so severe, and was accompanied by such irritability, that a state of comfortable intimacy could never extend through and beyond the period. This meant that in the course of a year, the cycle of adoration-panic-rage outburst-rejection-loneliness-reconciliation would repeat itself at least a dozen, perhaps nearly 20, times. This kind of cycle will often become discernible to the clinician working with a borderline patient whose relationships have the stormy or tumultuous quality depicted here.

From the standpoint of therapy, there are only two ways out of this disastrous cycle. If the patient can understand and work through the problems connected with trust, it may be possible to find a love partner whose trustworthiness (1) is valid and (2) can be recognized. This permits a life of stable harmony and is represented in Figure 2 by a point on the lower right: high intimacy times minimal mistrust. The other solution is reserved for patients who prove, over time, to be incapable of trusting a love partner. These patients need to be taught, if possible, to maximize pleasures of a more "narcissistic" sort, which do not depend on intimacy with another person. Some patients of this sort are able to derive enough enjoyment from casual acquaintances, travel, hobbies, reading, and so forth to live in stable solitude (upper left portion of the diagram). This is the solution to which many borderline schizophrenics gravitate, but one also sees in practice a number of mood-labile borderlines (including some whose early life was particularly traumatic) who need to be guided in this direction.

SEPARATION-INDIVIDUATION

Many who write on the dynamics of borderline conditions have emphasized the issue of separation and individuation. The work of Margaret Mahler (15) has been seminal in this regard. Important contributions were made earlier by Jacobson, and later in the syntheses elaborated by Kernberg (11). Greenacre (9) spoke of "focal symbiosis"—an intensely strong symbiosis between mother and child—as relevant to the psychopathology of the perversions and the borderline states. A number of authors have assumed that traumata in the separation-individuation phases outlined by Mahler underlie borderline psychopathology as it becomes manifest in late adolescence/early adulthood (17, 23). The latter have tended to underplay the importance of constitution as well as the role of other dynamics that might figure in the etiology of borderline conditions, such as those adumbrated in this chapter. In Masterson's view (17), the mothers of borderline patients have themselves often been borderline (p. 132). Now it is true that some mothers of children who later become borderline do react sharply to signs of independent thought and action, as Masterson suggests. Such children must either keep in line with mother's wishes (at the expense of self-fulfillment) or else oppose mother (at the risk of her abandoning them emotionally and at the risk of future depression). This theory is valid, in my opinion, only in a fraction of the cases (the fraction will vary from series to series). Furthermore, the theory is handicapped by the linearity of its construction: it presupposes a developmental path carved out along the original Freudian lines, from oral to anal to genital, and tries to situate the diagnostic entities we encounter in adult patients as stemming from traumata that create fixation points somewhere along that straight-line path. This theory, seductive in its simplicity, has led certain analytical writers into temptation. I refer to the temptation to assume causation where there is merely correlation or coexistence.

I find no convincing data to support the contention that even two out of three (let alone "all") mothers of future borderlines thwarted their children's efforts to effect a proper emotional separation. Among hospitalized female borderlines, for example, a history of incest or early sexual molestation is present in more than half the patients (8 of 14 in a series I recently evaluated in Brisbane, Australia; 60 percent of a larger series at New York Hospital/Westchester Division). In the remainder, and among the males, physical abuse or verbal humiliation (usually by the father) — or else early loss of either parent through death, abandonment, or divorce — was present in all but a few cases. These factors, which often involve "bad fathering," may well weigh heavier in the balance than "bad mothering." Finally, even when serious problems in separation/individuation do dominate the psychodynamic picture, the clinician must still assess the contributions of nature and nurture. There are indeed cases where maternal mishandling was so egregious as to acquire causative significance. But there are others where constitutional factors either overshadowed the mother's shortcomings or else overwhelmed the best efforts of a mother who Winnicott himself would have agreed was "good enough." There are children, in other words, constitutionally damaged in such a way as to be unable to tolerate the briefest and most benign separations to which two- and three-year-olds are routinely subjected by empathic and well-intentioned parents. The Spungen case alluded to above is a poignant example.

When nature and nurture elements are both highly unfavorable, the situation is of course not informative as to the importance of either component. The pathogenic quality of certain adverse "natures" shines through in those instances where the family environment has been, as best we can reconstruct, nurturing and well-attuned to the unique characteristics of the child. In my experience it is among children who have constitutional predisposition to bipolar illness that we find borderline conditions developing even in the absence of adverse family factors. (Perhaps one should say: absence of any readily discernible environmental factors — since in judging the family environment we are always at the mercy of recollections and impressions from the distant past.) Furthermore, these future bipolar or manic/irritable children tend, because of their extreme drivenness and demandingness, to set the calmest mother on edge — so that she, too, is reduced to the kind of crankiness, impatience, and stridor that characterize her "temperamental" offspring. The adult borderline patient, reflecting back on these early memories, may experience a "good-enough" mother (as she is indeed remembered by the healthier siblings) as a witch. This seemed to be the case in the following example:

Case H

A 36-year-old woman was referred for psychotherapy because of bulimia.

She had worked only sporadically after graduation from college, had never married, and, in recent years, had rarely gone out with men. Anorectic during her late teen years, she was chiefly bulimic since her twenties, maintaining normal weight through vomiting or periods of fasting. She was vain, hypercritical, and haughty; as a result, she had no close friends of either sex. She lived by herself, but tolerated being alone poorly and abused alcohol (mildly) to contain her anxiety. Her parents had provided her with a large trust fund for her support. Temperamentally, she oscillated between hypomania and dysthymia. She spoke too loudly and with a great pressure most of the time. She was also hypochondriacal and would check herself into various medical centers in distant cities, in hopes that a famous specialist could diagnose her ailments. Her irritability was such that she would phone her mother (who lived in a different part of the country) at all hours, to whom she would pour out her complaints. Often she pleaded with her mother to cancel other plans and pay her daughter a visit. If the mother was unable to do so, the patient became vituperative on the phone, would smash down the receiver — only to call the mother back half an hour later, apologizing tearfully for yelling at her.

The patient had a brother and a sister, both of whom were even-tempered as children and highly successful as adults. Their memories of their mother were quite at variance with the patient's: they remembered her as kindly, emotionally warm, and nurturing (to all her three children) — though worn thin by their sister, who created tension wherever she went. When the patient was out of the house, the other four got on comfortably. The neighborhood children rejected her — a tendency her father went to great lengths to combat, accompanying her to the playground and urging the other children to include his daughter in their games. Despite all these attentions, mother was usually, in the patient's recollection, an "uncaring bitch"; father, a "self-centered tyrant."

In the patient's immediate family there were no psychiatric disorders; among her aunts and uncles, there were several manic-depressives. In the absence of any evidence of abuse, gross parental mishandling, neglect, etc., it seems more reasonable to assign the larger share of her borderline psychopathology to constitutional factors (predisposition to manic-depression) rather than to environmental factors. Likewise, her failure to negotiate adequately the steps of separation and individuation seems more a reflection of innate handicap than of insensitive rearing: the minor frustrations her siblings tolerated with ease threw her into panic.

CONCLUDING REMARKS

Given the heterogeneity of borderline conditions and the large literature devoted to them, to summarize their dynamics is at best difficult (and at worst, presumptuous). To begin with, various combinations of constitutional disadvantage, of deprivation, overstimulation, or abuse conduce to establish a pattern of inordinate craving. Usually this is accompanied by irritability. Not all the aforementioned inciting factors need be present in any given case. Abuse, for example, may by itself emerge as a sufficient cause; so may an irritable temperament.

The craving is similar to what Rado wrote about under the rubric of "pharmacothymia," but may manifest itself in any number of ways — not merely as a dependency on drugs. The craving, no matter what means are employed to satisfy it (food, sex), stems from anxieties about basic security and acceptance (will I survive? am I loved at all?) rather than from the milder anxieties encountered among neurotic persons (viz., am I loved as much as the others in my family?).

One has the sense that something has "gone wrong" early in development — earlier than those phases we are disposed to call Oedipal — hence the many references by the earlier analytical writers (most notably, those of the British Object Relations School) to disturbances in the pre-Oedipal periods (of infancy and the toddler phase). The contributions of Melanie Klein, Fairbairn, and Guntrip concerning the "depressive" and "schizoid" positions in the first few months of life are a reflection of this concern to discover the trouble spot(s) in borderline development. Others have drawn attention to the separation/individuation phase as the band along the developmental continuum where this trouble occurred. As we have noted, these theoretical speculations are simplistic: a purely linear model assigning diagnostic entities to a particular phase of early development ignores the multiplicity of interacting pre- and postnatal factors that one must take into consideration. Nor is mother always the culprit. Sometimes it is father; sometimes Nature. One can thus speak of typical patterns in the psychodynamics of borderlines, but not of one uniform and ever-present pattern.

The borderline patient's *own* experience of something having gone (seriously) wrong is captured in Balint's concept (2) of the basic fault. Balint's *ocnophilic* and *philobatic* subtypes correspond closely to the depressive (clinging) and schizoid (going one's own way) positions — as these would manifest themselves later in the life course.

The *observer's* experience of the borderline personality deformations stemming from the above-mentioned factors is captured in Winnicott's concept of the false self, recently compartmentalized into the subtypes outlined by Gallwey.

The *symptoms* that accompany some borderline conditions some of the time (but not all borderline conditions all of the time) are what make up the bulk of the characteristics of the DSM-III definitions of borderline and (borderline schizophrenic) schizotypal personality disorders. The DSM definitions do justice neither to the admixture of traits and symptoms found in typical broadly defined borderline conditions nor to the descriptive foundation that these definitions supposedly reflect.

The Kernberg definition, because of its breadth, does not refer to any simple set of dynamic underpinnings. In addition, Kernberg acknowledges the role of "innate aggression" in (many) borderline states — a concept that overlaps considerably with my emphasis on constitutional irritability, especially in borderlines of the affective (especially bipolar) type. The subtypes sketched by Kernberg (depressive/masochistic, infantile, narcissistic, etc.) tend to show common psychodynamics, but even here one cannot claim a homogeneous pattern for each subtype.

Finally, unique to each borderline — indeed, to each human being — is a personal set of psychodynamics: the inner script. In working with borderline patients over many years one begins to discern a number of scripts typical of this population. Often these scripts represent dramatic and exaggerated versions of dynamics relevant to the normal population. In other instances one finds borderlines who have been burdened by experiences almost unknown to people in everyday life. In the early backgrounds of borderline persons there is an overabundance of loss, abuse, unrealistic expectation, jealousy, scandal, embarrassing secrets, and the like. In the adult lives of our borderline patients these themes are reenacted, often enough with the tables turned: yesterday's victim becoming today's aggressor.

REFERENCES

1. AKISKAL, H. (1981). Subaffective disorders: Dysthymic, cyclothymic and bipolar II disorders in the "borderline" realm. In M. H. Stone (Ed.), *Borderline disorders*. Philadelphia: W. B. Saunders. *Psychiatric Clinics of North America*, 4(1), 25–46.
2. BALINT, M. (1968). *The basic fault*. New York: Brunner/Mazel.
3. BURNHAM, D. L. (1969). *Schizophrenia and the need-fear dilemma*. New York: International Universities Press.
4. CAHILL, T. (1986). *Buried dreams*. New York: Bantam Books.
5. DEUTSCH, H. (1942). Some forms of emotional disturbance and their relationships to schizophrenia. *Psychoanalytic Quarterly*, 11, 301–321.
6. *Diagnostic and Statistical Manual of Mental Disorders* (Third edition) (DSM-III) (1980). Washington, D.C.: American Psychiatric Association.
7. FRANK, G. (1966). *The Boston strangler*. New York: New American Library.
8. GALLWEY, P. L. G. (1985). The psychodynamics of borderline personality. In D. P. Farrington & J. G. Dunn (Eds.), *Aggression and dangerousness* (pp. 127–152). New York: Wiley.

9. GREENACRE, P. (1959). On focal symbiosis. In L. Jessner & E. C. Pavenstedt (Eds.), *Dynamic psychopathology in childhood.* New York: Grune & Stratton.
10. GUNDERSON, J. G., & SINGER, M. T. (1975). Defining borderline patients: An overview. *American Journal of Psychiatry, 132,* 1–10.
11. KERNBERG, O. F. (1967). Borderline personality organization. *Journal of the American Psychoanalytic Association, 15,* 641–685.
12. KLUFT, R. (1985). *Multiple personality.* Washington, DC: American Psychiatric Association Press.
13. KNIGHT, R. P. (1953). Borderline states. *Bulletin of the Menninger Clinic, 17,* 1–12.
14. KULLGREN, G. (In press). Borderline diagnostik med. DSM-III och diagnostisk intervju forborderline. *Nord. Psyktr.-Tidsskr.*
15. MAHLER, M. S. (1971). A study of the separation-individuation process and its possible application to borderline phenomena in the psychoanalytic situation. *Psychoanalytic Study of the Child, 26,* 403–424.
16. MASTERS, B. (1985). *Killing for company.* New York: Stein & Day.
17. MASTERSON, J. F. (1981). *The narcissistic and borderline disorders.* New York: Brunner/Mazel.
18. MEWSHAW, M. (1980). *Life for death.* New York: Doubleday.
19. MOYER, K. E. (1974). Sex differences in aggression. In R. C. Friedman, R. M. Richart, & R. L. VandeWiele (Eds.), *Sex differences in behavior* (pp. 335–372). New York: Wiley.
20. PAYKEL, E. S. (1982). *The handbook of affective disorders.* New York: Guilford Press.
21. PERRY, J. C., & KLERMAN, G. L. (1978). The borderline patient. *Archives of General Psychiatry, 35,* 141–150.
22. RADO, S. (1956). *Psychoanalysis of behavior: Collected papers.* New York: Grune & Stratton.
23. RINSLEY, D. B. (1982). *Borderline and other self disorders.* New York: Aronson.
24. SANDLER, J. (1984). Personal communication.
25. SPUNGEN, D. (1983). *And I don't want to live this life.* New York: Villard Books.
26. STERN, A. (1938). Psychoanalytic investigation and therapy in the borderline group of neuroses. *Psychoanalytic Quarterly, 7,* 467–489.
27. STONE, M. H. (1977). The borderline syndrome: Evolution of the term, genetic aspects, and prognosis. *American Journal of Psychotherapy, 31,* 345–365.
28. STONE, M. H. (1982). Borderline conditions and the menstrual cycle. In R. Freidman (Ed.), *Behavior and the menstrual cycle* (pp. 317–344). New York: Dekker.
29. STONE, M. H., HURT, S., & STONE, D. K. (In press). The P.I. 500: Long-term follow-up of borderline inpatients meeting DSM-III criteria. *Journal of Personality Disorders.*
30. WILLI, J., & GROSSMAN, S. (1983). Epidemiology of anorexia in a defined region of Switzerland. *American Journal of Psychiatry, 140,* 564–567.
31. WILSON, J. Q., & HERRNSTEIN, R. J. (1985). *Crime and human nature.* New York: Simon & Schuster.
32. WINNICOTT, D. (1955). Clinical varieties of transference. In M. R. Kahn (Ed.), *Through paediatrics to psychoanalysis.* London: Hogarth.
33. WINNICOTT, D. (1965). *The maturational processes and the facilitating environment.* New York: International Universities Press.
34. ZILBOORG, G. (1941). Ambulatory schizophrenia. *Psychiatry, 4,* 149–151.

12

TOXIC PSYCHOSIS

Mark Zetin, M.D.,
Chris Stasiek, M.S.,
Editha A. C. Pangan, M.D.,

and

Stacey Warren, B.A.

*Department of Psychiatry and Human Behavior,
University of California, Irvine Medical Center,
Orange, California*

INTRODUCTION

Psychosis is by definition restricted to those disturbances of such magnitude that there is personality disintegration and loss of contact with reality, with hallucinations, delusions, or disordered thought processes. Psychoses may be of primary or functional origin, such as schizophrenia or mania. The organic disorders may be due to numerous causes. Psychosis is manifest by changes in behavior, emotional tone, and ideation. Behavior may be disorganized, assaultive, impulsive, asocial, and out of context of social norms and environmental cues. Emotional tone may be excited or dulled, euphoric or sad. Ideation may be disorganized with looseness of associations and misinterpretation of environmental events.

The functional psychoses, including schizophrenia and affective disorders, have classically been considered to be unassociated with well-defined neuropathology or chemical abnormalities, though recent studies have inconsistently indicated changes in ventricular/brain ratio on computerized tomography and changes in various spinal fluid metabolites of central monoamine neurotransmitters. The organic psychoses have various causes, including poisons or drugs, metabolic abnormalities, infections, and others. The differential diagnosis of functional from organic psychoses de-

231

pends highly on the clinician's sophistication in obtaining appropriate history and laboratory studies as well as physical examination and observation of response to treatment.

Toxic psychosis may include several types of syndromes with behavioral abnormalities, delirium (confusion), affective symptoms (depression or mania), paranoid symptoms, hallucinatory states, dementia or pseudo-dementia, and others. Toxins may be endogenous or exogenous. Endogenous toxins may occur with failure of organic systems to function normally, resulting in the body's inability to metabolize or excrete natural nutrients or metabolic products. Exogenous toxins are commonly drugs of abuse, such as alcohol, hallucinogens, stimulants, sedatives, or anticholinergics.

The focus of this chapter is on the differential diagnosis of exogenous toxic psychoses. Endogenous toxic psychoses are discussed briefly for completeness.

Several excellent reviews of organic mental disorders have been written, including those by Fauman (28), Hales and Hershey (43), Davidson (21), and Whitlock (113). The interested reader may wish to review these also.

RISK FACTORS

There are numerous risk factors for the development of toxic psychosis. These include, in general, the history of past psychiatric illness or brain injury, very old or young age, polypharmacy, substance abuse, and multiple medical illnesses, which may lead to increased vulnerability by decreasing drug clearance and other mechanisms. Similarly, environmental stressors such as hospitalization in an intensive-care unit may contribute to risk. Some individuals are genetically slow metabolizers of drugs and so may develop higher-than-average blood levels (21,113). Antihypertensive and cardiac drugs (113) and steroids (21) are especially common causes of organic mental disorders.

Whitlock (113) has pointed out the risk of vitamin malabsorption, especially of the B group, leading to depression or dementia. This may occur with anticonvulsants, cholestyramine, antituberculosis drugs, levodopa, antineoplastic drugs, and oral contraceptives. Another major risk factor is the interaction of alcohol intoxication or withdrawal with drugs such as sedatives, psychotropics, and antihistamines.

Whitlock estimates that adverse psychiatric reactions to drugs occur in 1 to 5 percent of patients (113). This estimate would be reduced if patients with preexisting psychiatric conditions were protected from drug exposure when not essential and would probably be increased if patients with mild or outpatient conditions were reported.

PATIENT EVALUATION

Fauman has elaborated a stepwise approach to the emergency psychiatric evaluation of organic mental disorders (28). The initial assessment includes the history and mental status examination. Important features of the history include past similar episodes and an observer's report of the evolution of the present episode, past psychiatric illness in the patient or family, recent and past medical illnesses, review of systems with emphasis on neurological symptoms, toxin exposure, history of prescribed, over-the-counter, and abusable drug use, and alcohol use. A mental status examination should include the usual observations and questioning on behavior, orientation, attention, affect, thought processes and content, perception, judgment, as well as careful evaluation of memory, language, and higher cortical functions. Vital signs are an important basic screening for medical problems.

Fauman's second level of evaluation includes physical examination, chest and skull x-rays, electrocardiogram, and laboratory screening (chemistry and electrolytes, complete blood count, urinalysis, drug screen, and blood alcohol level). His third level involves more specific tests, such as the electroencephalogram, glucocorticosteroid level, thyroid function tests, B_{12} and RBC folate, ceruloplasmin, antinuclear antibodies, erythrocyte sedimentation rate, cerebrospinal fluid evaluation, arterial blood gases, blood carbon monoxide, serum heavy metal levels, and syphilis serology. (Urine porphyrins might be added to this.) His fourth level of evaluation includes computerized axial tomography or nuclear magnetic resonance brain imaging.

At the risk of overstating the obvious, we would add to this list the importance of consultations with a neurologist and internist, contact with the patient's primary-care physician to obtain details of prescribed medications and medical history, and contact with the patient's family and employer to obtain details of changes in behavior, mood, clarity of thinking, and social habits and their duration and possible relation to abuse of alcohol or drugs. We would also emphasize the importance of inpatient evaluation free of all nonessential drugs and with determination of blood levels of all drugs for which this is available.

Acute onset of illness, lack of similar previous episodes, negative family history, hallucinatory experiences (especially taste, touch, smell, or visual), abnormal pupillary responses, nystagmus, slurred speech, incoordination, and abnormalities of vital signs all point toward toxic psychosis. Definitive diagnosis requires a history of exposure, demonstrable presence of the substance in the body, clearing of the illness with removal from exposure to the offending agent, and recurrence of the symptoms on rechallenge.

ENDOGENOUS TOXIC PSYCHOSES

The endogenous disorders associated with mental status changes and major, obvious medical illness that is easily discovered on routine laboratory screening include diabetic ketoacidosis, hepatic and renal failure, hyper- and hypoparathyroidism, hyper- and hypothyroidism, Cushing's and Addison's diseases, porphyria, and collagen vascular diseases, including systemic lupus erythematosus and periarteritis nodosa. The treatability of many of these conditions makes the use of a screening battery of laboratory examinations essential.

Parathyroid adenoma was the cause of syncope, muscle weakness, drowsiness, disorientation, confusion, paranoid thoughts, and auditory hallucinations in a 67-year-old woman with a history of hypertension and heart failure who had serum calcium of 11.7 mg/dl and phosphate of 2.7 mg/dl with normalization of calcium and mental status after removal of the tumor (58).

Thymomas may present with numerous clinical manifestations, including myotonic disorders, erythroblastic anomalies, Sjögren's syndrome, Cushing's disease, carcinoid syndrome, amenorrhea, severe proximal myopathy, depression, and acute psychosis (4).

A 19-year-old woman was brought to the emergency room because of strange behavior, lying on the floor with twitching eyes, hyperreligiosity, with normal physical and laboratory evaluation except potasium of 3.2 mEq/l, and negative toxicology, with rapid response to haloperidol and discharge. She died the day after discharge; autopsy revealed lymphocytic thymoma with cause of death attributed to respiratory failure due to myasthenia gravis. Antibody to central nervous system cholinergic receptors may account for the psychotic manifestations of myasthenic patients (4).

Adult neuronal ceroid lipofuscinosis (Kufs' disease) may present with episodic stuporous, excited, and hallucinatory psychotic states, mental retardation, generalized convulsions, and icthyosis vulgaris with a positive family history of the syndrome (105). This may be misdiagnosed as schizophrenia.

Abnormalities in calcium metabolism during pregnancy or parturition may be related to puerperal psychosis, which is more common in individuals with personal or family history of bipolar affective disorder (87).

Basal ganglia calcification may occur in puberty with adult manifestations of schizophreniform psychosis and extrapyramidal symptoms in a variety of clinical conditions, including postencephalitic psychosis, hepatolenticular degeneration (Wilson's disease), and Huntington's chorea. An X-linked dominant familial basal ganglia calcification has been associated with schizophreniform disorder in one family (30).

Aqueduct stenosis with hydrocephalus may present with schizophrenialike psychosis which does not respond to operative intervention (88).

WATER INTOXICATION

Water intoxication occurs when ingestion greatly exceeds excretion and produces a variety of neurobehavioral signs, including anxiety, agitation, confusion, psychosis, tremors, convulsions, stupor, coma, and even death. The encephalopathy may be a result of hyponatremia, intracellular potassium loss, brain edema, or a combination of all these factors. This syndrome may occur in patients with schizophrenia and inappropriate ADH release and might reflect dopaminergic supersensitivity induced by neuroleptic exposure (55,90).

ANTICHOLINERGIC DRUGS

These include neuroleptics, antidepressants, anti-Parkinsonian drugs, and antihistamines.

There are several groups of patients who are at risk for anticholinergic toxicity: those receiving benztropine or trihexyphenidyl for treatment of extrapyramidal side effects of neuroleptics, especially if these are given in conjunction with a tricyclic antidepressant; those taking over-the-counter sleeping or cold pills containing scopolamine or atropine or methapyriline; and those using scopolamine patches for control of vertigo or atropine occular solution.* Physostigmine is the specific antidote for central anticholinergic syndrome and is given in doses of 1–2 mg intramuscularly (i.m.).

Principal features of central anticholinergic syndrome include delirium, anxiety, hyperactivity, hallucinations, disorientation, seizures, tachycar-

---

*Many gastrointestinal medications are anticholinergic.

dia, mydriasis, facial flushing, decreased sweating, hyperpyrexia, decreased secretions, urinary retention, and decreased bowel motility, with the additional symptom of cardiac conduction and rhythm abnormalities in the case of tricyclic antidepressants (41). The elderly may be especially sensitive to the development of these symptoms.

Psychiatric Patients

Granacher and Baldessarini reported four cases (41). A 32-year-old male drug abuser with an overdose of about 750 mg of doxepin hydrochloride developed within four hours agitation, impaired recent memory, incoherent speech, dysarthria, ataxia, dry mucous membranes, sluggish pupils, and moderate tachycardia, with excellent response within 35 minutes of receiving physostigmine salicylate, 2 mg i.m. A 43-year-old woman with bipolar affective disorder, history of neuroleptic and electroconvulsive treatment, treated on lithium and amantadine for idiopathic spasmodic retrotorticollis, had benztropine, 15 mg, added (accidentally?) and developed tachycardia, dilated pupils, and confusion, and responded to physostigmine i.m. and a reduced dose of benztropine. A 23-year-old man with mental retardation receiving haloperidol, 6 mg, thioridazine, 300 mg, and benztropine, 6 mg, daily developed disorientation, agitation, visual hallucinations, dry mouth, tachycardia, and dilated unreactive pupils, which responded to physostigmine. A 23-year-old methadone maintenance patient presented with two days of confusion, disorientation, and delusions, with impaired recent memory, hypertension, tachycardia, slight fever, unreactive pupils, and dry mucous membranes; he was treated initially with haloperidol following which the family brought in an empty bottle that had contained 1000 mg of amitriptyline. Anticholinergic toxicity was diagnosed and he improved with physostigmine.

Woody and O'Brien reported three cases (115). A 24-year-old male schizophrenic was admitted with delirium, confusion, agitation, disturbance of memory, and visual and auditory hallucinations despite fluphenazine enanthate maintenance and rapidly improved off medications in the hospital. It was then determined that he had taken 12 benztropine tablets (1 mg) on the day of admission. A 24-year-old male heroin addict was admitted for detoxification and evaluation of fever and leukocyctosis, was treated with methadone, haloperidol, 6 mg/day, and benztropine, 4 mg/day, and developed loosening of associations, disturbance of memory, and visual and tactile hallucinations, which improved the day after benztropine and haloperidol were stopped. A 25-year-old male heroin addict with polydrug abuse took 36 mg of benztropine and 72 mg of haloperidol over two days and had restlessness, slurred speech, visual and tactile hallucinations, loose associations, and impaired recent and past memory, with responses to supportive therapy and amnesia for the period of intoxication.

Coid and Strang reported on mania secondary to procyclidine (Kemadrin) abuse in a polydrug abuser (18).

Aderhold and Muniz reported a 44-year-old woman taking estrogen replacement treatment and amitriptyline, 75 mg daily, for depression treated later with furazolidone, 300 mg daily, and adiphenoxylate for diarrhea (1). Furazolidone is a synthetic antimicrobial nitrofuran with monoamine oxidase-inhibiting properties. Four days after having these medications added, she developed blurred vision, perspiration, chills, hot flashes, restlessness, motor hyperactivity, persecutory delusions, auditory hallucinations, and visual illusions. Furazalidone was discontinued while continuing the other drugs, and 24 hours later the symptoms had cleared.

Hvizdos et al. reported a 52-year-old woman with no previous psychiatric history who was admitted for "strange behavior" and had poor responses to questions, poor judgment, delusions, and auditory hallucinations, low potassium, elevated blood urea nitrogen, slightly elevated T_3 (due to a minor thyroid-protein binding abnormality) and was diagnosed as having major depression with psychotic features for which she was treated with haloperidol, benztropine, and desipramine in increasing doses (49). On her 12th hospital day she developed visual hallucinations, incoherent speech, tachycardia, dry mouth, dilated pupils, and muscle twitching in her hands and feet. Haloperidol and desipramine were discontinued after high serum concentrations were found, and the patient improved.

Hussain and Murphy reported the case of a 25-year-old sociopathic substance abuser who developed disorientation, hallucinations, and violent behavior following an overdose on thioridazine, 1200 mg (48). Symptoms resolved with chlordiazepoxide and supportive care over two days.

Beszterczey and Pecknold reported a 21-year-old schizophrenic who was treated with chlorpromazine, 1200 mg daily, and benztropine, 4 mg daily, who developed visual hallucinations on the fifth hospital day, which resolved within 24 hours of stopping all medications (9).

Davies et al. reviewed cases of confusional reactions among 150 patients receiving the antidepressants imipramine or amitriptyline and found that these occurred in 13 percent of the total sample and 35 percent of those over 40 years of age (22). Age was a risk factor but sex, prior electroencephalographic (EEG) abnormality, and dosage did not affect incidence.

Episodes typically developed during the first two weeks of antidepressant treatment with an average dose of 125 mg daily (range 50–225 mg daily), with restlessness and sleep disturbance, progressing to agitation, disorientation, and insomnia, with delusions in some cases; 11 of the 20 patients who developed confusion were also receiving benztropine, 1–3 mg daily, and perphenazine prior to the onset of the confusion.

Goggin and Solomon reported a 40-year-old male chemist who was treated with thiothixene, 10 mg daily, and trihexyphenidyl, 10 mg daily, and then was started on doxepin for the treatment of "depressive neurosis . . . with psychotic trends and obsessive character" (38). He synthesized his own trihexyphenidyl and ingested 25 mg in six hours, without other drug abuse, and developed tachycardia, nausea, weakness, restlessness, and faintness.

Brodsky et al. reported on four bipolar patients and one schizoaffective patient who developed anticholinergic toxic psychosis with confusion and disorientation while taking usual doses of amitriptyline, chlorpromazine, or thioridazine, or trifluoperazine with benztropine (13). They felt that the hypersensitivity to antidepressants or neuroleptics that were high in anticholinergic activity might be a result of a defect in the cholinergic modulation of the noradrenergic system in bipolar patients and this could reflect a difference in the pathogenesis of bipolar disorder compared with schizophrenia.

Zetin reviewed several cases of toxic psychosis induced by phenothiazine administration in patients with chronic renal failure and noted that patients receiving chlorpromazine, promethazine, and diphenhydramine developed confusion, disorientation, paranoia, agitation, and visual and auditory hallucinations, with resolution two to eight days after discontinuing these drugs (119). Their clinical picture was that of central anticholinergic syndrome. Patients with renal failure are at risk for toxic psychosis because of higher free-drug levels, drug accumulation due to low dialyzability of phenothiazines, and exposure to polypharmacy.

Hasan and Mooney described a 62-year-old woman with a six-month history of depression who was treated in the hospital with amitriptyline, 150 mg, and thioridazine, 50 mg, and on hospital day 9 developed abdominal pain and nausea, which were treated with Donnatal (phenobarbital, hyoscyamine, atropine, and scopalamine) and an antacid (47). Within three hours she became disoriented, incoherent, and delusional, and she responded well to physostigmine, 2 mg subcutaneously. An 84-year-old woman presented with confusion, disorientation, and depression, and was treated with chlorpromazine and amitriptyline, 75 mg each daily, with increased confusion on the third day of treatment, resulting in the discontinuation of amitriptyline and reduction of chlorpromazine to 50 mg daily. Visual hallucinations were suspected and insomnia was noted, and promazine, 50 mg i.m., was given. Diphenhydramine was given for dystonic reaction. Physostigmine, 2 mg i.m., was given three times with immediate clearing of speech and thought.

El-Yousef et al. reported on three cases of central anticholinergic syndrome treated with double-blind injections of placebo or physostigmine salicylate, 4 mg i.m. (25). In all cases, placebo failed to cause improvement and physostigmine was effective. All patients had been on highly anticholinergic medication combinations, including thioridazine with benztropine; imipramine, perphenazine, and benztropine; and chlorpromazine with benztropine.

Nonpsychiatric Patients

Cowen reported on a 40-year-old woman with an overdose of promethazine causing unconsciousness, sluggish pain response, tachycardia, and dilated unreactive pupils (19). She was managed with gastric lavage and sodium bicarbonate. Six hours after admission she was rousable, restless, and aggressive, and over the next 24 hours she received chlorpromazine, 100 mg i.m. twice, and diazepam, 10 mg. Psychiatric consultation revealed her to be restless, agitated, confused, disoriented, and having visual hallucinations, with prompt improvement in mental status noted following physostigmine, 0.5 mg i.m.

Scopolamine patches and eyedrops have also been reported to cause central anticholinergic syndrome. Rodysill and Warren reported on a 76-year-old woman who developed bizarre behavior, hypertension, slowly reactive pupils, confusion, agitation, rambling pressured speech, visual hallucinations, and delusions eight hours after applying a transdermal scopolamine patch without removing the previously placed one (89). She was being treated for herpes zoster oticus with nausea and vertigo, and a similar episode of toxic psychosis had occurred 10 months earlier when she had been on multiple medications including transdermal scopolamine.

Hamborg-Petersen et al. reported on five children aged five to nine years who developed visual hallucinations, strange behavior, and restlessness 3 to 22 hours after .6–1.8 mg of scopolamine eyedrops (45). All recovered completely within 13 to 24 hours after the last instillation.

Nonprescription sleeping pills often include methapyriline, which is an antihistamine, and scopolamine. Both have central and peripheral anticholinergic properties. Allen et al. reported on 21 cases of over-the-counter hypnotic drug overdoses in patients aged 17 to 82 (mean 29.5) years (3). Ten cases involved psychosis with hallucinations, disorientation, delirium, confusion, agitation, or hyperactivity. Seven patients had tachycardia and three had mild hypertension. Only four patients were comatose; the rest were drowsy. Physostigmine was infrequently used in this series of patients.

Jones et al. reported on the occurrence of toxic psychosis with use of pheniramine p-aminosalicylate (Avil); visual and auditory hallucinations predominated and treatments were mixed or none (53). Several patients used the drug in doses of 6 to 37 tablets of 50 mg each to induce hallucinations, with common clinical features including cramps, dilated pupils, anorexia, ataxia, incoordination, and inactivity while hallucinating.

Ullman and Groh reported on two patients who had overdosed on Sominex and Sleep-Eze with Sominex (107). Both patients had dilated pupils, dry mucous membrances, hot dry skin, slight pyrexia, confusion, restlessness, and hallucinations, and responded well to physostigmine, 1 mg given twice. Four additional hypnotic overdose cases responded to double-blind physostigmine administration. These authors noted that Sominex, Sleep-Eze, Compoz, and Excedrin PM contain methapyrilene and salicylamide, and the first three contain scopolamine. Scopolamine is more difficult to detect on urine toxicology than the other ingredients because only 1 percent is excreted in the urine.

ANTIARRHYTHMIC DRUGS

Propranolol may cause a wide variety of psychiatric symptoms including depression, acute confusion, vivid dreams, nightmares, visual hallucinations, and schizophrenialike illnesses with vivid auditory hallucinations (113). Oxprenolol appears to be the highest-risk beta blocker for causing depression with 5 percent of patients developing this problem, which is comparable to the 6 percent risk for alpha-methyldopa (113).

Prakash et al. reported that propranolol-induced psychosis was considered in the case of a 25-year-old mentally retarded woman who had intermittent explosive disorder that had failed to respond to lithium, carbamazepine, and phenytoin, and who developed excitement, persecutory delusions, and auditory hallucinations on propranolol, 640 mg daily. The patient responded to dose reduction (83). Propranolol was being used in an attempt to control her psychiatric symptoms. She received fluphenazine decanoate, 50 mg i.m., and continued on propranolol, 400 mg daily. She became disoriented, confused, incoherent, but without hallucinations or delusions, and propranolol was gradually discontinued with resolution of the organic brain syndrome.

Kuhr reported a case of a 63-year-old woman with mitral valve disease, mitral valve replacement, and a pacemaker, taking digoxin, quinidine, and propranolol for several months (60). When propranolol was increased from 480 to 560–960 mg daily she developed visual hallucinations and disorientation. She was reduced to propranolol, 560 mg daily, and given haloperidol, 12 mg daily, with good results; nine days after discharge she was readmitted for cardiac problems. Propranolol was increased to 800 mg daily, and confusion and auditory and visual hallucinations unresponsive to neuroleptic medication occurred. These resolved following medication discontinuation, surgical transection of the bundle of His, and programmed pacemaker implantation with medication maintenance on digoxin alone. Her prolonged delirium cleared within two weeks of discontinuing propranolol.

Remick et al. reported a 50-year-old mildly mentally retarded woman with thyrotoxicosis, hypercalcemia, medication refusal, agitation, paranoia, irritability, lability, tachycardia, and systolic ejection murmur (85). She was treated with an ablative dose of radioactive iodine and discharged taking propranolol, 160 mg daily, and methimazole, 30 mg daily. She was readmitted a week later for irritability, agitation, lability, insomnia, disorientation, medication refusal, and because the peripheral manifestations of hyperthyroidism were stable, propranolol was tapered to 80 mg daily with improvement in mental status within 24 hours. She was later rechallenged with propranolol, 160 mg daily, and her mental status again transiently worsened, confirming the diagnosis of propranolol-induced toxic psychosis.

ANTIHYPERTENSIVE DRUGS

Paykel et al. reviewed the psychiatric side effects of antihypertensive drugs other than reserpine and noted that methyldopa was often associated with lethargy, drowsiness, fatigue, and that 5.7 percent of patients experienced depression (81). Clonidine caused sedation, drowsiness, lethargy, fatigue, but not depression. Propranolol and other beta blockers may cause depression, sedation, lightheadedness, confusion, and visual perceptual changes, as well as hypnagogic and hypnopompic visual hallucinations, which clear with complete wakefulness and are dose-dependent.

INFECTIONS

Toxic shock syndrome may present with psychosis. A 35-year-old woman presented on various occasions with delusions, confusion, paranoia, anorexia, cramping abdominal pain, diarrhea, asthenia, malaise, lethargy, insomnia, headaches, auditory hallucinations, fever, chills, headaches, hypotension, and abdominal tenderness. Pelvic examination revealed purulent malodorous discharge, and after removal of a tampon and treatment with oxacillin and Betadine douches she progressively improved (63).

Mononucleosis presented as acute catatonic schizophrenia in a 16-year-old girl who had motor inhibition, confusion, delusions of impending harm, self-derogation, fever of 38°C, and infrequent jerks of the legs and arms with loss of strength and deep tendon reflexes in the right upper extremity after two weeks of neuroleptic treatment. She had an elevated erythrocyte sedimentation rate, positive Monospot, heterophil antibodies titer of 1 : 28, and occasional atypical lymphocytes in her peripheral blood smear, with mild slowing on EEG. Low-dose neuroleptic and psychotherapy were provided, and by four months the psychosis and brachial neuritis resolved (93).

Mycoplasma pneumoniae encephalitis was suspected of causing psychosis in a nine-year-old girl with fever, unproductive cough, and blisters on the lips two weeks prior to admission for restlessness, irritability, tiredness, slow thinking and moving, thought blocking, auditory hallucinations, choreiform movements, and impaired diadochokinesis with EEG and cerebrospinal fluid (CSF) examinations consistent with encephalitis and psychiatric symptoms suggestive of schizophreniform disorder. Serum complement fixation revealed a negative and then 1 : 64 positive reaction to *M. pneumoniae*, but CSF did not contain antibodies to the organism. She developed nocturnal sweating, quadriceps atrophy, and was treated at five months with trimipramine; she began recovering at six months, with full recovery by one year (37).

Epstein-Barr virus was suspected to have triggered psychosis in a 45-year-old male physician with a history of bipolar affective disorder and alcohol abuse who presented with overactivity, suspiciousness, guardedness, difficulty focusing in the interview, fever, tachycardia, and hypertension, with fever going up to 105°F a few days after admission despite chlordiazepoxide, chlorpromazine, and lithium treatment. Monospot test and heterophil antibody tests were positive; EEG and liver-spleen scan were normal and CSF cultures were negative (57).

Antituberculosis drugs share the general neurotoxic potential of causing depression and peripheral neuropathy and may aggravate preexisting schizophrenia (113).

Sharma et al. reported on a 16-year-old boy with moderately advanced pulmonary tuberculosis and no history of mental disorder who was treated with streptomycin, .75 gm daily, isoniazid, 300 mg daily, and thiacetazone, 150 mg daily (97). On the 2nd hospital day he was restless, violent, confused, and incoherent; he recovered within a week of these drugs being stopped and receiving pyridoxine and sedation. On the 8th hospital day he was given streptomycin and isoniazid was added and increased to 300 mg daily, and on day 16 he developed psychotic symptoms, which resolved seven days after stopping isoniazid. On the 24th hospital day, he was started on ethambutal, 800 mg daily, ethionamide, and PAS, and the next day he was irritable, talkative, confused, and violent and was improved three days following drug discontinuation. Ethionamide was proven to be the offending agent because he was able to tolerate ethambutal and PAS fairly well.

Murray reported a 57-year-old female with orbital cellulitis due to coagulase-negative *Staphylococcus*, which was treated with cephalothin, 1 gm every four hours, heparin i.v., and probenecid, 500 mg four time daily, with development on the 2nd and 3rd hospital day of headache and jerking of limbs, which persisted after discontinuation of the antibiotic and probenecid on the 4th day (72). Diphenylhydantoin was started. She became confused and agitated and had headache, neck and shoulder pain, and paranoid ideation and then auditory and visual hallucinations. Trifluoperazine, 15 mg daily, and benztropine, 3 mg daily, were started on the 6th day, and she was then treated with penicillin with no adverse effects and no subsequent drug rechallenge was done.

Saker et al. reported the case of a 46-year-old woman with hypertension and uremia due to probable analgesic nephropathy who later developed congestive heart failure with fever, blood pressure 160/90, aortic diastolic murmur, plasma creatinine 13 mg/100 cc, and urea 285 mg/100 cc. (94). She required peritoneal dialysis and cephalothin for bacterial endocarditis. After two weeks of parenteral antibiotic, therapy was changed to oral cephalexin, 1 gm twice daily, with a high level of 120 μg/cc after a total dose of 5 gm over three days. On the 4th day of cephalexin therapy, she was euphoric, overactive, had a grand mal seizure for which she was given diazepam i.v., and she remained confused, disoriented, and suffered from paranoid delusions. CSF was normal but EEG was abnormal. She gradually improved and cephalexin, 250 mg every other day, was continued.

Weisholtz et al. reported on three cases of quinacrine-induced psychosis (110). A 37-year-old male homosexual who had been treated with metronidazole for 10 days for giardiasis was then given oral quinacrine, 300 mg daily, and tetracycline, 1.5 gm daily, and eight days later developed lightheadedness and anxiety, followed by confusion, disorientation, inappropriate affect, looseness of associations, delusions, but no hallucinations or disorientation, with no physical or EEG or blood chemistry abnormalities. Diazepam i.m. helped briefly, but the patient became anxious, euphoric, pressured, and had ideas of reference and paranoia, and had auditory hallucinations, for which chlorpromazine was given with resolution of the psychosis over the next eight days. A 37-year-old woman with giardiasis received quinacrine, 300 mg daily, and became restless, anxious, insomnic, agitated, and developed auditory hallucinations three days after starting medication. The drug was stopped, and the irritability, fever, flushing, and urinary incontinence noted were resolved within two days. A 33-year-old woman with a one-year history of giardiasis received quinacrine, 300 mg daily, and five days later developed anxiety, abdominal cramps, confusion, agitation, and visual hallucinations, and was well within 12 hours of stopping medication.

Lindenmayer and Vargas reported the case of a 16-year-old boy with intestinal parasites found on preemployment physical who received quinacrine, 300 mg daily, and became restless, talking incessantly, then became incoherent and disoriented, and began hallucinating by four days of therapy (66). Physical and laboratory evaluation were remarkable only for elevated alkaline phosphatase and creatine phosphokinase. He was hospitalized, treated with supportive therapy and haloperidol, and developed waxy flexibility and muteness, which gradually resolved over 18 days of hospitalization.

Chloroquine is used in the treatment of malaria and rheumatoid arthritis (113). Good and Shader reviewed chloroquine toxicity and noted that this could include psychosis, personality change, depression, and delirium (40). Psychotic symptoms developed after 2–6 gm at about four days of treatment. Hydroxychloroquine and amodiaquine have similar psychological side effects. Antimalarial drugs given to rheumatoid arthritis patients were noted to cause tiredness, depression, claustrophobia, inferiority feelings, insomnia, suspiciousness, and depression, which sometimes required antidepressant or ECT therapy. These symptoms generally resolved after drug discontinuation.

Sato et al. reviewed 21 cases of injectable methamphetamine-induced psychosis admitted to 10 mental hospitals in individuals who were not suffering from schizophrenia or major affective disorder (96). All patients had used the drug for at least a month, and the average duration of use was 6.6 years; drug use started at average age of 24.8 years and age average at hospitalization was 31.5 years. All had reexperienced psychosis after reexposure to drug following abstinence of at least a month, and history was verified by another observer who knew the patient. The recurrence of the acute paranoid psychosis appeared rapidly, following one to six injections of 5–120 mg, implying a sensitization process. Sato et al. described cases with paranoid (persecutory and jealous) delusions, visual and auditory hallucinations, and rapid recurrence with reexposure after a period of abstinence. Neuroleptic maintenance appeared to have some protective effect against psychosis on reexposure.

Janowsky and Risch reviewed cases of amphetamine-induced psychosis under controlled conditions in nonschizophrenic subjects (52). They found that Schneiderian 1st-rank symptoms of schizophrenia do occur in experimental psychostimulant psychosis.

Lake et al. described a 21-year-old patient who had a three-week manic episode with euphoric mood, pressured speech, and grandiose ideation induced by "black beauties" (generally containing caffeine, ephedrine, and phenylpropanolamine), with a personal history of depression but no mania (61). He had a family history of bipolar affective disorder.

Waters and Lapierre described cases of secondary mania occurring in a 44-year-old man who had begun a 15-day course of a decongestant containing phenylephrine, hydrocodone, and diphenylpyraline with symptoms occurring at 10 days on this medication (109). Another patient, a 62-year-old woman with alcoholism and acute increase of her long-term bronchodilators Tedral SA (theophylline, ephedrine, and phenobarbital) and Primatene (theophylline, isophedrine, and methapyrilene), developed her 1st manic episode. Both patients responded rapidly to haloperidol.

Roxanas and Spalding reported the case of a 26-year-old male epileptic drug abuser who presented with paranoid delusions, auditory and visual hallucinations, in a setting of clear consciousness and intact intellect, following ingestion of 750 mg of ephedrine over three days (92). He had subtherapeutic phenytoin and normal EEG on admission and rapidly responded to low-dose trifluoperazine and phenytoin, 300 mg daily. Another case involved a 26-year-old man with several months of odd behavior and aggressive outbursts who had taken 300 mg of ephedrine three days prior to admission and became aggressive. He presented with auditory hallucinations and delusions of persecution and grandeur, and four days after admission became aggressive after taking 900 mg of ephedrine with very slow response to neuroleptics over the next six weeks. A 30-year-old woman with marked change in behavior over two years presented with accelerated speech, tangential thinking, paranoid delusions, and talking to herself, but denying auditory hallucinations, consistent with acute schizophrenic psychosis aggravated by her excessive use of ephedrine (Tedral). She responded well to thiroidazine, and two years later it was learned that she had improved off of phenothiazines with a change from Tedral to cromoglycic acid (Intal) for her asthma. The authors note the similarity of ephedrine-induced psychosis to that induced by amphetamine and to schizophrenia.

Wetli and Mittleman reported on the "body packer syndrome" in 10 cocaine smugglers traveling after taking large quantities of the drug in balloons, condoms, or plastic bags (112). Ingestion was oral, rectal, or intravaginal. Patients had agitated behavior, grand mal seizures, respiratory collapse, mydriasis, acute toxic psychosis, and coma prior to death.

HALLUCINOGENS

Yago et al. reported on 145 consecutive psychiatric emergency patients seen in Los Angeles County in a 48-hour period (116). Phencyclidine (PCP) assay was performed using gas capillary gas chromatographic nitrogen detector method, which is sensitive and specific. PCP was found in 63 patients, and 53 charts were available for review, which revealed over half the patients having the following symptoms: auditory hallucinations, sleep disturbance, paranoid delusions, hostility and negativism, confused thinking, disorientation, and anxiety. The patients were 67 percent males and had mean age of 24 years; only 32 percent reported PCP use. Some patients experienced visual or haptic hallucinations. The nearly pathognomonic findings were nystagmus, hypertension, pyrexia, dissociative states, and hyperreflexia.

Jacob and Carlen reported on nine cases of PCP intoxication with agitation, severe behavior disorder, paranoid ideation, and amnesia for the episode, with resolution taking 2 to 13 days (51). A 33-year-old man (Case 2) with THC ingestion two days prior to admission presented in a catatonic mute state with rigidity, decreased response to pain, hyperreflexia, and excessive salivation, followed by echolalia, euphoria, confusion, disorientation, agitation, hallucinations, and short attention span; urine and blood samples were positive for PCP. He improved over the next six to nine days with diazepam i.v. A 20-year-old male (Case 8) presented comatose, rigid, with pulse of 120 and blood pressure of 150/100, apnea, cyanosis, and PCP present in blood. He awoke after 14 hours with slurred speech, echolalia, and decreased response to pain; his subsequent course involved periods of mental lucidity alternating with periods of agitation, confusion, disorientation, hallucinations, and paranoia. Chorpromazine was used for behavioral control, and after a period of depression he was completely recovered by the 12th hospital day with no memory for the period of toxic psychosis.

Griffin et al. reviewed the cases of 153 patients admitted with PCP intoxication and found the most frequent symptoms to be aggression, bizarre behavior, anxiety, paranoia, hallucinations, delusions, and affective disturbance (42).

Garey noted that PCP psychosis consists of three phases, including an initial violent aggressive disorganized phase, a restless combative phase, and finally personality reintegration and restoration of normal behavioral and thought patterns from one week to 12 to 18 months (34). Neurological symptoms occurring in some patients are nystagmus, variable pupil size with depressed light reflex, diminished pain response, slurred speech, tremors, increased deep-tendon reflexes, clonus, muscle weakness, and, at higher doses, respiratory depression, coma, decreased muscle tone, status epilepticus, and death.

Chopra reviewed 200 cases of chronic cannabis dependence in a predominantly male sample and defined three groups of patients (15). Group I (37 percent of subjects) had little or no personality problems or history of mental illness and presented with euphoria, excitation, hallucinations, delusions, negative attitudes, alternate laughing and weeping, paranoia, depersonalization from a few hours to a few days, and had good prognosis for recovery when drug was withdrawn. Group II (58 percent of subjects) were psychopaths, delinquents, and hypochondriacs, who manifested disorientation, anxiety, morbid delusions, schizophrenic, depressive, or manic or paranoid symptoms from a few days to a few months with frequent relapses and poor prognosis, many showing "ambulatory psychosis" after long-term drug withdrawal. Group III (5 percent of subjects) had a history of psychosis and most manifested acute intoxication with talkativeness, indifference about the future and family, were calm but had violent reactions to small provocations, and schizophrenia-like and confusional reactions occurred with poor prognosis and chronic psychotic states.

Palsson et al. reported on 11 hospitalized patients with psychosis associated with cannabis use without preexisting psychosis or mixed substance abuse (78). Symptoms were mixed with affective, schizophrenia-like, confusion, and aggressive features of variable duration.

Rottanburg et al. reported on hypomanic and agitated features in 20 psychotic inpatient males with high urinary cannabinoid levels, and noted that they had less affective flattening, auditory hallucinations, incoherence, and hysteria than matched controls (91).

Ifabumuyi and Jeffries reported on drug-induced psychosis with prolonged hallucinogen use and noted both schizophrenia-like and organic features, with depression, anxiety, panic, depersonalization, illusions, hallucinations, and paranoid ideas that may respond to "talking down" or go on to resemble a "drug-induced schizophrenia" of variable response to major tranquilizers and/or ECT (50). These acute vivid symptoms are in contrast to another pattern of response with complex convoluted thinking, loose associations, paranoia, philosophical content, marked vagueness, limited insight, and flat affect that occurs following prolonged hallucinogen use and responds poorly to major tranquilizers. The 1st course of illness is illustrated in a 22-year-old woman with an eight-year history of hallucinogen use who presented with bizarre visual and tactile hallucinations, loose associations, lability, and depersonalization, with poor response to chlorpromazine and abnormal EEG attributed to it and some response to diphenylhydantoin. The 2nd course of illness is illustrated in a 23-year-old male "psychopathic personality" who had an eight-year history of hallucinogen and other drug abuse and presented with auditory hallucinations, visual misperceptions, loose associations, fragmented thoughts, but full orientation. Over a period of five years, trials of trifluoperazine, 25 mg daily, and then thioridazine, up to 600 mg daily, followed by seven ECT treatments failed to alleviate the symptoms, but there was improvement with diphenylhydantoin, 200 mg daily, for 10 weeks.

ALCOHOL

Kosbab and Kuhnley described pathological intoxication as occurring in people with low alcohol tolerance who develop hours to days of excitement and aggressive, dangerous, homicidal reactions, with persecutory ideas occurring commonly (59). The condition terminates with sleep and there is usually amnesia for the episode. A 22-year-old man drank one bottle of malt liquor and became violent, felt that "his thoughts were talking to him," and on recovery was embarrassed at the events for which he was amnesic and acknowledged multiple life problems. A similar episode had occurred two years earlier. EEG, physical, and laboratory examinations were normal.

WERNICKE-KORSAKOFF SYNDROME

Wernicke's encephalopathy involves abrupt onset of oculomotor disturbances (nystagmus or gaze palsy), cerebellar ataxia, and mental confusion (73).

Bowerman reviewed the Korsakoff syndrome and noted that the four essential elements include memory defects for recent events, retrograde amnesia, disorientation, and confabulation (11). Lack of insight and initiative are also part of the syndrome. The syndrome is often associated with alcoholism, avitaminosis, and polyneuritis. The amnesia may be fluctuating and cause the patient to be unable to give a complete history of his illness. Differential diagnosis includes thiamine deficiency due to malabsorption, malignancy, and other factors (73).

DISULFIRAM

Disulfiram is used to prevent a return to drinking in alcoholic patients. The most commonly noted psychiatric side effects have included delirium, depression (with risk of suicide attempts), and mania or hypomania (113). Acute catatonia has been reported. High-dose treatment especially in the elderly with liver impairment appears to increase the risk of toxicity (113).

Stuller et al. described disulfiram (Antabuse) psychosis in two patients (104). The first, a 27-year-old man, had noted confusion and anxiety seven months prior to admission when taking disulfiram for one and one-half weeks. One week prior to admission he was restarted on it in a dose of 500 mg daily, and he presented confused, unable to concentrate, anxious, impulsive, labile, with loose associations and disorientation and auditory hallucinations. He was started on haloperidol, and the disulfiram was discontinued, with improvement over the next three days and discharge on no drugs. Six-month follow-up revealed no further problems. A 42-year-old man with a 20-year history of alcoholism, mood swings, and a self-inflicted gunshot wound to the head was treated with lithium, phenytoin, and disulfiram and presented for hospitalization amnesic and with auditory hallucinations, with therapeutic drug levels, and with resolution of the symptoms within two days of stopping disulfiram.

MINOR TRANQUILIZERS AND SEDATIVE-HYPNOTICS

Minor tranquilizers, including benzodiazepines, barbiturates, and other sedative-hypnotics, remain a major cause of reversible dementia in the elderly (113). Prolonged excretion and resulting accumulation of these drugs in the elderly, especially with the inappropriate choice of the very long-acting agent flurazepam for nighttime sedation, may cause many iatrogenic dementias. Abrupt cessation of benzodiazepines, like that of alcohol, may produce anxiety, irritability, tremor, sweating, insomnia, incoherent thinking, blurred vision, sensory hypersensitivity, and, of course, convulsions (113).

Mellor and Jain described 10 inpatients who were dependent on diazepam, 60–120 mg daily, for the previous 3 to 14 years and who were treated with chlorpromazine, hydroxyzine, or placebo during withdrawal (70). Withdrawal symptoms were frequent initially, fell, then rose again at three weeks, before finally declining. Throughout withdrawal patients had tremor, anorexia, insomnia, and myoclonus. During the first 10 days patients had toxic psychosis similar to delirium tremens. During the 3rd and 4th weeks symptoms such as sensory perceptions being heightened or lowered, photophobia, hyperacusis, and abnormalities of cutaneous sensation occurred. Tremor, myoclonus, and relief of symptoms by a test dose of the drug permit diazepam withdrawal to be distinguished from anxiety.

ANTICONVULSANTS

Psychosis of epilepsy is an important topic reviewed in depth elsewhere by Monroe, Parnas et al., and Flor-Henry (29,71,79,80). Our review focuses on cases of anticonvulsant toxicity.

Franks and Richter reported several cases of anticonvulsant toxicity (31). A 25-year-old with childhood encephalitis, major motor seizures, chronic organic brain syndrome, and long-term treatment with phenytoin, 300 mg daily, primidone, 750 mg daily, and diazepam, 20 mg daily, presented with loose associations, intact memory and orientation, ataxia, equivocal horizontal nystagmus, and initial levels of phenytoin, 25 μg/ml (therapeutic 10–20), and primidone, 36 μg/ml (therapeutic 15–30), with improvement following dose decreases of the drugs. A 23-year-old woman with borderline mental retardation, childhood onset of psychomotor seizures, treatment with primidone, 650 mg daily, carbamazepine, 600 mg daily, and clonazepam, 10 mg daily, took an inadvertent overdose of clonazepam and presented with bizarre behavior, slurred speech, moderate slow-wave activity, but no epileptic focus on EEG, and clearing on discontinuation of all medications. She was restarted on carbamazepine, 600 mg daily, for psychomotor seizure control, and her psychosis worsened, with increased bizarre motor behavior and lability, loose associations, paranoid delusions, and auditory hallucinations with intact memory and orientation. Toxic psychosis was suspected, medication was reduced, and the patient improved within a week. A 47-year-old man with borderline mental retardation with idiopathic major motor seizure disorder starting in infancy had been treated with phenytoin, 300 mg daily, and primidone, 750 mg daily, and was admitted with frequent spells of choreoathetoid movements and autistic thinking; he had low drug levels and normal EEG and CT scan. He was given haloperidol for worsening psychosis, and repeat drug levels revealed phenytoin level, 43 μg/ml, and primidone level, 6 μg/ml. The psychosis cleared following reduction of phenytoin, and it was discovered later that he had been taking his anticonvulsants erratically and so had unstable blood levels.

Wessely et al. reported on manifestations of diphenylhydantoin intoxication in five patients and noted that all had cerebellar signs, two had polyneuropathy, and one had itching (111).

OPIATES

Pentazocine appears to be more frequently associated with adverse psychiatric effects than most opiates, with hallucinations, vivid dreams, delusions, depression, depersonalization, and derealization having been reported (113).

Harris and Harper reported the case of a 38-year-old woman taking Distalgesic (dextropropoxyphene HCl and paracetamal) who overdosed on this following a two-year period of depression and back pain (46). On the 3rd hospital day she was given mianserin, 30 mg daily, and on the 8th day she developed auditory hallucinations and confusion, which continued despite stopping mianserin, but resolved by the 10th day and did not recur when mianserin was restarted. The psychosis was attributed to withdrawal from the narcotic.

LEVODOPA

Levodopa is widely used in the treatment of Parkinson's disease and is associated with side effects, including confusion, overactivity, depression, paranoid psychosis, mania or hypomania, and increased sexual drive (102,113). Bromocriptine and amantadine may cause similar problems (102,113).

Klawans states that levodopa-induced psychosis can occur early in the course of treatment in individuals with a previous history of mental disorders or after several years of treatment in patients with no previous history of mental disorders (56). Early psychosis usually occurs within a few weeks of starting levodopa and usually in schizophrenics, either off antipsychotics with idiopathic Parkinsonism or on antipsychotics with drug-induced Parkinsonism. Psychotic symptoms are reversed by withdrawal of levodopa. Late psychosis occurs after years of treatment in patients with Parkinsonism without previous psychiatric disorders or dementia and occurs in association with other manifestations of levodopa use, such as dreams that are vivid or terrifying and stereotyped hallucinations, which are most often nocturnal, nonthreatening, recurrent, and predominantly visual. A pure paranoid delusional disorder may also occur. Confusional psychosis may be due to anticholinergic anti-Parkinsonian drugs or amantadine, which should be stopped. Levodopa should then be stopped, and the psychosis usually clears within days following its withdrawal; the drug may then be restarted in about half the previous dose. Neuroleptics are to be avoided as they worsen Parkinsonism.

AMANTADINE

Amantadine may cause hallucinations and acute confusion, probably owing to its release of dopamine or presynaptic uptake inhibition (113).

STEROIDS

Lewis and Smith reported on 14 cases of steroid-induced psychosis and reviewed the literature on this phenomenon (63). They found that about 5 percent of steroid-treated patients develop psychiatric symptoms, including depression and mania (the most common manifestations), psychosis, and delirium. Patients at highest risk are females, have systemic lupus erythematosus, and/or are receiving high doses of prednisone.

Ducore et al. reported two cases of adolescents with acute lymphoblastic leukemia who developed acute psychotic episodes after induction therapy including prednisone and displayed regressive behavior, incontinence, fluctuating levels of activity, and delusions, which cleared within a few weeks of tapering steroids but required chlorpromazine for initial management (23).

INDOMETHACIN

Indomethacin may cause headache, vertigo, ataxia, and psychiatric side effects, including hallucinations, paranoid psychoses, and depression, more frequently than other nonsteroidal antiinflammatory drugs (113).

Tollefson and Garvey reported the case of an 83-year-old woman with no past psychiatric history who received indomethacin, 150 mg daily, for the treatment of acute gouty arthritis; on the 6th day of treatment she became acutely agitated, delusional, hypervigilant, electively mute, labile, without hallucinations or disorientation (106). The indomethacin was discontinued, and haloperidol, 10 mg daily, was started, with resolution of the paranoid psychosis over the next seven days.

CIMETIDINE

Cimetidine may cause confusion and depression in some patients (113).

Adler et al. described a 51-year-old man who underwent aortofemoral bypass and was given cephalothin, meperidine, hydroxyzine, and then cimetidine for gastrointestinal bleeding (2). Over the next one to two days he developed belligerence, agitation, visual and auditory hallucinations, and paranoia. These all resolved within 36 hours of discontinuing the cimetidine.

Barnhart and Bowden described a 58-year-old man who underwent cholecystectomy and received cimetidine with acute development of confusion, visual hallucinations, and bizarre speech which did not respond to chlordiazepoxide or magnesium pemoline, but cleared within 24 hours of discontinuing these drugs (8). A 58-year-old chronic schizophrenic taking perphenazine, amitriptyline, Maalox, and Donnatal for peptic ulcer developed bleeding, which was treated with cimetidine, 900 mg daily, as an outpatient. On the 2nd day of cimetidine, she developed confusion and disorientation, which cleared after 24 hours medication-free and did not recur after restarting all medications except cimetidine.

BACLOFEN

Baclofen is used to control muscle spasm, especially in multiple sclerosis, and causes depression in some patients. It may aggravate schizophrenia and withdrawal may cause hallucinations (113).

CARBON MONOXIDE

Carbon monoxide poisoning may occur as a result of intentional or accidental inhalation of automobile exhaust, from fires, or as a result of using indoor heating or cooking devices without adequate ventilation (77). It is a colorless, odorless gas which displaces oxygen from hemoglobin and thus causes hypoxia, as well as ischemia and cellular asphyxia. Acute poisoning may present with headache, dyspnea on exertion, angina, nausea, dizziness, ataxia, syncope, convulsions, and coma, and arterial blood gasses and skin color may be normal. Physical signs of smoke inhalation suggest the diagnosis in fire victims. Sequelae in survivors may include Parkinsonism, mutism, agnosia, apraxia, visual impairment, amnestic/confabulatory state, psychosis, personality deterioration, and memory impairment. "Affective incontinence" involving irritability, impulsiveness, and uncontrollable crying may occur.

METALS

Yung's excellent review of metals in medicine and psychiatry reports neurotoxicity with arsenic, antimony, lead, mercury, thallium, nickel, and lithium (118). Poisoning with copper occurs in Wilson's disease, and poisoning with iodine may result in thyrotoxicosis. Manganese poisoning may resemble Parkinsonism. Vanadium poisoning may appear as symptoms of mania or depression (74). Davidson points out that bismuth salts have been used for gastric disorders and are associated with headache, insomnia, asthenia, mental sluggishness, confusion, visual, auditory, and gustatory hallucinations, hostility, and excitement, which may progress to myoclonic jerks, ataxia, dysarthria, convulsions, coma, and death (21).

CONCLUSIONS

While there are no pathognomonic findings that alert a clinician performing an initial evaluation of a psychotic patient that toxic psychosis is present, there are several indicators that deserve attention. The clinical history should be obtained from at least one or two other observers because the acutely psychotic patient can generally be assumed to be an unreliable informant. The most important questions to ask of the family member or primary-care physician concern the history of past similar episodes, acuteness of onset and duration of the present episode, exposure to prescribed, over-the-counter, or abusable drugs, and pattern of alcohol use. The most important findings on mental status examination include impaired orientation, memory, and concentration, with hallucinations occurring in modalities other than auditory. Fluctuations in mental status from clear to confused, cooperative to hostile, and mood lability all point toward toxic psychosis. Physical findings of abnormal vital signs and neurological examination indicate physiological disturbance that may be toxic in origin. Laboratory examination may be basic or highly sophisticated, but screening toxicology is essential. Observation free of all nonessential drugs in the hospital allows the body to clear most toxins completely and can be of great diagnostic value. General principles of treatment of toxic psychosis include elimination of all nonessential medications, hospitalization for supportive care, and rechallenging with the suspected causative agent in the hospital if the patient has strong medical indications for ongoing use of the drug. Finally, observation of worsening mental status during treatment with *any* drug should be cause for suspicion that the drug, rather than the disease for which it is being given, may be the cause of toxic psychosis.

REFERENCES

1. ADERHOLD, R. M., & MUNIZ, C. E. (1970). Acute psychosis with amitriptyline and furazolidone. *Journal of the American Medical Association, 213*, 2080.
2. ADLER, L. E., SADJA, L., & WILETS, G. (1980). Cimetidine toxicity manifested as paranoia and hallucinations. *American Journal of Psychiatry, 137*, 1112.
3. ALLEN, M. D., GREENBLATT, D. J., & NOEL, B. J. (1979). Self-poisoning with over-the-counter hypnotics. *Clinical Toxicology, 15*, 151.
4. ANANTH, J., DAVIES, R., & KERNER, B. (1984). Single case study psychosis associated with thymoma. *Journal of Nervous and Mental Disorders, 172*, 556.
5. ANGRIST, B., & VAN KAMMEN, D. P. (1984). CNS stimulants as tools in the study of schizophrenia. *Trends in Neurosciences, 7*, 388.
6. ARNESON, G. A. (1979). More on toxic psychosis with cimetidine. *American Journal of Psychiatry, 136*, 1348–1349.
7. AXELSSON, R., MARTENSSON, E., & ALLING, C. (1982). Impairment of the blood-brain barrier as an aetiological factor in paranoid psychosis. *British Journal of Psychiatry, 141*, 273.
8. BARNHART, C. C., & BOWDEN, C. L. (1979). Toxic psychosis with cimetidine. *American Journal of Psychiatry, 136*, 725.
9. BESZTERCZEY, A., & PECKNOLD, J. C. (1971). Toxic psychosis induced by high-dosage chlorpromazine therapy (Letter to the Editor). *Canadian Medical Association Journal, 104*, 884.
10. BIGLER, E. D. (1979). Neuropsychological evaluation of adolescent patients hospitalized with chronic inhalant abuse. *Clinical Neuropsychiatry, first quarter*, 8.
11. BOWERMAN, W. M. (1982). Korsakoff revisited. *Orthomolecular Psychiatry, 11*, 140.
12. BOWERS, M. B., & SWIGAR, M. E. (1983). Vulnerability to psychosis associated with hallucinogen use. *Psychiatry Research, 9*, 91.
13. BRODSKY, L., SHAH, A., & CASENAS, E. (1984). Two distinct "paradoxical" reactions to neuroleptics. *Psychiatric Journal of the University of Ottawa, 9*, 61.

14. CHAPEL, J. L., & HUSAIN, A. (1978). The neuropsychiatric aspects of carbon monoxide poisoning. *Psychiatric Opinion*, March, *15*(3), 33.
15. CHOPRA, G. S. (1971). Marijuana and adverse psychotic reactions: Evaluation of different factors involved. *Bulletin on Narcotics*, *23*, 15.
16. CHOPRA, G. S., & SMITH, J. W. (1974). Psychotic reactions following cannabis use in East Indians. *Archives of General Psychiatry*, *30*, 24.
17. COID, J. (1979). Mania a potu: A critical review of pathological intoxication. *Psychological Medicine*, 9, 709.
18. COID, J., & STRANG, J. (1982). Mania secondary to procyclidine ('Kemadrin') abuse. *British Journal of Psychiatry*, *141*, 81.
19. COWEN, P. J. (1979). Toxic psychosis with antihistamines reversed by physostigmine. *Postgraduate Medical Journal*, *55*, 556.
20. DANIELSON, D. A., PORTER, J. B., LAWSON, D. H., SOUBRIE, C., & JICK, H. (1981). Drug-associated psychiatric disturbances in medical inpatients. *Psychopharmacology*, *74*, 105.
21. DAVIDSON, K. (1981). Diagnoses not to be missed: Toxic psychosis. *British Journal of Hospital Medicine*, November, *26*(5), 530–537.
22. DAVIES, R. K., TUCKER, G. J., HARROW, M., & DETRE, T. P. (1971). Confusional episodes and antidepressant medication. *American Journal of Psychiatry*, *128*, 127.
23. DUCORE, J. M., WALLER, D. A., EMSLIE, G., & BERTOLONE, S. J. (1983). Acute psychosis complicating induction therapy for acute lymphoblastic leukemia. *Journal of Pediatrics*, September, *103*(3), 477.
24. DYSKEN, M. W., MERRY, W., & DAVIS, J. M. (1978). Anticholinergic psychosis. *Psychiatric Annals*, *8*, 30/452.
25. EL-YOUSEF, M. K., JANOWSKY, D. S., DAVIS, J. M., & SEKERKE, J. (1973). Reversal of antiparkinsonian drug toxicity by physostigmine: A controlled study. *American Journal of Psychiatry*, *130*, 141.
26. EVANS, D. L. (1981). Cimetidine-associated toxic psychosis. *American Journal of Psychiatry*, *139*, 1262.
27. EVANS, D. L., EDELSOHN, G. A., & GOLDEN, R. N. (1983). Organic psychosis without anemia or spinal cord symptoms in patients with vitamin B_{12} deficiency. *American Journal of Psychiatry*, *140*, 218.
28. FAUMAN, M. A. (1983). The emergency psychiatric evaluation of organic mental disorders. *Psychiatric Clinics of North America*, *6*, 233.
29. FLOR-HENRY, P. (1983). Determinants of psychosis in epilepsy: Laterality and forced normalization. *Biological Psychiatry*, *18*, 1045.
30. FRANCIS, A. F. (1979). Familial basal ganglia calcification and schizophreniform psychosis. *British Journal of Psychiatry*, *135*, 360–362.
31. FRANKS, R. D., & RICHTER, A. J. (1979). Schizophrenia-like psychosis associated with anticonvulsant toxicity. *American Journal of Psychiatry*, *136*, 973.
32. FUDENBERG, H. H., WHITTEN, H. D., CHOU, Y. K., ARNAUD, P., SHUMS, A. A., & KHANASARI, N. K. (1984). Sigma receptors and autoimmune mechanisms in schizophrenia: Preliminary findings and hypotheses. *Biomedicine and Pharmacotherapy*, *38*, 285.
33. GARDNER, E. R., & HALL, R. C. W. (1982). Psychiatric symptoms produced by over-the-counter drugs. *Psychosomatics*, *23*, 187.
34. GAREY, R. E. (1979). PCP (phencyclidine): An update. *Journal of Psychedelic Drugs*, *11*, 265.
35. GARRIOTT, J. C. (1975). Propylhexadrine—A new dangerous drug? *Clinical Toxicology*, *8*, 665.
36. GIANNINI, A. J., & CASTELLANI, S. (1982). A manic-like psychosis due to khat (*catha edulis* forsk.). *Journal of Toxicology—Clinical Toxicology*, *19*, 455.

37. GILLBERG, C. (1980). Schizophreniform psychosis in a case of mycoplasma pneumoniae encephalitis. *Journal of Autism and Developmental Disorders, 10,* 153.

38. GOGGIN, D. A., & SOLOMON, G. F. (1979). Trihexyphenidyl abuse for euphorigenic effect. *Clinical Research Reports, 136,* 459.

39. GOLDSTEIN, D. J., & KEISER, H. R. (1983). A case of episodic flushing and organic psychosis: Reversal by opiate antagonists. *Annals of Internal Medicine, 98,* 30.

40. GOOD, M. I., & SHADER, R. I. (1982). Lethality and behavioral side effects of chloroquine. *Journal of Clinical Psychopharmacology, 2,* 40.

41. GRANACHER, R. P., & BALDESSARINI, R. J. (1975). Physostigmine. *Archives of General Psychiatry, 32,* 375.

42. GRIFFIN, P. T., GAREY, R. E., DAUL, G. C., & GOETHE, J. W. (1983). Sex and race differences in psychiatric symptomatology in phencyclidine psychosis. *Psychological Reports, 52,* 263.

43. HALES, R. E., & HERSHEY, S. C. (1984). Psychopharmacologic issues in the diagnosis and treatment of organic mental disorders. *Psychiatric Clinics of North America, 7,* 817.

44. HALL, R. C. W., POPKIN, M. K., & McHENRY, L. E. (1977). Angel's trumpet psychosis: A central nervous system anticholinergic syndrome. *American Journal of Psychiatry, 134,* 312.

45. HAMBORG-PETERSEN, B., NIELSEN, M. M., & THORDAL, C. (1984). Toxic effect of scopolamine eye drops in children. *Acta Ophthalmologica, 62,* 485.

46. HARRIS, B., & HARPER, M. (1979). Psychosis after dextropropoxyphene. *Lancet, 2,* 743.

47. HASAN, M. K., & MOONEY, R. P. (1979). Reversible toxic psychosis. *AFP,* December, *20,* 89.

48. HUSSAIN, M. A., & MURPHY, J. (1971). Thioridazine-induced toxic psychosis. *Canadian Medical Association Journal, 104,* 884.

49. HVIZDOS, A. J., BENNETT, J. A., WELLS, B. G., RAPPAPORT, K. B., & MENDEL, S. A. (1983). Anticholinergic psychosis in a patient receiving usual doses of haloperidol, desipramine and benztropine. *Clinical Pharmacy, 2,* 174.

50. IFABUMUYI, O. I., & JEFFRIES, J. J. (1976). Treatment of drug-induced psychosis with diphenylhydantoin. *Canadian Psychiatric Association Journal, 21,* 565.

51. JACOB, M. S., & CARLEN, P. L. (1981). Phencyclidine ingestion: Drug abuse and psychosis. *International Journal of Addictions, 16,* 749.

52. JANOWSKY, D. S., & RISCH, C. (1979). Amphetamine psychosis and psychotic symptoms. *Psychopharmacology, 65,* 73.

53. JONES, I. H., STEVENSON, J., JORDAN, A., CONNELL, H. M., HETHERINGTON, H. D. G., & GIBNEY, G. N. (1973). Pheniramine as an hallucinogen. *Medical Journal of Australia, 1,* 382.

54. KATO, M. (1983). A bird's eye view of the present state of drug abuse in Japan. *Drug and Alcohol Dependence, 11,* 55.

55. KHAMNEI, A. K. (1984). Psychosis, inappropriate antidiuretic hormone secretion, and water intoxication. *Lancet, 1,* 963.

56. KLAWANS, H. L. (1978). Levodopa-induced psychosis. *Psychiatric Annals, 8,* 447/19.

57. KLEIN, R. F., BETTS, R., HORN, R., & SULLIVAN, J. L. (1984). Acute psychosis in a 45-year-old man with bipolar disorder and primary Epstein-Barr virus infection: A case report. *General Hospital Psychiatry, 6,* 13.

58. KLEINFELD, M., PETER, S., & GILBERT, G. M. (1984). Delirium as the predominant manifestation of hyperparathyroidism: reversal after parathyroidectomy. *Journal of the American Geriatrics Society, 32,* 689.

59. KOSBAB, F. P., & KUHNLEY, E. J. (1978). Pathological intoxication. *Psychiatric Opinion,* December, *15*(12), 35.

60. KUHR, B. M. (1979). Prolonged delirium with propanolol. *Journal of Clinical Psychiatry, 40,* 194.

61. LAKE, C. R., TENGLIN, R., CHERNOW, B., & HOLLOWAY, H. C. (1983). Psychomotor stimulant-induced mania in a genetically predisposed patient: A review of the literature and report of a case. *Journal of Clinical Psychopharmacology, 3*, 97.
62. LAUX, G., & PURYEAR, D. A. (1984). Benzodiazepines—Misuse, abuse and dependency. *American Family Physician, 30*, 139.
63. LEWIS, D. A., & SMITH, R. E. (1983). Steroid-induced psychiatric syndromes. *Journal of Affective Disorders, 5*, 319.
64. LEWIS, J. E. (1983). Toxic shock syndrome manifested as psychosis. *Southern Medical Journal, 76*, 245.
65. LIEBOWITZ, M. R., NEUTZEL, E. J., BOWSER, A. E., & KLEIN, D. F. (1978). Phenelzine and delusions of parasitosis: A case report. *American Journal of Psychiatry, 135*, 1565.
66. LINDENMAYER, J., & VARGAS, P. (1981). Toxic psychosis following use of quinacrine. *Journal of Clinical Psychiatry, 42*, 162.
67. LIVANAINEN, M., & SAVOLAINEN, H. (1983). Side effects of phenobarbital and phenytoin during long-term treatment of epilepsy. *Acta Neurologica Scandinavica, 68*, 49.
68. MCALLISTER, C. J., SCOWDEN, E. B., & STONE, W. J. (1978). Toxic psychosis induced by phenothiazine administration in patients with chronic renal failure. *Clinical Nephrology, 10*, 191.
69. MCCARRON, M. M., SCHULZE, B. W., THOMPSON, G. A., CONDER, M. C., & GOETZ, W. A. (1981). Acute phencyclidine intoxication: Clinical patterns, complications, and treatment. *Annals of Emergency Medicine, 10*, 290/9.
70. MELLOR, C. S., & JAIN, V. K. (1982). Diazepam withdrawal syndrome: Its prolonged and changing nature. *Canadian Medical Association Journal, 127*, 1093.
71. MONROE, R. R. (1982). Limbic ictus and atypical psychoses. *Journal of Nervous and Mental Disorders, 170*, 711.
72. MURRAY, G. (1974). Toxic paranoid reaction to cephalothin. *Drug Intelligence and Clinical Pharmacy, 8*, 71.
73. NAKADA, T., & KNIGHT, R. T. (1981). Alcohol and the central nervous system. *Medical Clinics of North America, 68*, 121.
74. NAYLOR, G. J., & SMITH, A. H. W. (1981). Vanadium: A possible aetiological factor in manic depressive illness. *Psychological Medicine, 11*, 249.
75. NICHOLI, A. M. (1984). Phencyclidine hydrochloride (PCP) use among college students: Subjective and clinical effects, toxicity, diagnosis, and treatment. *Journal of the American College of Health, 32*, 197.
76. OKA, E., YAMATOGI, Y., ICHIBA, N., TERASAKI, T., KOHNO, C., YOSHIDA, H., MATSUDA, M., & OHTAHARA, S. (1983). Psychotic symptoms in childhood epilepsy—An electroencephalographic study. *Folia Psychiatric Neurologica Japan, 37*, 239.
77. OLSON, K. R. (1984). Carbon monoxide poisoning: Mechanisms, presentation, and controversies in management. *Journal of Emergency Medicine, 1*, 233.
78. PALSSON, A., THULIN, S. O., & TUNVING, K. (1982). Cannabis psychoses in south Sweden. *Acta Psychiatrica Scandinavica, 66*, 311.
79. PARNAS, J., & KORSGAARD, S. (1982). Epilepsy and psychosis. *Acta Psychiatrica Scandinavica, 66*, 83.
80. PARNAS, J., KORSGAARD, S., KRAUTWALD, O., & JENSEN, P. S. (1982). Chronic psychosis in epilepsy: A clinical investigation of 29 patients. *Acta Psychiatrica Scandinavica, 66*, 282.
81. PAYKEL, E. S., FLEMINGER, R., & WATSON, J. P. (1982). Psychiatric side effects of antihypertensive drugs other than reserpine. *Journal of Clinical Psychopharmacology, 2*, 14.
82. PRADHAN, S. N. (1984). Phencyclidine (PCP): Some human studies. *Neuroscience and Behavioral Reviews, 8*, 493.
83. PRAKASH, R., CAMPBELL, T. W., & PETRIE, W. M. (1983). Psychoses with propranolol: A case report. *Canadian Journal of Psychiatry, 28*, 657.

84. RAINEY, J. M. (1977). Disulfiram toxicity and carbon disulfide poisoning. *American Journal of Psychiatry, 134,* 371.
85. REMICK, R., O'KANE, J., & SPARLING, T. G. (1981). A case report of toxic psychosis with low-dose propranolol therapy. *American Journal of Psychiatry, 138,* 850.
86. RENAULT, P. F., SCHUSTER, C. R., FREEDMAN, D. X., SIKIC, B., NEBEL DE MELLO, D., & HALARIS, A. (1974). Repeat administration of marihuana smoke to humans. *Archives of General Psychiatry, 31,* 95.
87. RILEY, D. M., & WATT, D. C. (1985). Hypercalcemia in the etiology of puerperal psychosis. *Biological Psychiatry, 20,* 479.
88. ROBERTS, J. K. A., TRIMBLE, M. R., & ROBERTSON, M. (1983). Schizophrenic psychosis associated with aqueduct stenosis in adults. *Journal of Neurology, Neurosurgery, and Psychiatry, 46,* 892.
89. RODYSILL, K. J., & WARREN, J. B. (1984). Transdermal scopolamine and toxic psychosis. *Lancet, 1,* 561.
90. ROSENBAUM, J. K., ROTHMAN, J. S., & MURRAY, G. B. (1979). Psychosis and water intoxication. *Journal of Clinical Psychiatry, 40,* 287.
91. ROTTANBURG, D., ROBINS, A. H., BEN-ARIE, W., TEGGIN, A., & ELK, R. (1982). Cannabis-associated psychosis with hypomanic features. *Lancet, 2,* 1364.
92. ROXANAS, M. G., & SPALDING, J. (1977). Ephedrine abuse psychosis. *Medical Journal of Australia, 2,* 639.
93. RUBIN, R. L. (1978). Adolescent infectious mononucleosis with psychosis. *Journal of Clinical Psychiatry, 39,* 773.
94. SAKER, B. M., MUSK, A. W., HAYWOOD, E. F., & HURST, P. E. (1973). Reversible toxic psychosis after cephalexin. *Medical Journal of Australia, 1,* 497.
95. SALZMAN, B. (1982). Opiates and severely disturbed patients. *Annals of the New York Academy of Sciences, 398,* 58.
96. SATO, M., CHEN, C., AKIYAMA, K., & OTSUKI, S. (1983). Acute exacerbation of paranoid psychotic state after long-term abstinence in patients with previous methamphetamine psychosis. *Biological Psychiatry, 18,* 429.
97. SHARMA, G. S., GUPTA, P. K., JAIN, N. K., SHANKER, A., & NANAWATI, V. (1979). Toxic psychosis to isoniazid and ethionamide in a patient with pulmonary tuberculosis. *Tubercle, 60,* 171.
98. SMIRNIOTOPOULOS, J. G., MURPHY, F. M., SCHELLINGER, D., KURTZKE, J. F., & BORTS, F. T. (1984). Cortical blindness after metrizamide myelography. *Archives of Neurology, 41,* 224.
99. SMITH, J. M. (1980). Abuse of the antiparkinson drugs: A review of the literature. *Journal of Clinical Psychiatry, 41,* 351.
100. SNOW, S. S., LOGAN, T. P., & HOLLENDER, M. H. (1980). Nasal spray 'addiction' and psychosis: A case report. *British Journal of Psychiatry, 136,* 297.
101. STANDISH-BARRY, H. M. A. S., & SHELLY, M. A. (1983). Toxic neurological reaction to lithium/thioridazine. *Lancet, 1,* 771.
102. STASIEK, C., & ZETIN, M. (1985). Organic manic disorders. *Psychosomatics, 26,* 394.
103. STEVENS, J. R. (1982). Risk factors for psychopathology in individuals with epilepsy. *Advances in Biological Psychiatry, 8,* 56.
104. STULLER, S., BELL, K., READ, S., & ANANTH, J. (1983). Antabuse psychosis. *Psychiatry Journal of the Univerity of Ottawa, 8,* 179.
105. TOBO, M., MITSUYAMA, Y., IKARI, K., & ITOI, K. (1984). Familial occurrence of adult-type neuronal ceroid lipofuscinosis. *Archives of Neurology, 41,* 1091.
106. TOLLEFSON, G. D., & GARVEY, M. J. (1982). Indomethacin and prostaglandins: Their behavioral relationships in an acute toxic psychosis. *Journal of Clinical Psychopharmacology, 2,* 62.
107. ULLMAN, K. C., & GROH, R. H. (1972). Identification and treatment of acute psychotic

state secondary to the usage of over-the-counter sleeping preparations. *American Journal of Psychiatry, 128*, 1244.

108. VENKATESAN, J., BALAN, V., & SURESH, T. R. (1983). Toxic delirious state due to accidental ingestion of datura. *Indian Journal of Psychiatry, 25*, 338.

109. WATERS, B. G. H., & LAPIERRE, Y. D. (1981). Secondary mania associated with sympathomimetic drug use. *American Journal of Psychiatry, 138*, 837.

110. WEISHOLTZ, S. J., McBRIDE, A., MURRAY, M. W., & SHEAR, M. K. (1982). Quinacrine-induced psychiatric disturbances. *Southern Medical Journal, 73*, 359.

111. WESSELY, V., MAYR, N., BINDER, H., & KLINGER, D. (1981). Neurologische ausfallserscheinungen bei diphenylhydantoin-intoxikation (fallberichte und ubersicht) [Neurological signs in diphenylhydantoin intoxication]. *Wiener Klinische Wochenschrift, 93*, 315.

112. WETLI, C. V., & MITTLEMAN, R. E. (1981). The "body packer syndrome" — Toxicity following ingestion of illicit drugs packaged for transportation. *Journal of Forensic Science, 26*, 492.

113. WHITLOCK, F. A. (1981). Adverse psychiatric reactions to modern medication. *Australia and New Zealand Journal of Psychiatry, 15*, 87.

114. WILCOX, J. A. (1983). Psychoactive properties of benztropine and trihexyphenidyl. *Journal of Psychoactive Drugs, 15*, 319.

115. WOODY, G. E., & O'BRIEN, C. P. (1974). Anticholinergic toxic psychosis in drug abusers treated with benztropine. *Comprehensive Psychiatry, 15*, 439.

116. YAGO, K. B., PITTS, F. N., BURGOYNE, R. W., ANILINE, O., YAGO, L. S., & PITTS, A. F. (1981). The urban epidemic of phencyclidine (PCP) use: Clinical and laboratory evidence from a public psychiatric hospital emergency service. *Journal of Clinical Psychiatry, 42*, 193.

117. YESAVAGE, J. A., & FREMAN, A. M., III (1978). Acute phencyclidine (PCP) intoxication: Psychopathology and prognosis. *Journal of Clinical Psychiatry, 39*, 664.

118. YUNG, C. Y. (1984). A synopsis on metals in medicine and psychiatry. *Pharmacology, Biochemistry and Behavior, 21*, 41.

119. ZETIN, M. (1980). Letter to the Editor. *Clinical Nephrology, 12*, 95.

13

ALZHEIMER'S DISEASE

ANTHONY F. JORM, PH.D.

Senior Research Fellow,
NH & MRC Social Psychiatry Research Unit,
Australian National University,
Canberra, Australia

INTRODUCTION

In 1907 Alzheimer described the case of a 51-year-old woman who initially showed personality change, followed soon after by increasing memory impairment and disturbances of reading, writing, and oral language (4). After several years the woman died. At autopsy, Alzheimer described the presence of senile plaques and neurofibrillary tangles in the patient's brain. These are regarded as the neuropathological hallmarks of the disease that now bears Alzheimer's name.

From Alzheimer's initial report until the 1970s, Alzheimer's disease was regarded as a rare presenile dementia. The common senile dementias of the elderly were generally thought to be due to cerebral atherosclerosis. However, with the important neuropathological work of Tomlinson, Blessed, and Roth (101) it was clearly established that Alzheimer-type changes were a major factor in producing senile dementia. With this realization, the term *senile dementia of the Alzheimer type (SDAT)* became established. More recently, there has been a tendency to ignore the arbitrary distinction between presenile and senile forms altogether, and to use the term *Alzheimer's disease* to refer to the disorder at any age. The result has been that in the space of two decades Alzheimer's disease has been transformed from a rare disorder affecting the middle-aged to the most prevalent severe psychiatric condition in the elderly.

DIAGNOSIS

Difficulties of diagnosis are a significant stumbling block to progress in understanding Alzheimer's disease. Neuropathological evidence from a biopsy or autopsy is necessary for the disorder to be diagnosed with certainty. Clinical diagnosis can only indicate probable Alzheimer's disease.

Approaches to Diagnosis

Two contrasting approaches to clinical diagnosis can be distinguished. The first is diagnosis of Alzheimer's disease by exclusion of other alternatives. The main diagnostic alternatives are multiinfarct dementia and mixed Alzheimer/multiinfarct dementia, although there are a myriad of other less likely possibilities. DSM-III-R (6) uses the exclusionary approach with its diagnostic criteria for primary degenerative dementia (which includes Alzheimer's and Pick's diseases). A recent Finnish study on the prevalence of dementia compared the results of such an exclusionary diagnostic approach with neuropathological diagnoses (74). Clinical diagnosis of Alzheimer's disease was correct in 69 percent of cases, while 28 percent of other dementias were incorrectly diagnosed as Alzheimer's disease. Particular problems were caused by patients who had a combination of Alzheimer's disease and multiinfarct dementia. They tended to be diagnosed as having either one of these disorders or the other. This mixed group represents a generally difficult problem for clinical diagnosis by exclusion. For example, with the popular Ischemic Score (44) for the diagnosis of multiinfarct dementia, a low score effectively excludes multiinfarct dementia but a high score can be due to either multiinfarct dementia or a mixed dementia (66).

A contrasting approach to clinical diagnoses of Alzheimer's disease involves a search for positive neuropsychological features of the disorder (17,28,43). According to advocates of this approach, Alzheimer's disease has unique features that allow it to be differentiated from other forms of dementia. Cummings and Benson (28) have presented the strongest case for this approach with their distinction between cortical and subcortical dementias. Alzheimer's and Pick's diseases are held to involve cortical neuropsychological changes, in particular aphasia, apraxia, and agnosia, which allow them to be differentiated from the dementias due to, say, Huntington's disease and Parkinson's disease, which involve subcortical features. According to Cummings and Benson, multiinfarct dementia can involve subcortical or cortical features, depending on the site of the infarction, and for this reason can be difficult to differentiate from Alzheimer's disease on neuropsychological grounds alone. As yet, the success of the positive diagnostic approach to Alzheimer's disease has not been evaluated against neuropathological diagnoses. However, one study that did use cortical signs as an aid to clinical diagnoses of Alzheimer's disease found that 82 percent of these patients have the neuropathological features of Alzheimer's disease at autopsy, and no cases of multiinfarct dementia were found among them (98). Perhaps the major problem with regarding Alzheimer's disease as a cortical dementia is that there are reports that many patients who are believed to have Alzheimer's disease do not exhibit cortical features, particularly in the earlier stages of the disorder (15,64).

NINCDS-ADRDA Work Group Diagnostic Criteria

Until recently there have been no widely accepted diagnostic criteria for Alzheimer's disease. Recently, however, the U.S. National Institute of Neurological and Communicative Disorders and the Alzheimer's Disease and Related Disorders Association set up a work group on the diagnosis of Alzheimer's disease. The work group proposed criteria to standardize clinical diagnosis, which should receive broad acceptance (69). These criteria allow for diagnosis of possible, probable, and definite Alzheimer's disease. Definite Alzheimer's disease requires neuropathological evidence, while possible and probable Alzheimer's disease require varying degrees of clinical evidence. Possible Alzheimer's disease is basically diagnosed by excluding all other causes of dementia, while probable Alzheimer's disease requires a number of positive diagnostic features as well. The criteria for probable Alzheimer's disease are listed in Table 1. As yet, there are no data on the extent to which different clinicians' diagnoses agree when using these criteria or on the validity of the criteria as assessed against neuropathological evidence. Nevertheless, they represent a significant step toward diagnostic consistency.

BRAIN ABNORMALITIES

Over the past decade there have been enormous advances in our understanding of brain changes in Alzheimer's disease, including the regional distribution of plaques and tangles, the pattern of cell loss, and, most of all, the neurotransmitter deficits involved in the disorder.

Plaques and Tangles

Senile plaques consist of a core of the abnormal protein amyloid surrounded by degenerating nerve terminals. The other classic neuropathological changes are neurofibrillary tangles, which are composed of bundles

Table 1
NINCDS-ADRDA Work Group Criteria
for the Diagnosis of Probable Alzheimer's Disease (69)

I. The criteria for the clinical diagnosis of PROBABLE Alzheimer's disease include:

dementia established by clinical examination and documented by the Mini-Mental Test, Blessed Dementia Scale, or some similar examination, and confirmed by neuropsychological tests;

deficits in two or more areas of cognition;

progressive worsening of memory and other cognitive functions;

no disturbance of consciousness;

onset between ages 40 and 90, most often after age 65; and

absence of systemic disorders or other brain diseases that in and of themselves could account for the progressive deficits in memory and cognition.

II. The diagnosis of PROBABLE Alzheimer's disease is supported by:

progressive deterioration of specific cognitive functions such as language (aphasia), motor skills (apraxia), and perception (agnosia);

impaired activities of daily living and altered patterns of behavior;

family history of similar disorders, particularly if confirmed neuropathologically; and

laboratory results of:

normal lumbar puncture as evaluated by standard techniques;

normal pattern of nonspecific changes in EEG, such as increased slowwave activity; and

evidence of cerebral atrophy on CT with progression documented by serial observation.

III. Other clinical features consistent with the diagnosis of PROBABLE Alzheimer's disease, after exclusion of causes of dementia other than Alzheimer's disease, include:

plateaus in the course of progression of the illness:

associated symptoms of depression, insomnia, incontinence, delusions, illusions, hallucinations, catastrophic verbal, emotional, or physical outbursts, sexual disorders, and weight loss;

(continued)

Table 1
(Continued)

---

other neurologic abnormalities in some patients, especially with more advanced disease and including motor signs such as increased muscle tone, myoclonus, or gait disorder;

seizures in advanced disease; and

CT normal for age.

IV. Features that make the diagnosis of PROBABLE Alzheimer's disease uncertain or unlikely include:

sudden, apoplectic onset;

focal neurologic findings such as hemiparesis, sensory loss, visual field deficits, and incoordination early in the course of the illness; and

seizures or gait disturbances at the onset or very early in the course of the illness.

Reprinted with permission from McKhann et al. (69), p. 939.

of paired filaments wound around each other in a helical pattern. They occur within nerve cells and gradually take over much of the cell space. The number of plaques and tangles observed at autopsy is known to be strongly correlated with the severity of the dementia before death (12,108).

The distribution of plaques and tangles is not uniform throughout the brain. The hippocampus is universally affected in Alzheimer's disease, leading Ball and his colleagues (8) to propose that the disorder should be defined as a hippocampal dementia. The finding of hippocampal involvement provides an explanation of the great difficulty Alzheimer patients have in new learning, since hippocampal lesions are well known to produce problems of this sort. Cortical involvement is also common, but not always found. The parietal, temporal, and frontal areas are most affected, with the occipital and motor regions being largely spared (19). These cortical changes presumably underlie the neuropsychological defects, such as aphasia, apraxia, and agnosia, which are often reported by clinicians. Recent work has shown that the olfactory bulb can be affected (32), a finding that ties in with reports of deficient odor recognition by Alzheimer patients (94).

Neurotransmitter Deficits

Probably the most exciting discovery about Alzheimer's disease in recent years has been the role of cholinergic deficiencies in the disorder. The enzyme choline acetyltransferase, which is involved in the synthesis of the neurotransmitter acteylcholine, has been found to be reduced in Alzheimer's disease. Furthermore, the amount of reduction in choline acetyltransferase is correlated with both plaque counts and the degree of cognitive impairment. The enzyme acetylcholinesterase, which breaks down the neurotransmitter, has also been found to be reduced, but the muscarinic cholinergic receptors on neurons receiving cholinergic innervation are not (81). There is also some evidence that cholinergic axons are involved in the formation of plaques (97), providing a link between the neuropathological and neurochemical changes in Alzheimer's disease.

A cholinergic deficit in Alzheimer's disease provides an explanation of some of the cognitive deficits seen in the disorder. Drachman and Leavitt (30) have shown that when normal volunteers are given the anticholinergic drug scopolamine, they show transient deficits in memory and problem solving similar to those seen in early Alzheimer's disease.

Although acetylcholine is the neurotransmitter that has received most attention, it is not the only one affected in Alzheimer's disease. There has been much recent interest in the neuropeptide somatostatin. Somatostatin receptors are reported to be lost from the cortex (10) and cortical somatostatin neurons are associated with plaques and tangles (75,87). The possible contribution of somatostatin deficits to the clinical features of Alzheimer's disease is as yet unknown.

Neuronal Loss

Loss of neurons from specific regions of the brain has been reported for Alzheimer's disease. An important recent finding is that there is a loss of those cells connecting the hippocampus with other regions, such as the association areas of the cortex, the basal forebrain, the thalamus, and the hypothalamus (56). The result is that the hippocampus is isolated from other areas of the brain, producing the significant memory impairment characteristic of Alzheimer's disease.

Another region showing notable cell loss in Alzheimer's disease is the nucleus basalis of Meynert (107). Cholinergic neurons from this small area of the basal forebrain project to the hippocampus and to cortical regions. In fact, the nucleus basalis is believed to be the major source of cortical cholinergic innervation. Coyle et al. (27) have proposed that the cholinergic deficit of Alzheimer's disease results from a specific loss of cells from the nucleus basalis. More recent work has shown that, while there is marked loss of cells from this region in Alzheimer's disease, there is also some loss in other types of dementia, particularly in dementia associated with Parkinson's disease (89). Such a deficit may therefore not be unique to Alzheimer's disease.

Brain Imaging

A number of researchers have applied computerized tomography (CT) scanning to Alzheimer's disease. When a quantitative analysis is carried out, CT scans appear to have some diagnostic value (3,29), but overall the results have not been exciting. However, positron emission tomography (PET), which indexes brain metabolic function rather than structural changes, has provided more interesting findings. Consistent with recent neuropathological findings of regional differences in plaques and tangles, PET studies have shown differences between cortical regions in the living brains of Alzheimer patients. The temporal and parietal regions show decreased glucose metabolism, while the sensory and motor areas are relatively spared (11,34). The frontal cortex has also been reported to be less affected (34). Importantly, the degree of metabolic reduction is strongly correlated with psychological tests of cognitive function. PET therefore appears to offer a useful in vivo technique for monitoring regional brain changes.

Subtypes of Alzheimer's Disease

The distinction between presenile and senile forms of Alzheimer's disease around the arbitrary dividing age of 65 has largely been abandoned. However, there is an increasing amount of evidence for differences in the neurochemical, neuropathological, and clinical features of the disorder as a function of age of onset. Early-onset Alzheimer's disease tends to have a faster course and produces a more severe dementia. At autopsy, there appear to be deficits in several neurotransmitter symptoms, while with later-onset cases a more purely cholinergic deficit is seen (90). Neuronal loss from the nucleus basalis is greater, as is the reduction in the enzyme choline acetyltransferase. Clinically, language disorder is more often seen with early-onset Alzheimer's disease (93). These differences have led Bondareff (14) to propose that there are two distinct subtypes of Alzheimer's disease. In neurochemical studies, the most commonly used dividing age between the two hypothesized subtypes seems to be death before or after 80. Although there are undoubtedly differences between early- and late-onset cases, it has been disputed whether there are really two distinct subtypes (59). There appears to be no evidence of a distinct break between the two, but rather a continuous gradation. Furthermore, much of the evidence in favor of subtypes comes from autopsy studies. It is likely that early-onset cases usually die of the dementia and so reveal the features of its final stages, while late-onset cases often die of intercurrent illnesses and so are exhibiting the features of earlier stages of the disorder. Only by longitudinal studies of early- and late-onset cases with comparisons at equivalent stages of the disorder will it be possible to obtain definite evidence for or against subtypes.

EPIDEMIOLOGY

A decade ago very little was known about the epidemiology of Alzheimer's disease, but it is now a fast-growing area of inquiry.

Prevalence of Alzheimer's Disease

Although there are many studies of the prevalence of dementia, it is difficult to give figures specifically on the prevalence of Alzheimer's disease. Some dementia prevalence studies do attempt a clinical diagnosis of the type of dementia, but without neuropathological confirmation the figures they provide could be misleading. A further problem is that the neuropathological and cognitive changes of Alzheimer's disease blend into those of normal aging, without a discrete break between the two. Thus, prevalence rates will vary as a function of where the cutoff is placed between dementia and normal aging. Nevertheless, some interesting data come from a study of plaques and tangles in an autopsy study of 199 cases (71). Taking cases reported as having many plaques and tangles at autopsy, we get the results shown in Table 2. Most notable is the sharp rise in neuropathological features of Alzheimer's disease with age at death.

Neuropathological studies also indicate that Alzheimer's disease is the major cause of dementia in the elderly. Table 3 shows the results of the larger studies. Taken together, these indicate that it accounts for around

Table 2
Frequency of Many Plaques and
Tangles in an Autopsy Series (71)

Age	Frequency (%)
<55	0
55–64	2.6
65–74	4.5
75–84	19.6
85 +	45.5

half the cases of dementia in its own right and perhaps another fifth of cases in combination with multiinfarct dementia. It is notable, however, that all these studies deal with Western European samples. Whether Alzheimer's disease is as common in the rest of the world is unknown. In fact, there are data from prevalence studies using clinical diagnosis which cast doubt on any general assertion that Alzheimer's disease is the most common cause of dementia in the elderly. Table 4 shows the results obtained in field studies or case register studies which have attempted a differentiation between Alzheimer's disease and multiinfarct dementia on clinical grounds. Whereas all but one of the Western European studies report Alzheimer's disease to be the more common, all the Soviet and Japanese studies report multiinfarct dementia to be more common. Given the difficulties of clinical diagnosis, it must be asked whether these results are simply a reflection of national differences in diagnostic practice. In the case of the Japanese, at least, this does not appear to be the case. Their published criteria appear to be remarkably similar to those used in Western European studies (62). Furthermore, consistent with a high rate of multiinfarct dementia, Japan is known to have a high incidence of stroke compared to other countries (1). The Soviet studies are more problematic and may reflect either diagnostic differences or a rising occurrence of cerebrovascular disease in that country (25).

A further notable feature of the studies listed in Table 4 is a sex difference in the relative prevalence of Alzheimer's disease and multiinfarct dementia. Of the 13 studies that give a breakdown by sex, 10 report Alzheimer's disease to be more common than multiinfarct dementia in women, while only two report it to be more common than multiinfarct demen-

Table 3
Percentage of Demented Patients with Alzheimer's Disease at Autopsy

Author	Year	Country	Number of Patients	% Alzheimer	% Multiinfarct	% Mixed	% Other
Tomlinson et al.[101]	1970	Britain	50	50	12–18	8–18	14
Todorov et al.[100]	1975	Switzerland	682	32	19	37	12
Jellinger[57]	1976	Austria	1009	50	22	14	14
Wilcock & Esiri[108]	1982	Britain	59	78	0	22	0
St. Clair & Whalley[92]	1983	Britain	89	52	30	18	0
Mölsä et al.[74]	1984	Finland	58	50	17	10	22
Averages				52	17	19	10

Table 4

Most Common Dementia in Prevalence Studies Differentiating
Alzheimer's Disease and Multiinfarct Dementia on Clinical Grounds

Author	Year	Most Common Dementia
	Western Europe	
Primrose (84)	1962	AD
Kay et al. (63)	1964	AD
Åkesson (2)	1969	AD
Bollerup (13)	1970	MID
Broe et al. (18)	1976	AD
Gurland et al. (42)	1981	AD
Mölsä et al. (73)	1982	AD
Pinessi et al. (82)	1984	AD
Sulkava et al. (99)	1985	AD
	United States	
Gurland et al. (42)	1983	AD
	U.S.S.R.	
Sternberg & Gawrilowa (96)	1978	MID
Gavrilova (36)	1984	MID
	Japan	
Kaneko (study 1) (61)	1975	MID
Kaneko (study 2) (61)	1975	MID
Karasawa et al. (62)	1982	MID
Hasegawa et al. (49)	1983	MID
Hasegawa et al. (48)	1984	MID

AD = Alzheimer's disease; MID = multiinfarct dementia.

tia in men. Even the Japanese and Soviet studies, with their higher rates of multiinfarct dementia, show this sex difference.

Risk Factors for Alzheimer's Disease

Although numerous risk factors have been proposed for Alzheimer's disease, to date only five have been replicated in two or more independent studies. These confirmed risk factors are: old age, a family history of dementia, Down's syndrome, a family history of Down's syndrome, and head trauma.

Old age. Old age is without doubt the most important risk factor for Alzheimer's disease. As shown in Table 2, the presence of plaques and tangles at autopsy becomes dramatically more frequent with advancing age. Field studies and case register studies that have studied the incidence of Alzheimer's disease using clinical diagnosis have likewise shown a sharp increase with age (2,45,73,77). However, there is some evidence that incidence may decline in extreme old age (90 + years). The incidence of clinically diagnosed Alzheimer's disease has been reported to decrease at this age (45), as has the incidence of senile plaques (70) and neurofibrillary tangles (79).

Family history of dementia. Parents and siblings of Alzheimer's disease patients are known to have a greater risk of developing the disorder (50,53,105). Undoubtedly, the most important study in this area is that of Heston (50) in Minnesota, which involves the families of a large number of autopsy-proven cases of Alzheimer's disease. He has reported risk to parents of cases as being 15 to 23 percent and the risk to siblings as 10 to 14 percent. However, the risk to relatives varies greatly with the age of onset of the dementia. Risk to siblings varies from around 40 percent for cases where onset is in the forties to around 10 percent for cases of onset after 80. The risk to offspring is of course of greatest relevance for clinical purposes, but is not yet known because it requires longitudinal study of at-risk offspring into old age.

Down's syndrome. Plaques and tangles are found to occur in virtually all patients with Down's syndrome dying over the age of 40, but are uncommon in other cases of mental retardation (111). Whether middle-aged Down's sufferers have a clinical dementia in the usual sense is hard to say. In one recent study, only a minority of middle-aged Down's cases showed signs of dementia before death, although all had plaques and tangles at autopsy (110). However, dementia may manifest differently in someone who is already mentally retarded.

Family history of Down's syndrome. Sufferers from Alzheimer's disease have been reported to have an excess of Down's syndrome among family members (50,53). However, Down's syndrome is not a common condition, so the incidence among relatives is still rather small. Some studies have not replicated the effect (5,105), perhaps because a large sample is required to detect an increased incidence of a rare condition. It is also notable that the studies reporting the excess of Down's have dealt with early-onset cases, for which we have already seen that familial factors are more important.

A further intriguing link between Alzheimer's disease and Down's syndrome has been provided by a recent study on fingerprint patterns in Alzheimer's disease (103). Alzheimer's patients were found to have more ulnar loops than normal controls. Much previous work with Down's syndrome has shown that they too have an excess of this fingerprint pattern. Interestingly, the Alzheimer patients in this study were a mixture of early- and late-onset cases. If the excess of ulnar loops in Alzheimer's disease can be confirmed, it may prove to be a general risk factor for the disorder.

One early report claimed that Alzheimer's disease patients tended to have older mothers (22). If confirmed, this would provide a further link with Down's syndrome, because increased maternal age is the prime risk factor for Down's. However, many studies have now failed to replicate the original work, so we can safely dismiss it as a risk factor (26,31,53,105).

Head trauma. Several recent studies have shown that Alzheimer's disease patients are more likely to have suffered an incident of head trauma earlier in life (5,54,76). Often this head trauma occurred several decades before the onset of the dementia. It was generally due to a car accident and was serious enough to result in loss of consciousness. The discovery of this risk factor is of great practical importance, because it is the first confirmed risk factor that is amenable to preventative action.

ETIOLOGICAL THEORIES

An etiological theory must account for the neuropathological and neurochemical changes seen in Alzheimer's disease and the confirmed risk factors for the disorder. To date, no single theory adequately meets these requirements. Most theories have proposed a single etiological factor, but it is likely that the etiology of Alzheimer's disease is multifactorial. Nevertheless, simple theories need to be pushed to their limits before being abandoned for more complex alternatives. Three of the major single-factor theories are discussed here: the genetic theory, the toxic-exposure theory, and the viruslike particle theory.

The Genetic Theory

Family histories of Alzheimer's disease are compatible with a genetic account of the disorder. Indeed, there may be a small group of early-onset Alzheimer's disease cases for which single gene effects are important. However, in the majority of cases only a multifactorial genetic account appears viable. One view is that plaques and tangles are a normal feature of aging, but in some individuals genetic influences produce these changes at an earlier age than usual and these patients are regarded as having Alzheimer's disease (111).

The finding that Down's syndrome always results in early-onset Alzheimer's disease provides a clue as to the genetic mechanisms that could be involved. Down's syndrome involves an extra supply of the genes on chromosome 21, with the result that the products of these genes may be overproduced. Heston (51) has suggested that some product of the genes on chromosome 21 is important to the development of Alzheimer's disease.

It has been proposed by Heston and White (52) that Down's syndrome and Alzheimer's disease may occur within the same families owing to a basic deficit of neurotubules and neurofilaments. These are long, threadlike structures running parallel to the length of neurons. They are thought to play a role in transport of chemicals around the cell. Neurotubules are also believed to be important to the orientation and separation of chromatids during meiosis. Defective neurotubules may predispose to Down's syndrome by producing nondisjunction of chromosomes during meiosis. Similarly, defective neurofilaments may be the source of neurofibrillary tangles in Alzheimer's disease.

A genetic theory can account for most of the confirmed risk factors for Alzheimer's disease, but does not readily explain head trauma. This is clearly an environmental event predisposing to Alzheimer's disease. Cases of identical twins discordant for Alzheimer's disease have also been reported (55), further implicating environmental factors. Clearly, a genetic theory can provide only a partial account of Alzheimer's disease.

The Toxic-Exposure Theory

It is possible that a toxic substance could produce selective destruction of neurons in certain regions of the brain (e.g., the nucleus basalis) and so produce Alzheimer's disease. A strong boost for such a possibility comes from the recent finding that the chemical MPTP can selectively destroy cells in the substantia nigra and so produce Parkinson's disease (65). The effects of this chemical were originally observed because it was a contaminant of synthetic heroin and Parkinson's disease subsequently appeared in relatively young users of the drug. However, MPTP can be absorbed through inhalation and skin contact, and early Parkinson's effects have been reported in industrial chemical workers who were briefly exposed to it.

Could there be similar toxic exposures producing Alzheimer's disease? The candidate receiving most attention has been aluminum. There are two pieces of evidence implicating aluminum. First, when injected into certain animal species aluminum produces tangles. Second, neurons affected by tangles in Alzheimer's disease patients contain increased aluminum, whereas unaffected neurons do not (80).

Despite this evidence, there are many reasons for rejecting the aluminum hypothesis. For a start, the tangles produced in animals by aluminum exposure are different from those found in Alzheimer's disease. Also, kidney dialysis patients can develop a type of dementia believed to be caused by exposure to aluminum in the large quantities of water used during dialysis. However, this dementia is different from Alzheimer's disease. Finally, antacids are the major dietary source of aluminum (not cookware, as generally believed) (95), but Alzheimer's disease patients are no more likely to have taken such antacids than normal elderly people (54). Although aluminum is unlikely to be a cause of Alzheimer's disease, it is possible that neurons containing neurofibrillary tangles are more likely to accumulate aluminum. Consequently, some authorities advise that Alzheimer's disease patients should avoid aluminum-containing antacids (95).

Despite the weight of evidence against aluminum as a culprit, there may well be unknown toxic substances that produce the disorder. An intriguing finding that suggests the possibility of a toxic exposure is that cases of Alzheimer's disease in Edinburgh have been found to cluster in certain areas of the city rather than be randomly distributed (106).

As with the genetic theory, a toxic exposure appears incapable of explaining all the known facts about Alzheimer's disease. Rather, it must be regarded as a possible component of a multifactorial account.

The Viruslike Particle Theory

Following the demonstration that neurological diseases such as kuru, scrapie, and Creutzfeldt-Jakob disease are transmissible by viruslike particles, there has been interest in whether Alzheimer's disease might be as well (35). Although there have been many attempts to transmit Alzheimer's disease to other species, these have been unsuccessful so far. Such negative results do not necessarily mean, however, that a transmissible agent is not involved. Alternative explanations are that the agent affects only humans or that the incubation period is so long that animals do not live long enough to manifest the disease (85). Clearly, if Alzheimer's disease is transmissible, it is not highly infectious, for otherwise professionals dealing with sufferers would have shown notable excesses of the disease themselves.

If a viruslike particle is involved, then the spread of neuropathological changes through the brain might provide clues as to its mode of entry. Ulrich (102) has studied the early spread of tangles by examining the brains of normal individuals dying in late middle age. At this age, he found them limited to the base of the brain, consistent with the possibility that an agent entered from the nasopharyngeal cavity and spread via neuronal pathways. Another suggestion is that the olfactory bulb is the starting point for the spread of the disease (33).

Prusiner (85) has attempted to explain plaques within the context of a transmissible particle theory. He speculates that the amyloid found at the core of plaques is actually an accumulation of the transmissible particles. There is, of course, no evidence to support this speculation as yet.

The viruslike particle theory accounts for a number of the confirmed risk factors for Alzheimer's disease. Old age as a risk factor would be explained in terms of the long incubation period of such agents, with only the elderly having lived long enough to show its effects. Family histories of dementia are, of course, explained by transmission between family members. The occurrence of Alzheimer's disease in Down's cases is harder to explain, but one suggestion is that just as Down's sufferers are particularly susceptible to conventional infections, their disorder may also allow a commonly occurring viruslike particle to enter the brain and cause Alzheimer's disease (110).

MANAGEMENT

The management of Alzheimer's disease is a complex area which cannot be fully covered in a chapter such as this. Instead, recent research on selected aspects of the topic will be described.

Detection of Dementia

The first step toward management of Alzheimer's disease is a recognition that a dementia is present. Often this task will fall to the general practitioner. It is widely believed, following Williamson's (109) classic work, that general practitioners are poor at detecting dementia in their patients. Williamson found that the Scottish general practitioners he studied correctly detected only 13 percent of their demented patients. However, subsequent research, which is less well known, shows much better results. In a study in Wales, general practitioners detected 60 percent of cases (78), and in a recent German study 44 percent were correctly detected (104). Furthermore, both studies indicate that general practitioners rarely misdiagnose a normal elderly person as demented. Nevertheless, brief psychological screening instruments such as the Mini-Mental State do somewhat better than this at detecting cases of dementia (7). In view of the success of such instruments, it has been argued that the usefulness of mass screening programs for dementia should be further explored (24).

Community and Residential Care Options

Although it is generally considered desirable to maintain the demented elderly in the community as long as possible, they can often be a significant strain on the family members who care for them. Not surprisingly, a high rate of psychiatric disturbance among caregivers has been reported (37). Unfortunately, support from other family members and professional help were found not to relieve this stress. However, day hospital attendance does seem to provide some relief to the demented person's family (39) even though it does not appear to reduce the need for eventual residential care (9,41). The aspect of the demented person's behavior that is most difficult to tolerate is not the cognitive impairment, but passive, withdrawn behavior or unstable mood (40). Not surprisingly, deficits that demand the time of the caregiver are seen as causing more problems than those that do not intrude so directly. These include demanding attention, interfering with personal social life, being unable to be left alone, being unsafe outside alone, and lack of concern for personal hygiene (38). When attempts have been made to reduce residential care for the demented in favor of community care, increases in family strain have been reported (67,91).

Very little evaluative work has been done comparing the effectiveness of different kinds of care for the demented. However, one British study compared matched groups of elderly patients in day centers, day hospitals, wards, and local authority homes (68). No differences were found in mortality or in dementia, but improvements in dependency were more noticeable in day centers and local authority homes.

Pharmacological Treatments

Drugs such as Hydergine have been traditionally used to treat dementia on the rationale that they act as vasodilators and improve blood flow. With the discovery that most cases of senile dementia are due to Alzheimer's disease rather than atherosclerosis, this rationale has been discredited. However, in recent years it has been recognized that these drugs also act as metabolic enhancers, providing a rationale for their continued use. Indeed, there is evidence that these metabolic enhancers do have some small effect on dementia, although improvement seems to be greater in mood than for cognitive function (23). It has also been suggested that improvement is greater for Alzheimer's disease than for multiinfarct dementia (86).

The discovery of a cholinergic deficit in Alzheimer's disease has given great hope that a rational treatment involving cholinergic enhancement can be developed. Three main approaches have been tried. The first is precursor loading, which attempts to increase acetylcholine levels by administration of choline or lecithin (a dietary source of choline). The second is to administer an anticholinesterase such as physostigmine or THA. The aim here is to increase the neurotransmitter by inactivating the enzyme acetylcholinesterase. The third major approach is a combination of precursor loading and anticholinesterase. Results of these cholinergic enhancement treatments have generally been disappointing. However, when the combination approach has been tried with individually tailored dosages for each patient, some encouraging effects have been reported (60). There are a number of problems with attempts at cholinergic enhancement. The most serious is that it may be difficult to improve the function of neurons for which presynaptic degeneration is occurring. Another is that other neurotransmitter systems (e.g., somatostatin) are affected in Alzheimer's disease, so only limited effects can be expected by attempts to enhance the function of a single system.

Psychological Interventions

The aim of psychological interventions is not to treat the disorder causing the dementia, but to ameliorate its effects. Such interventions can be placed into two broad classes. The first kind aims to give demented people skills that enable them to function better in their environment. An example of this approach is training in memory-encoding strategies (16) or in use of a diary to retain personal information and daily appointments (46). Such approaches require the active involvement of the demented person and may have limited potential because the capacity for new learning is impaired early in Alzheimer's disease.

The alternative kind of approach is to change the person's environment to suit his capabilities better. Such interventions have proved more profitable. Even simple environmental manipulations such as providing recreational materials and providing encouragement in their use seem to improve activity levels (20,58). By far the most popular approach of this sort has been reality orientation. Ideally, this program should involve attempts by staff to use every interaction with demented residents as an opportunity to decrease confusion by providing information as to person, place, and time. In addition, reality orientation involves daily classes where orientation knowledge is taught to small groups. Although many evaluation studies have been carried out on reality orientation, nearly all have been restricted to classroom reality orientation without the 24-hour staff interaction component. The results of classroom reality orientation have been very limited, but when 24-hour reality orientation is included, the effects are much better (21,47). Even if reality orientation can be effective, the appropriateness of its goals has been questioned. It has been argued that it is more important for a demented person to have self-care skills like dressing, bathing, and toileting than to know what day or month it is (83).

Another environmental approach is the token economy which involves staff giving tokens for appropriate social interaction, self-care, or work. These tokens can then be exchanged for extra food or privileges. In one evaluation, a token economy was found to produce improvements in bizarre behaviors and incontinence among some demented patients. However, equal improvements were produced simply by improving the general institutional milieu. This was done by providing more activities and social stimulation, increasing opportunities for choices by patients, and promoting to staff the view that they are there to work for the patient's benefit (72).

Trends in the Need for Services

Because Alzheimer's disease and other forms of dementia become increasingly prevalent with age, countries experiencing demographic shifts toward an older population will show the greatest increase in the number of demented citizens in coming years. Although there is a strong trend toward an aging population across all developed countries, some are undergoing a faster demographic shift than others. Rocca et al. (88) have used United Nations population projections for the period 1980–2000 to estimate the extent of increase in dementia in a number of countries. They estimated that the percentage increase will be much greater in some countries (Italy 40 percent, United States 42 percent, Japan 77 percent) than in others (France 9 percent, Britain 12 percent, Sweden 15 percent). Applying this approach to other English-speaking countries, Australia, Canada, and New Zealand will also be among the countries showing rapid increases. We would expect most of these cases to be Alzheimer's disease. Expansion of services will consequently need to be greater in these countries.

ACKNOWLEDGMENTS

Thanks are due to A. S. Henderson and A. Korten for comments on an earlier draft of this manuscript.

REFERENCES

1. Aho, K., Harmsen, P., Hatano, S., Marquardsen, J., Smirnov, V. E., & Strassen, T. (1980). Cerebrovascular disease in the community: Results of a WHO collaborative study. *Bulletin of the World Health Organization, 58*, 113.
2. Åkesson, H. O. (1969). A population study of senile and arteriosclerotic psychoses. *Human Heredity, 19*, 546.
3. Albert, M., Naeser, M. A., Levine, H. L., & Garvey, A. J. (1984). CT density numbers in patients with senile dementia of the Alzheimer's type. *Archives of Neurology, 41*, 1264.
4. Alzheimer, A. (1907). On a peculiar disease of the cerebral cortex. Reprinted in R. H. Wilkins, & I. A. Brody, (1969). Neurological classics XX: Alzheimer's disease. *Archives of Neurology, 21*, 109.
5. Amaducci, L. A., Fratiglioni, L., Rocca, W. A., Fieschi, C., Livrea, P., Pedore, D., et al. (1985). Risk factors for Alzheimer's disease (AD): A case-control study on an Italian population. *Neurology, 35*, 277.
6. American Psychiatric Association (1987). *Diagnostic and Statistical Manual of Mental Disorders*. (3rd ed. Revised). Washington, DC: American Psychiatric Association.
7. Anthony, J. C., Le Resche, L., Niaz, U., Von Korff, M. R., & Folstein, M. F. (1982). Limits of the "Mini-Mental State" as a screening test for dementia and delirium among hospital patients. *Psychological Medicine, 12*, 397.
8. Ball, M. J., Fisman, M., Hachinski, V., Blume, W., Fox, A., Kral, V. A., Kirshen, A. J., & Fox, H. (1985). A new definition of Alzheimer's disease: A hippocampal dementia. *Lancet, 1*, 14.
9. Ballinger, B. R. (1984). The effects of opening a geriatric psychiatry day hospital. *Acta Psychiatrica Scandinavica, 70*, 400.
10. Beal, M. F., Mazurek, M. F., Tran, V. T., Chattha, G., Bird, E. D., & Martin, J. B. (1985). Reduced numbers of somatostatin receptors in the cerebral cortex in Alzheimer's disease. *Science, 229*, 289.
11. Benson, D. F., Kuhl, D. E., Hawkins, R. A., Phelps, M. E., Cummings, J. L., & Tsai, S. Y. (1983). The fluorodeoxyglucose 18F scan in Alzheimer's disease and multi-infarct dementia. *Archives of Neurology, 40*, 711.

12. BLESSED, G., TOMLINSON, B. E., & ROTH, M. (1968). The association between quantitative measures of dementia and senile change in the cerebral grey matter of elderly subjects. *British Journal of Psychiatry, 114,* 797.
13. BOLLERUP, T. R. (1975). Prevalence of mental illness among 70-year-olds domiciled in nine Copenhagen suburbs. *Acta Psychiatrica Scandinavica, 51,* 327.
14. BONDAREFF, W. (1983). Age and Alzheimer disease. *Lancet, 1,* 1447.
15. BREITNER, J. C. S., & FOLSTEIN, M. F. (1984). Familial Alzheimer dementia: A prevalent disorder with specific clinical features. *Psychological Medicine, 14,* 63.
16. BRINKMAN, S. D., SMITH, R. C., MEYER, J. S., VROULIS, G., SHAW, T., GORDON, J. R., & ALLEN, R. H. (1982). Lecithin and memory training in suspected Alzheimer's disease. *Journal of Gerontology, 37,* 4.
17. BROE, G. A. (1985). Investigating dementia. *Bulletin of the Postgraduate Committee in Medicine, University of Sydney, 41,* 39.
18. BROE, G. A., AKHTAR, A. J., ANDREWS, G. R., CAIRD, F. I., GILMORE, A. J. J., & McLENNAN, W. J. (1976). Neurological disorders in the elderly at home. *Journal of Neurology, Neurosurgery & Psychiatry, 39,* 362.
19. BRUN, A., & ENGLUND, E. (1981). Regional pattern of degeneration in Alzheimer's disease: Neuronal loss and histopathological grading. *Histopathology, 5,* 549.
20. BURTON, M. (1980). Evaluation and change in a psychogeriatric ward through direct observation and feedback. *British Journal of Psychiatry, 137,* 566.
21. CITRIN, R. S., & DIXON, D. N. (1977). Reality orientation: A milieu therapy used in an institution for the aged. *Gerontologist, 17,* 39.
22. COHEN, D., EISDORFER, C., & LEVERENZ, J. (1982). Alzheimer's disease and maternal age. *Journal of the American Geriatric Society, 30,* 656.
23. COLE, J. O., & LIPTZIN, B. (1984). Drug treatment of dementia in the elderly. In D. W. Kay & G. D. Burrows (Eds.), *Handbook of studies on psychiatry and old age.* Amsterdam: Elsevier.
24. COOPER, B., & BICKEL, H. (1984). Population screening and the early detection of dementing disorders in old age: A review. *Psychological Medicine, 14,* 81.
25. COOPER, R. (1981). Rising death rates in the Soviet Union: The impact of coronary heart disease. *New England Journal of Medicine, 304,* 1259.
26. CORKIN, S., GROWDON, J. H., & RASMUSSEN, S. L. (1983). Parental age as a risk factor in Alzheimer's disease. *Annals of Neurology, 13,* 674.
27. COYLE, J. T., PRICE, D. L., & DELONG, M. R. (1983). Alzheimer's disease: A disorder of cortical cholinergic innervation. *Science, 219,* 1184.
28. CUMMINGS, J. L., & BENSON, D. F. (1983). *Dementia: A clinical approach.* Boston: Butterworths.
29. DAMASIO, H., ESLINGER, P., DAMASIO, A. R., RIZZO, M., HUANG, H. K., & DEMETER, S. (1983). Quantitative computed tomographic analysis in the diagnosis of dementia. *Archives of Neurology, 40,* 715.
30. DRACHMAN, D. A., & LEAVITT, J. (1974). Human memory and the cholinergic system: A relationship to aging? *Archives of Neurology, 30,* 113.
31. ENGLISH, D., & COHEN, D. (1985). A case-control study of maternal age in Alzheimer's disease. *Journal of the American Geriatric Society, 33,* 167.
32. ESIRI, M. M., & WILCOCK, G. K. (1984). The olfactory bulbs in Alzheimer's disease. *Journal of Neurology, Neurosurgery & Psychiatry, 47,* 56.
33. FERRY, G. (1985). Dementia research sheds new light on old brains. *New Scientist,* August 22, 33.
34. FOSTER, N. L., CHASE, T. N., MANSI, L., BROOKS, R., FEDIO, P., PATRONAS, N. J., & DI CHIRO, G. (1984). Cortical abnormalities in Alzheimer's disease. *Annals of Neurology, 16,* 649.
35. GAJDUSEK, D. C. (1977). Unconventional viruses and the origin and disappearance of kuru. *Science, 197,* 943.

36. GAVRILOVA, S. I. (1984). Demonstrability of mental disorders in late middle and old age (Russian). *Zh. Nevropat. Psikhiat.*, *84*, 911.
37. GILLEARD, G. J., BELFORD, H., GILLEARD, E., WHITTICK, J. E., & GLEDHILL, K. (1984). Emotional distress amongst the supporters of the elderly mentally infirm. *British Journal of Psychiatry*, *145*, 172.
38. GILLEARD, C. J., GILLEARD, E., GLEDHILL, K., & WHITTICK, J. (1984). Caring for the elderly mentally infirm at home: A survey of supporters. *Journal of Epidemiology & Community Health*, *38*, 319.
39. GILLEARD, C. J., GILLEARD, E., & WHITTICK, J. E. (1984). Impact of psychogeriatric day hospital care on the patient's family. *British Journal of Psychiatry*, *145*, 487.
40. GREENE, J. G., SMITH, R., GARDINER, M., & TIMBURY, G. C. (1982). Measuring behavioural disturbance of elderly demented patients in the community and its effects on relatives: A factor analytic study. *Age & Ageing*, *11*, 121.
41. GREENE, J. G., & TIMBURY, G. C. (1979). A geriatric psychiatry day hospital service: A five-year review. *Age & Ageing*, *8*, 49.
42. GURLAND, B., COPELAND, J., KURIANSKY, J., KELLEHER, M., SHARPE, L., & DEAN, L. L. (1983). *The mind and mood of aging.* London: Croom Helm.
43. GUSTAFSON, L., & NILSSON, L. (1982). Differential diagnosis of presenile dementia on clinical grounds. *Acta Psychiatrica Scandinavica*, *65*, 194.
44. HACHINSKI, V. C., ILIFF, L. D., ZILHKA, E., DU BOULAY, G. H., MCALLISTER, V. L., MARSHALL, J., RUSSELL, R. W. R., & SYMON, L. (1975). Cerebral blood flow in dementia. *Archives of Neurology*, *32*, 632.
45. HAGNELL, O., LANKE, J., RORSMAN, B., ÖHMAN, R., & ÖJESJÖ, L. (1983). Current trends in the incidence of senile and multiinfarct dementia. *Arch. Psychiat. Nervenkr.*, *233*, 423.
46. HANLEY, I. G., & LUSTY, K. (1984). Memory aids in reality orientation: A single-case study. *Behavioral Research & Therapy*, *22*, 709.
47. HARRIS, C. S., & IVORY, P. B. C. B. (1976). An outcome evaluation of reality orientation therapy with geriatric patients in a state mental hospital. *Gerontologist*, *16*, 496.
48. HASEGAWA, K., HONIMA, A., SATO, H., AOBA, A., IMAI, Y., YAMAGUCHI, N., & ITAMI, A. (1984). The prevalence study of age-related dementia in the community (Japanese). *Geriatric Psychiatry*, *1*, 94.
49. HASEGAWA, K., IWAI, H., AMAMOTO, H., SATO, H., SHUKUTANI, K., HONMA, A., YUN, M., KARASAWA, A., KAWASHIMA, K., & YAMADA, O. (1983). The epidemiological study on the psychogeriatric disorders (Japanese). *N. Shinfuku Memorial Volume for Retirement.*
50. HESTON, L. L. (1981). Genetic studies of dementia: With emphasis on Parkinson's disease and Alzheimer's neuropathology. In J. A. Mortimer & L. M. Schuman (Eds.), *The epidemiology of dementia.* New York: Oxford University Press.
51. HESTON, L. L. (1984). Down's syndrome and Alzheimer's dementia: Defining an association. *Psychiatric Development*, *4*, 287.
52. HESTON, L. L., & WHITE, J. (1978). Pedigrees of 30 families with Alzheimer disease: Associations with defective organization of microfilaments and microtubules. *Behavior Genetics*, *8*, 315.
53. HEYMAN, A., WILKINSON, W. E., HURWITZ, B. J., SCHMECHEL, D., SIGMON, A. H., WEINBERG, T., HELMS, M. J., & SWIFT, M. (1983). Alzheimer's disease: Genetic aspects and associated clinical disorders. *Annals of Neurology*, *14*, 507.
54. HEYMAN, A., WILKINSON, W. E., STAFFORD, J. A., HELMS, M. J., SIGMON, A. H., & WEINBERG, T. (1984). Alzheimer's disease: A study of epidemiological aspects. *Annals of Neurology*, *15*, 335.
55. HUNTER, R., DAYAN, A. D., & WILSON, J. (1972). Alzheimer's disease in one monozygotic twin. *Journal of Neurology, Neurosurgery & Psychiatry*, *35*, 707.
56. HYMAN, B. T., VAN HOESEN, G. W., DAMASIO, A. R., & BARNES, C. L. (1984). Alz-

heimer's disease: Cell-specific pathology isolates the hippocampal formation. *Science, 225,* 1168.

57. JELLINGER, K. (1976). Neuropathological aspects of dementias resulting from abnormal blood and cerebrospinal fluid dynamics. *Acta Neurologica Belgica, 76,* 83.

58. JENKINS, J., FELCE, D., LUNT, B., & POWELL, L. (1977). Increasing engagement in activity of residents in old people's homes by providing recreational materials. *Behaviour Research & Therapy, 15,* 429.

59. JORM, A. F. (1985). Subtypes of Alzheimer's dementia: A conceptual analysis and critical review. *Psychological Medicine, 15,* 543.

60. JORM, A. F. (1985). Effects of cholinergic enhancement therapies on memory function in Alzheimer's disease: A meta-analysis of the literature. *Australia & New Zealand Journal of Psychiatry, 20,* 237.

61. KANEKO, Z. (1975). Care in Japan. In J. G. Howells, (Ed.), *Modern perspectives in the psychiatry of old age.* Edinburgh: Churchill Livingstone.

62. KARASAWA, A., KAWASHIMA, K., & KASAHARA, H. (1982). Epidemiological study of the senile in Tokyo metropolitan area. *Proceedings of World Psychiatric Association regional symposium.* Kyoto, Japan: World Psychiatric Association, p. 285.

63. KAY, D. W. K., BEAMISH, P., & ROTH, M. (1964). Old age mental disorders in Newcastle upon Tyne. Part I: A study of prevalence. *British Journal of Psychiatry, 110,* 146.

64. KNESEVICH, J. W., TORO, F. R., MORRIS, J. C., & LA BARGE, E. (1985). Aphasia, family history, and longitudinal course of senile dementia of the Alzheimer type. *Psychiatry Research, 14,* 255.

65. LANGSTON, J. W. (1985, February). MPTP and Parkinson's disease. *Trends in Neurosciences, 8,* 79–83.

66. LISTON, E. H., & LA RUE, A. (1983). Clinical differentiation of primary degenerative and multi-infarct dementia: A critical review of the evidence. Part II: Pathological studies. *Biological Psychiatry, 18,* 1467.

67. LOUDON, J. M., HONNEYMAN, F. D., & BANNERJEE, M. (1977). Another style of psychogeriatric service. *British Journal of Psychiatry, 130,* 522.

68. MACDONALD, A. J. D., MANN, A. H., JENKINS, R., RICHARD, L., GODLOVE, C., & RODWELL, G. (1982). An attempt to determine the impact of four types of care upon the elderly in London by the study of matched groups. *Psychological Medicine, 12,* 193.

69. MCKHANN, G., DRACHMAN, D., FOLSTEIN, M., KATZMAN, R., PRICE, D., & STADLANE, E. M. (1984). Clinical diagnosis of Alzheimer's disease: Report of the NINCDS-ADRDA Work Group under the auspices of Department of Health and Human Services Task Force on Alzheimer's Disease. *Neurology, 34,* 939.

70. MATSUYAMA, H. (1983). Incidence of neurofibrillary change, senile plaques, and granulovacuolar degeneration in aged individuals. In B. Reisberg (Ed.), *Alzheimer's disease: The standard reference.* New York: Free Press.

71. MILLER, F. D., HICKS, S. P., D'AMATO, C. J., & LANDIS, J. R. (1984). A descriptive study of neuritic plaques and neurofibrillary tangles in an autopsy population. *American Journal of Epidemiology, 120,* 331.

72. MISHARA, B. (1978). Geriatric patients who improve in token economy and general milieu treatment programs: A multivariate analysis. *Journal of Consulting & Clinical Psychology, 46,* 1340.

73. MÖLSÄ, P. K., MARTTILA, R. J., & RINNE, U. K. (1982). Epidemiology of dementia in a Finnish population. *Acta Neurologica Scandinavica, 65,* 541.

74. MÖLSÄ, P. K., PALJÄRVI, L., RINNE, U. K., & SÄKÖ, E. (1984). Accuracy of clinical diagnosis in dementia. *Acta Neurologica Scandinavica, 69* (Suppl. 98), 232–233.

75. MORRISON, J. H., ROGERS, J., SCHERR, S., BENOIT, R., & BLOOM, F. E. (1985). Somatostatin immunoreactivity in neuritic plaques of Alzheimer's patients. *Nature, 314,* 90.

76. MORTIMER, J. A., FRENCH, L. R., HUTTON, J. T., & SCHUMAN, L. M. (1985). Head injury as a risk factor for Alzheimer's disease. *Neurology, 35*, 264.
77. NILSSON, L. V. (1984). Incidence of severe dementia in an urban sample followed from 70 to 79 years of age. *Acta Psychiatrica Scandinavica, 70*, 478.
78. PARSONS, P. L. (1965). Mental health of Swansea's old folk. *British Journal of Preventive and Social Medicine, 19*, 43.
79. PERESS, N. S., KANE, W. C., & ARONSON, S. M. (1978). Central nervous system findings in a tenth decade autopsy population. *Progress in Brain Research, 40*, 473.
80. PERL, D. P., & BRODY, A. R. (1980). Alzheimer's disease: X-ray spectrometric evidence of aluminum accumulation in neurofibrillary tangle-bearing neurons. *Science, 208*, 297.
81. PERRY, E. K., TOMLINSON, B. E., BLESSED, G., BERGMANN, K., GIBSON, P. H., & PERRY, R. H. (1978). Correlation of cholinergic abnormalities with senile plaques and mental test scores in senile dementia. *British Medical Journal, 2*, 1457.
82. PINESSI, L., RAINERO, I., ASTEGGIANO, G., FERRERO, P., TARENZI, L., & BERAMASCO, B. (1984). Primary dementias: Epidemiological and sociomedical aspects. *Italian Journal of Neurological Science, 5*, 51.
83. POWELL-PROCTOR, L., & MILLER, E. (1982). Reality orientation: A critical appraisal. *British Journal of Psychiatry, 140*, 457.
84. PRIMROSE, E. J. R. (1962). *Psychological illness: A community study.* London: Charles C Thomas.
85. PRUSINER, S. B. (1984). Some speculations about prions, amyloid, and Alzheimer's disease. *New England Journal of Medicine, 310*, 661.
86. REISBERG, B. (1981). Empirical studies in senile dementia with metabolic enhancers and agents that alter blood flow and oxygen utilization. In J. Crook and S. Gershon (Eds.), *Strategies for the development of an effective treatment for senile dementia.* New Canaan, CT: Mark Powley Associates.
87. ROBERTS, G. W., CROW, T. J., & POLAK, J. M. (1985). Location of neuronal tangles in somatostatin neurones in Alzheimer's disease. *Nature, 314*, 92.
88. ROCCA, W. A., AMADUCCI, L. A., & SCHOENBERG, B. S. (1984). Projected demographic trends for the elderly population between 1980 and 2000: Implications for senile dementia prevalence. *Proceedings of the scientific meeting of the World Federation of Neurology Research Committee on Neuroepidemiology.* Boston: WFN Research Committee on Neuroepidemiology.
89. ROGERS, J. D., BROGAN, D., & MIRRA, S. S. (1985). The nucleus basalis of Meynert in neurological disease: A quantitative morphological study. *Annals of Neurology, 17*, 163.
90. ROSSOR, M. N., IVERSEN, L. L., REYNOLDS, G. P., MOUNTJOY, C. Q., & ROTH, M. (1984). Neurochemical characteristics of early and late onset types of Alzheimer's disease. *British Medical Journal, 288*, 961.
91. SAINSBURY, P., & GRAD DE ALARCON, J. (1970). The psychiatrist and the geriatric patient: The effects of community care on the family of the geriatric patient. *Journal of Geriatric Psychiatry, 4*, 23.
92. ST. CLAIR, D., & WHALLEY, L. J. (1983). Hypertension, multi-infarct dementia and Alzheimer's disease. *British Journal of Psychiatry, 143*, 274.
93. SELTZER, B., & SHERWIN, I. (1983). A comparison of clinical features in early- and late-onset primary degenerative dementia: One entity or two? *Archives of Neurology, 40*, 143.
94. SERBY, M., CORWIN, J., CONRAD, P., & ROTROSEN, J. (1985). Olfactory dysfunction in Alzheimer's disease and Parkinson's disease. *American Journal of Psychiatry, 142*, 781.
95. SHORE, D., & WYATT, R. J. (1983). Aluminum and Alzheimer's disease. *Journal of Nervous & Mental Disorders, 171*, 553.

96. STERNBERG, E., & GAWRILOWA, S. (1978). Über klinischepidemiologische Untersuchungen in der sowjetischen Aterspsychiatrie. *Nervenarzt, 49*, 347.

97. STRUBLE, R. G., CORK, L. C., WHITEHOUSE, P. J., & PRICE, D. L. (1982). Cholinergic innervation in neuritic plaques. *Science, 216*, 413.

98. SULKAVA, R., HALTIA, M., PAETAU, A., WIKSTRÖM, J., & PALO, J. (1983). Accuracy of clinical diagnosis in primary degenerative dementia: Correlation with neuropathological findings. *Journal of Neurology, Neurosurgery & Psychiatry, 46*, 9.

99. SULKAVA, R., WIKSTRÖM, J., AROMAA, A., RAITASALO, R., LEHTINEN, V., LAHTELA, K., & PALO, J. (1985). Prevalence of severe dementia in Finland. *Neurology, 35*, 1025.

100. TODOROV, A. B., GO, R. C. P., CONSTANTINIDIS, J., & ELSTON, R. C. (1975). Specificity of the clinical diagnosis of dementia. *Journal of the Neurological Sciences, 26*, 81.

101. TOMLINSON, B. E., BLESSED, G., & ROTH, M. (1970). Observations on the brains of demented old people. *Journal of the Neurological Sciences, 11*, 205.

102. ULRICH, J. (1985). Alzheimer changes in nondemented patients younger than sixty-five: Possible early stages of Alzheimer's disease and senile dementia of Alzheimer type. *Annals of Neurology, 17*, 273.

103. WEINREB, H. J. (1985). Fingerprint patterns in Alzheimer's disease. *Archives of Neurology, 42*, 50.

104. WEYERER, S. (1983). Mental disorders among the elderly: True prevalence and use of medical services. *Archives of Gerontology & Geriatrics, 2*, 11.

105. WHALLEY, L. J., CAROTHERS, A. D., COLLYER, S., DE MEY, R., & FRACKIEWICZ, A. (1982). A study of familial factors in Alzheimer's disease. *British Journal of Psychiatry, 140*, 249.

106. WHALLEY, L. J., & HOLLOWAY, S. (1985). Non-random geographical distribution of Alzheimer's presenile dementia in Edinburgh, 1953–76. *Lancet, 1*, 578.

107. WHITEHOUSE, P. J., PRICE, D. L., STRUBLE, R. G., CLARK, A. W., COYLE, J. T., & DE LONG, M. R. (1982). Alzheimer's disease and senile dementia: Loss of neurons in the basal forebrain. *Science, 215*, 1237.

108. WILCOCK, G. K., & ESIRI, M. M. (1982). Plaques, tangles and dementia. *Journal of the Neurological Sciences, 56*, 343.

109. WILLIAMSON, J., STOKOE, I. H., GRAY, S., FISHER, M., SMITH, A., McGHEE, A., & STEPHENSON, E. (1964). Old people at home: Their unreported needs. *Lancet, 1*, 1117.

110. WISNIEWSKI, K. E., WISNIEWSKI, H. M., & WEN, G. Y. (1985). Occurrence of neuropathological changes and dementia of Alzheimer's disease in Down's syndrome. *Annals of Neurology, 17*, 278.

111. WRIGHT, A. F., & WHALLEY, L. J. (1984). Genetics, ageing and dementia. *British Journal of Psychiatry, 145*, 20.

14

SUBCORTICAL DEMENTIAS

GEORGE W. PAULSON, M.D.

and

STEVEN J. HUBER, PH.D.

The Ohio State University College of Medicine,
Department of Neurology, Columbus, Ohio

INTRODUCTION

Subcortical dementia (SCD) is a recently emerging concept that is of value educationally as well as a research hypothesis, even if the concept is misleading when carried to logical extremes. The logical extreme for the concept may suggest that only either cortical or subcortical regions are concerned with dementia, or that all subcortical lesions cause dementia. In fact, dementia might result from limbic, lobar, or quite focal (thalamic) lesions. All psychiatrists and neurologists have experienced changes in labels and nomenclature. During the lifetime of most of the American readers of this chapter the label "chronic brain syndrome" has become passé, and "dementia" now sounds more satisfactory, even more scientific. Chronic brain syndrome became obsolete at the same time that similar labels such as "chronic congestive heart failure" or "chronic obstructive pulmonary disease" became terms quite well accepted by American internists.

Dementia refers to progressive intellectual deterioration that has replaced normal mental function. It is clear that a variety of diseases can cause dementia and that the nature and severity of the dementia vary widely among underlying disease processes. It is logical to classify dementia syndromes by localization, the most parsimonious approach since symptoms are often more dependent on the area of damage than on the etiology of the damage. This chapter focuses on the distinction between cortical and subcortical dementia syndromes, with emphasis placed on the controversial concept of SCD. SCD is more than a simple renaming of a previously described phenomenon and may represent a clinically distinct type of dementia different from the well-described dementia syndromes associated with primarily cortical degeneration.

Cortical Dementia

Cortical dementia is classically associated with degenerative disorders of the cerebral cortex, and dementia of the Alzheimer type (DAT) is the most common example of cortical dementia. Initial symptoms of DAT often involve memory. Amnestic memory is affected severely and deteriorates steadily throughout the course of the disease. With progressive cortical degeneration, impairments of higher-order associative function become evident. There is impairment of both expressive and comprehensive language (aphasia), and patients often misname common objects or fail to remember the name of acquaintances (anomia). Disturbances of perceptual interpretation (agnosia) and deficits in perceptual motor activity (apraxia) are also common in the course of DAT.

The cortical atrophy in DAT is often diffuse, with predominant areas of degeneration in the frontal lobes and hippocampal gyri. Neurofibrillary tangles and senile plaques are classic in DAT, and their prevalence can correlate with severity of dementia (5,53). The lateral ventricles are often enlarged, especially in the frontal and temporal poles, but this is rarely of diagnostic significance early in the disease (10).

There is increasing awareness that for the diagnosis of Alzheimer's disease, as of this time, there is nothing better than careful clinical assessment. Computerized-tomography (CT) scan may reveal atrophy and certainly rules out other disorders such as tumor. The electroencephalogram (EEG) is abnormal at least as often as CT, but mild slowing on EEG can be associated with many nonspecific disorders, including normal aging. By combining clinical and laboratory studies to rule out other more treatable disorders, clinicians are probably correct in 85 percent of the cases diagnosed as DAT.

Subcortical Dementia

Albert, Feldman, and Willis (3) were among the first to introduce the concept of SCD. This concept was derived from their analysis of the intellectual disturbance in progressive supranuclear palsy (PSP), a disease associated with a predominantly subcortical pathology (1). Patients with PSP have gait disturbance, expressionless facies, and impaired ocular movement, especially with downward gaze. Emotional disturbances are also seen, including forced laughter or crying similar to that of pseudobulbar palsy. Changes in personality and affective changes such as apathy and depression may appear. In the study of Albert, Feldman, and Willis (3), the intellectual disturbance was characterized by impairment in memory and pronounced slowing of mentation, but no disturbance in language, perception, or apraxia. Thus patients with PSP lacked the characteristic changes of the cortical dementia seen in DAT; this pattern was termed SCD.

Subcortical dementia suggests levels, implies a clinical distinction from cortical dementia, and may suggest a dementia resulting from degeneration of basal ganglia or brain stem that is unique in presentation. Many of our concepts related to levels reflect back to the writings of Hughlings Jackson (29) and his concept of "dissolution" of the nervous system. If one area is damaged, a region previously suppressed or inhibited by the damaged area becomes more apparent or distorted in its function. Jackson's concepts came from even earlier ideas of Herbert Spencer, including the philosophy of levels in society. Prior to any Victorian concepts of levels in society, or in the nervous system, the Greeks spoke of the golden mean. Some sort of golden mean, homeostasis, or balance between regions has been employed and reemployed by medicine to interpret physiological and clinical phenomena. Homeostasis itself implies too much, too little, or too rapidly changing (18,46), and certainly many of our interpretations of function in the nervous system rely on the idea of a balance or of the interrelationship between levels. Any discussion of the anatomy of emotion, for example, is likely to include observations on frontal lobe injury, defects generated by medial temporal insults, or a discussion of the coordination between limbic and cortical regions. The cortical/subcortical distinction in "dementia" refers to a balance between predominantly cortical and subcortical degeneration, and the presumed differential clinical outcome.

In addition to concepts of balance between areas, one can conceive of localization of behavioral phenomena in three axes (52). There is (1) a vertical axis for localization, which includes arousal, attention, memory, and associations, (2) a horizontal axis, which includes an anterior area for executive control and a posterior center for intellectual control, and (3) a lateral axis with the left hemisphere primarily concerned with language and the right hemisphere with nonlanguage functions such as visuospatial processing and the total Gestalt. It is thus no surprise that we use and reuse the concept of levels, homeostasis, and balance; and a new concept that suggests a relationship between regions can be rapidly assimilated into clinical medicine. "Subcortical dementia" is a new concept, becoming assimilated, and implies levels.

CLINICAL CHARACTERISTICS OF SCD

Table 1 lists some of the neurological diseases in which there could be SCD. The distinguishing features between SCD and disorders that cause cortical dementia are listed in Table 2. Motor deficits are prominent in most of the conditions in which SCD occurs. For example, in Wilson's disease one may observe a fatuous expression, tremor, and rigidity. Patients with Parkinson's disease (PD) classically have rigidity and akinesia. Huntington's disease (HD) is usually associated with chorea. Patients who have dementia due to subcortical insults following head injury often have slowed mental function, as well as prominent spasticity. It is possible that multiple sclerosis (MS) is another variety of SCD, and most patients with MS have motor deficits.

Mental status is clearly distinct in cortical and subcortical syndromes. Cortical dementia is assumed to be more severe and to progress at a more rapid rate than the subcortical syndromes. The nature of the intellectual dysfunction is also distinct. The hallmarks of cortical dementia — aphasia, agnosia, and apraxia — are typically absent in subcortical disorders. Let us now look individually at some of the conditions that may be manifestations of SCD.

Huntington's Disease

HD has, from the time that George Huntington first described it in 1872 (28), been associated with the genetic trait, chorea (and in a few, rigidity), as well as mental deterioration. Aphasia is not usually present, but in late stages the patients may become almost mute — although remaining aware. Woody Guthrie, the American folk singer, seemed to understand the people around him and to respond to kindness even in the terminal phase of HD (21). Speech may be marred by stops and starts, or be interrupted by clicks in the throat, or by jerky and inappropriate motor behavior. It is the impulsivity, lack of general bodily care, and movement disorder that usually lead to custodial care. Depression and suicidal efforts have all been emphasized by those who have written about the disease, and in earlier times patients were commonly classed as schizophrenic.

Table 1
Subcortical Dementing
Disorders

Progressive supranuclear palsy
Huntington's disease
Parkinson's disease
Wilson's disease

Intellectual decline in HD has classically been associated with cortical degeneration, particularly in the frontal regions, and the movement disorder was assumed to reflect striatal degeneration (12). McHugh and Folstein (39) provided an extensive examination of the nature of the intellectual changes in patients with HD. They found prominent slowing of mentation, impairment of memory, personality or affective changes in-

Table 2
Distinguishing Features of Cortical and Subcortical Dementia

Characteristics	Subcortical	Cortical
Mental state		
Language	Normal	Aphasia
Memory	Forgetful	Amnestic
Visuospatial skills	Impaired (moderate)	Impaired (severe)
Cognition	Impaired (slowed, forgetfulness, impaired problem-solving strategy)	Impaired (severe, amnesia, agnosia, apraxia, acalculia)
Personality	Depressed or apathetic	Normal (unaware, lack of insight)
Motor system		
Posture	Impaired (stopped, twisted)	Normal
Gait	Impaired (ataxic)	Normal
Movement	Impaired (chorea, rigidity, tremor)	Normal
Speech	Impaired (dysarthria, hypophonia)	Normal
Activity	Impaired (slow)	Normal

cluding apathy and depression, but no associative dysfunction such as
aphasia, agnosia, or apraxia. Based on their findings, they suggested HD
may be another example of subcortical dementia.

Parkinson's Disease

PD has also been described as being consistent with the concept of SCD
(2,4,17,36). Of all the degenerative disorders of the central nervous system
associated with dementia, PD may be the most complex. In his classic
work, Parkinson (45) described a clinical syndrome characterized by trem-
or, akinesia, and rigidity, with "the senses and intellects being uninjured."
However, Charcot (15) suggested that "at a given time the mind becomes
clouded and the memory is lost" (p. 159), and most clinicians feel that
intellectual impairment forms an integral part of the disease in many of
the patients. Recent neuropsychological studies indicated significant intellectual impairment in patients with PD as compared to age-matched controls (14,31,32,35,42,49). PD patients have been shown to have impairment of visuospatial skills (7–9,48), impairment in memory (24,48,54,55),
and significant depression (11,14,25,37,42,50,56). The nature of the intellectual impairment in PD, including that due primarily to a lack of cortical features, has been clinically described as another example of SCD.

The estimates of dementia in PD vary widely, and the frequency may
depend on what phase of the disease or what population group is studied.
Many clinicians suspect that 15 to 20 percent of patients suffer from mental
defects very early in the course of the disorder. Lieberman et al. (31)
suggested that there is a subgroup of patients with PD who not only develop dementia early, but for whom standard levodopa or anticholinergic
medication is less likely to be helpful. Some such patients may have
"*Parkinson plus*" and include cases of DAT with extrapyramidal features
(47), as well as conditions such as Shy-Drager syndrome, PSP, and
striatonigral degeneration, all of which may resemble PD. Overt cortical
atrophy has been reported in PD for several decades. Boller et al. (7) and
Hakim and Mathieson (23) found pathological changes in the cortex of
some patients with PD to be indistinguishable from DAT (senile plaques
and neurofibrillary tangles). PD patients with prominent cortical degeneration also tend to be more severely demented.

Patients with PD are commonly depressed; indeed depression may be an
initial feature of the disease. Even if the patient with PD is not depressed,
the somatic changes (sex, sleep, appetite, facies, activity) of depression are
very similar to those noted in PD. Finally, and a nagging concern for all

clinicians, the drugs most effective in PD often also produce hallucinations and confusion. It has even been suggested that the use of levodopa will rapidly accelerate the intellectual decline in PD patients with severe dementia (31,51). Even when patients are not demented, even without drugs, the classic akinesia in PD may look like the abulia of frontal lobe disease.

Wilson's Disease

The psychological aspects of Wilson's disease have been less well studied than the motor phenomena (40). There have been no specific studies of Wilson's disease as a form of SCD. Mental changes, including decline in school performance and affective disorders, are common. Clinicians may see patients for psychosis, but the motor phenomena are so dramatic that changes in mentation are usually ignored. Tremor can be severe, and rigidity (particularly, as in HD in children) can be present in limbs and the facial musculature. Resemblance to multiple sclerosis led to the label pseudosclerosis in the past century, and patients with Wilson's disease are still occasionally misdiagnosed as having a demyelinative disorder. Therapy is known both to lessen the motor disability and to improve mental function.

Brain Trauma

Trauma is probably the greatest crippler of the brain of the previously well young population. Trauma clearly affects both cortical and subcortical areas. As in other examples of SCD, brain-injured patients manifest abnormalities in motor function. Slowness, frequently combined with spasticity, is a characteristic of some of the more severely handicapped brain-injured patients, many of whom also lack "motivation." The pathology in this group is mixed and includes patients who have had penetrating wounds, infections, hematomata, and so forth. Many of the patients with residual defects in intellectual function after trauma have sustained multiple petechiae, tears, and sheering effects in the white matter. Widespread lesions in the association pathways lead to residual spasticity and often a persistent slowness in function.

Another example of the effect of trauma is "dementia pugilistica." Classically the "punch-drunk" person has a shuffling gait, slurred speech, and slowed verbal and intellectual performance. Some ex-boxers have had dilated ventricles and a cavum septum pellucidum that probably resulted from repeated subcortical and cortical insults that disrupt association pathways.

Multiple Sclerosis

In as many as 5 percent of patients, multiple sclerosis (MS) may present with intellectual deficits (58). After patients are severely affected by the disease, most experience deterioration in cognitive function. To the clinician the change is poorly defined and is linked with motor incapacity that has prompted dependence and withdrawal from employment. Family members are often keenly aware of the mental changes and the patient's emotional vulnerability can be prominent. The classic euphoria associated with MS is more a pattern of tangential and inappropriate thought than a true veneer of happiness. Most patients, at one time or another, are in fact depressed. Magnetic resonance imaging (MRI) studies, a flood of which have now been reported (20,34), document the common phenomenon of multiple lesions but reveal only a partial clinical or cognitive correlation with the number and size of the lesions. Patients may have severe MS but only a handful of crucially placed lesions, or may have multiple lesions on MRI although they look well. Dementia, in our recent study, did not correlate with plaque size or number but was often evident when the corpus callosum had become thinned — presumably reflecting the loss of association pathways that traverse the callosum. Neuropsychological performance of patients with MS defined as demented was consistent with the concept of subcortical dementia.

Multiinfarct Dementia

Multiinfarct Dementia (22) has been variously described and does not mean the same phenomena we used to label, so sloppily, "chronic brain syndrome associated with arteriosclerosis." The CT scan and MRI have made it possible to diagnose multiinfarct dementia before autopsy. Small "lacunar" infarctions may occur in patients with hypertension, diabetes, or cardiac disease (43). Some of these patients have clumsy hands and are dysarthric or display a purely motor or purely sensory loss, and many are mentally slowed. In addition, patients can have major repeated "minor" infarctions, which lead to so much loss of cortical tissue that there is insidious decline in intellectual function. As many as 50 percent of patients who develop a clear-cut major cerebral infarction are discovered to have had another more silent infarction at an earlier time. This phenomenon is particularly true for embolic processes, some of which affect small as well as large vessels.

In addition to multiinfarct dementia, whether due to small lacunae or to larger infarctions, and in addition to movement disorders, there are a host of other processes, including toxic, metabolic, and infectious disturbances, that affect both cortical and subcortical areas. For this reason it is obvious that the precise behavioral phenomenology noted in any one case of SCD can be expected to vary greatly.

As can be noted from the above discussion of separate diseases, a great complexity is present in the concept of SCD, certainly a greater variety of diseases than was initially suggested. It is possible that between the diseases associated with SCD there are different characteristics of mental disturbance produced by each disorder. Even though the nature of dementia in subcortical syndromes is similar, they may be quite different in terms of severity. In addition, the nature of specific characteristics that define subcortical dementia may be quite different for separate diseases. Depression is an early feature of PD, but the somatic aspects of depression and of PD are so similar that definition becomes difficult. Sexual dysfunction, restless sleep, change in appetite, and reduced activity are common somatic complaints of patients with PD.

Even among patients with the same disease, there can be striking differences. As seen in PD, a subgroup has dementia early, characterized by extensive cortical degeneration similar to DAT; medications used to treat PD may be ineffective and exacerbate mental illness for these patients (31,51). All medicines used for PD, both anticholinergic drugs and levodopa, can produce mental confusion. Above and beyond all the features of deterioration in PD and the effects of therapy there is a suggestion that some patients who develop Parkinsonism may have an underlying preexisting obsessive compulsive personality or other unique psychological features that predispose to the illness and even to depressive states. This may also represent a separate patient group. How can one expect all these subtleties of PD to be subsumed under any single label such as SCD?

IS THERE A DIFFERENCE BETWEEN SUBCORTICAL AND CORTICAL DEMENTIA?

There is some neurochemical evidence that suggests a distinction between dementia of PD and that in DAT. The primary neurochemical change in PD is a loss of dopamine from nigrostriatal pathways. In DAT the cholinergic system is primarily involved and results in loss of acetylcholine in the cerebral cortex. Loss of dopamine is mild in patients with DAT

(13), and the cholinergic system is often hyperactive in patients with PD (26). Mortimer and his associates (44) demonstrated a correlation between degree of intellectual impairment and motoric impairment (bradykinesia and rigidity) in patients with PD. This finding suggests a common mechanism related to movement and intellectual function, and there is a suggestion that levodopa, which is so effective to treat PD, may also improve intellectual performance (24,33). Levodopa has no effect on intellectual performance in patients with DAT (30,41).

Another striking difference between cortical and subcortical syndromes relates to neurological and motoric findings. Patients with subcortical syndromes typically have extensive motor abnormalities. Posture may be stooped and twisted; gait is often ataxic; and tremor, chorea, and dystonia are common. Most subcortical disorders affect speech articulation and cause dysarthia. This is in sharp contrast to findings of patients with DAT, where there is usually a lack of neurological abnormality. Patients with DAT, until very late stages, have a normal general neurological examination (16). Posture is erect, gait is crisp and unaffected, there are no visual field defects, and the patient is alert with retention of social graces. In fact, family members often report that the patient appears to be in better health, and may even look younger, than he has for many years. Aside from the obvious and severe loss of intellectual capability, patients with DAT usually manifest no physical findings.

Objective Confirmation of Subcortical Dementia

It is uncertain that laboratory tests of various types will be helpful for the separation of cortical from subcortical disorders. EEG may reflect cortical electrical function but does not distinguish most of the diseases that cause SCD. CT scan will show major changes such as infarction or tumor, but minor deterioration is less obvious. It is probably true that MRI, and when available the PET scan, will be more useful than CT. MRI is becoming the method of choice to demonstrate the plaques of multiple sclerosis. Many older individuals who don't have MS will show small punctate areas throughout the white matter and gray matter, perhaps representing fluid around vessels and shrinkage of the tissue close by. As of this time, however, there is no specific diagnostic laboratory test for most of the various conditions called SCD, and SCD remains, along with cortical dementia, a clinical impression. Logically the distinction might best be sought via psychological testing, but this work remains fragmented.

Mayeux et al. (38) and Whitehouse (57) suggested that SCD lacks clinical validation and has a questionable pathological basis. Quantitative neuropsychological assessment may reveal no distinctive pattern for SCD. These authors have suggested that the pattern of dementia in diseases such as PD and HD may result from a combination of both cortical and subcortical degeneration. The pattern of psychological testing, the selection of patients, and the interpretation of results are all open for discussion. Intellectual impairment is to be expected in each and every case of DAT, but this may not be the case for all types of subcortical disorders.

So, is SCD accepted? Certainly not completely. According to Mayeux et al. (38), SCD is not truly distinctive, perhaps even inaccurate, and use of the terms cortical and subcortical for the description of dementia is at best "problematic." We agree with Mayeux that cortical degeneration does occur in HD, and cortical degeneration also certainly can occur in PD. Furthermore, the changes noted in the nucleus basalis of Meynert and in the locus ceruleus in DAT are in fact subcortical, not cortical, in location.

Whitehouse (57) has strongly suggested that there are not sufficient clinical, neuropathological, or neurochemical studies to support the concept of SCD and states that adequate systematic studies have not been performed. Nevertheless, Whitehouse also notes that different types of dementia seem self-evident to clinicians even though precise or scientific characterization is difficult. The concept of a subcortical, in addition to a cortical, dementia has stimulated considerable interest and does raise the chance to reclassify the dementias. For example, perhaps all dementias can be classified into two categories, those with major physical features and those without. Both Mayeux and Whitehouse emphasize that even though substantial clinical evidence supports the distinction between cortical and subcortical dementia, the distinction remains uncertain owing to lack of carefully controlled neuropsychological studies that directly compare patients with presumed cortical and subcortical dementia.

The study provided by Mayeux and his associates (38) is a major improvement over previous research related to the cortical/subcortical distinction. Patients with PD and DAT were directly compared on neuropsychological performance, and distinctions were examined. These researchers compared performance on a lengthened version of the Mini-Mental State Examination (19). Their approach was to match the patient groups in terms of overall intellectual deterioration, determined by total score on their version of the Mini-Mental State Examination, and to examine whether there was a distinct pattern of neuropsychological deficits in terms of performance on subtest measures. The basic finding was that the two patient groups could not be characterized by qualitative neuropsychological differences, and the authors concluded that the concept of subcortical dementia is of questionable validity. While this is an important paper, it can be criticized for several reasons. First, the Mini-Mental State Examination is not specifically designed to detect differences between dementing syndromes. The procedure was designed to confirm the presence and assess the severity of dementia. Thus, it is possible that both patient groups achieved low scores on this mental status scale for different reasons.

Another problem with this research was the attempt to match the patient groups in terms of dementia severity, as defined by total scores on the Mini-Mental State Examination. We recognize that because dementia is often progressive, it is generally appropriate to match patient groups prior to examination of qualitative differences in various syndromes of dementia. This approach may not, however, be appropriate or adequate to evaluate the cortical/subcortical hypothesis. One of the previously recognized features of SCD is that "the intellectual impairment is more mild . . . than (in) the cortical dementias" (17, p. 874). Thus, matching patient groups in terms of intellectual severity does not allow examination of one critical aspect of the concept. Two other problems exist in the effort to match DAT and PD patients for severity of dementia. First is the issue of what constitutes an appropriate measure of dementia severity. Mayeux and associates (38) used the total score on their version of the Mini-Mental State Examination to equate patient groups. This procedure may reduce the likelihood of detecting differences in subtest performance since the patient groups had essentially the same total score. When their patient groups were compared while retaining functional disability appropriate to each disease, their results suggested qualitative neuropsychological differences between patient groups. A second problem is the likelihood that the more severely demented PD patients may have mixed Parkinsonism and Alzheimer's dementia, thereby blurring any possible neuropsychological distinctions. Boller et al. (6) found more severely demented PD patients to have pathological findings indistinguishable from those of patients with DAT.

We recently completed an investigation of the possible distinction between cortical and subcortical dementia by comparing patients with DAT, PD, and normal controls and used a neuropsychological test battery specifically designed to evaluate the proposed clinical differences (27). This battery included measures of overall mental functions, memory, language, apraxia, attention, visuospatial skills, and a scale for depression.

The results were quite different from the previous report of Mayeux and his associates (38). Severity of overall intellectual impairment, as measured by the Mini-Mental State Examination, was greater for patients with DAT compared to PD. Patients with PD and DAT were impaired in relation to controls on measures of cognition, memory, and visuospatial skills, but the severity of these deficits was significantly greater in DAT patients. Both patient groups had higher depression scores compared to controls. Unlike the PD patients, patients with DAT were significantly impaired on all measures of language and praxis.

In summary, the work by Cummings, Benson, and Albert suggests that SCD is a useful as well as an emerging concept, and many other authors confirm their opinion. SCD is a clinical syndrome characterized by slowness of mental processing, impairment in memory, disturbance of visuospatial skills, apathy, and perhaps depression. Though first recognized in PSP and HD, the concept has now been extended to PD, Wilson's disease, several forms of degeneration or calcification of the basal ganglia, multiinfarct dementia, and perhaps also the dementia syndrome of depression. Multiple sclerosis and head trauma may produce similar intellectual disturbances. The lesions primarily involved are in basal ganglia, white matter, and the brain stem nuclei. The clinical characteristics differ significantly from the dementia of DAT, where the cerebral and cortical involvement produces aphasia, amnesia, agnosia, and apraxia, and motor deficits are more common in SCD.

The best overall current summary may be that of Benson (4): "It is obvious that the clinical features alone provide a clear distinction for two types of dementia. . . . on the basis of the striking clinical differences acceptance of the two types of dementia would appear mandatory" (p. 189). The basic clinical differences between cortical and subcortical dementia seem clear. The distinction in terms of neurochemical, psychological, and pathological differences is less clear, however, and awaits future research. In addition, the specific characteristics of the many subcortical syndromes have not as yet been clearly delineated. The role of medication in terms of dementia related to subcortical disorders is also unknown. We feel the basic clinical distinction is sound and provides a useful framework for research related to these important clinical issues.

REFERENCES

1. ADAMS, R. D., & VICTOR, M. (1981). *Principles of neurology*. New York: McGraw-Hill.
2. ALBERT, M. (1978). Subcortical dementia. In R. Katzman, R. D. Terry, & K. L. Bick (Eds.), *Alzheimer's disease: Senile dementia and related disorders*. New York: Raven Press.

3. ALBERT, M. L., FELDMAN, R. G., & WILLIS, A. L. (1974). The subcortical dementia of progressive supranuclear palsy. *Journal of Neurology, Neurosurgery & Psychiatry*, 37, 121-130.

4. BENSON, D. F. (1983). Subcortical dementia: A clinical approach. In R. Mayeux & W. G. Rosen (Eds.), *The dementias: Advances in neurology*, vol. 38. New York: Raven Press.

5. BLESSED, G., TOMLINSON, B. E., & ROTH, M. (1968). The association between quantitative measures of dementia and of senile change in the cerebral grey matter of elderly subjects. *British Journal of Psychiatry, 114*, 797-811.

6. BOLLER, F., MIZUTANI, T., ROSESSMANN, U., et al. (1980). Parkinson's disease dementia, and Alzheimer's disease: Clinicopathological correlations. *Annals of Neurology, 7*, 329-335.

7. BOLLER, F., PASSATIUME, D., KEEFE, N. C., et al. (1984). Visuospatial impairments in Parkinson's disease. *Archives of Neurology, 41*, 485-490.

8. BOWEN, F., HOEHN, M. M., & YAHR, M. D. (1972). Parkinsonism: Alterations in spatial orientations as determined by a route-walking task. *Neuropsychologia, 10*, 355-361.

9. BOWEN, F. P. (1976). Behavioral alterations in patients with basal ganglia lesions. In M. D. Yahr (Ed.), *The basal ganglia* (pp. 169-177). New York: Raven Press.

10. BRADSHAW, J. R., THOMSON, J. L., & CAMPBELL, M. J. (1983). Computed tomography in the investigation of dementia. *British Medical Journal, 22*, 277-280.

11. BROWN, G. L., & WILSON, W. P. (1972). Parkinsonism and depression. *Southern Medical Journal, 65*, 540-545.

12. BRUYN, G. W. (1969). Huntington's chorea. In P. J. Vinken & G. W. Bruyn (Eds.), *Handbook of clinical neurology*, vol. 6: Diseases of the Basal Ganglia. New York: Wiley Interscience.

13. CARLSSON, A., GOTTFRIES, C. G., SVENNERHOLM, L., et al. (1980). Neurotransmitters in human brain analyzed post mortem: Changes in normal aging, senile dementia and chronic alcoholism. In U. K. Rinne, M. Klinger, & G. Stamm (Eds.), *Parkinson's disease: Current progress, problems and management* (pp. 121-133). New York: Elsevier North Holland.

14. CELESIA, G. G., & WANAMAKER, W. M. (1972). Psychiatric disturbance in Parkinson's disease. *Disorders of the Nervous System, 33*, 577-583.

15. CHARCOT, J. M. (1875). Quoted in Boller, *Journal of Clinical Neuropsychology, 2*, 157-172, 1980.

16. CUMMINGS, J. L., & BENSON, D. F. (1983). *Dementia: A clinical approach*. Woburn, MA: Butterworths.

17. CUMMINGS, J. L., & BENSON, D. F. (1984). Subcortical dementia: Review of an emerging concept. *Archives of Neurology, 41*, 874-879.

18. DAVIS, H. (1950). Homeostasis of cerebral excitability. *Electroencephalography & Clinical Neurophysiology, 2*, 243.

19. FOLSTEIN, M. F., FOLSTEIN, S. E., & McHUGH, P. R. (1975). "Mini-Mental State": A practical guide for grading the mental state of patients for the clinician. *Journal of Psychiatry Research, 12*, 189-198.

20. GEBARSKI, S. S., GABRIELSON, T. O., GILMAN, S., et al. (1985). The initial diagnosis of multiple sclerosis: Clinical impact of resonance imaging. *Annals of Neurology, 17*, 469-474.

21. GUTHRIE, M. Personal communications.

22. HACHINSKI, V. C., LASSEN, N. A., & MARSHALL, J. (1974). Multi-infarct dementia: A cause of mental deterioration in the elderly. *Lancet, 3*, 207-210.

23. HAKIM, A. M., & MATHIESON, G. (1979). Dementia in Parkinson disease: A neuropathologic study. *Neurology* (New York) 29, 1209-1214.

24. HALGIN, R., RIKLAN, M., & MISIAK, H. (1977). Levodopa, Parkinsonism, and recent memory. *Journal of Nervous Mental Disorders, 164*, 268-272.

25. HORN, S. (1974). Some psychological factors in Parkinsonism. *Journal of Neurology, Neurosurgery & Psychiatry, 37*, 27–31.
26. HORNYKIEWICZ, O. (1982). Brain neurotransmitter changes in Parkinson's disease. In C. D. Marsden & S. Fahn (Eds.), *Movement disorders* (pp. 41–58). Boston: Butterworths.
27. HUBER, S. J., SHUTTLEWORTH, E. C., PAULSON, G. W., et al. (1986). Cortical vs subcortical dementia: Neuropsychological differences. *Archives of Neurology, 43*, 392–394.
28. HUNTINGTON, G. (1872). On chorea. *Medical Surgical Reports, 26*, 317.
29. JACKSON, J. H. (1931). Selected writings of John Hughlings Jackson. J. Taylor (Ed.), vol. II. London: Hodden & Stoughton.
30. KRISTENSEN, V., OLSEN, M., & THEILGAARD, A. (1977). Levodopa treatment of presenile dementia. *Acta Psychiatrica Scandinavica, 55*, 41–51.
31. LIEBERMAN, A., DZIATOLOWSKI, M., KUPERSMITH, M., et al. (1979). Dementia in Parkinson's disease. *Annals of Neurology, 6*, 355–359.
32. LORANGER, A. W., GOODELL, H., LEE, J. E., et al. (1972). Intellectual impairments in Parkinson's syndrome. *Brain, 95*, 405–412.
33. LORANGER, A. W., GOODELL, H., LEE, J. E., et al. (1972). Levodopa treatment in Parkinson's syndrome. *Archives of General Psychiatry, 26*, 163–168.
34. LUKES, S. A., CROOKS, L. E., AMINOFF, M. J., et al. (1983). Nuclear magnetic resonance imaging in multiple sclerosis. *Annals of Neurology 13*, 592–601.
35. MARTIN, W. E., LOEWENSON, R. B., RESCH, J. A., et al. (1973). Parkinson's disease: Clinical analysis of 100 patients. *Neurology, 23*, 783–790.
36. MAYEUX, R., & STERN, Y. (1983). Intellectual dysfunction and dementia in Parkinson's disease. In R. Mayeux & W. G. Rosen (Eds.), *The dementias: Advances in neurology*, vol. 38. New York: Raven Press.
37. MAYEUX, R., STERN, Y., ROSEN, J., & LEVENTHAL, J. (1981). Depression, intellectual impairment, and Parkinson disease. *Neurology, 31*, 645–650.
38. MAYEUX, R., STERN, Y., ROSEN, J., et al. (1983). Is "subcortical dementia" a recognizable clinical entity? *Annals of Neurology, 14*, 278–283.
39. MCHUGH, P. R., & FOLSTEIN, M. F. (1975). Psychiatric syndromes of Huntington's chorea: A clinical and phenomenological study. In B. F. Benson & D. Blumer (Eds.), *Psychiatric aspects of neurological disease*. New York: Grune & Stratton.
40. MENKS, J. H. (1984). Disorders of mental metabolism. In L. P. Rowland (Ed.), *Merritt's textbook of neurology*. Philadelphia: Lea & Febiger.
41. MEYER, J. S., WELCH, K. M. A., OESHMUKH, V. D., et al. (1977). Neurotransmitter precursor amino acids in the treatment of multi-infarct dementia and Alzheimer's disease. *Journal of the American Geriatric Society, 25*, 289–298.
42. MINDHAM, R. H. S. (1970). Psychiatric symptoms in Parkinsonism. *Journal of Neurology, Neurosurgery & Psychiatry, 33*, 188–191.
43. MOHR, J. P. (1986). Lacunes. In H. J. M. Barrett, B. M. Stein, J. P. Mohr, & F. M. Yatsu (Eds.), *Stroke: Pathophysiology, diagnosis, and management, vol. 1*. London: Churchill Livingston.
44. MORTIMER, J. A., PIRROZZULO, F. J., HANSCH, E. C., et al. (1982). Relationship of motor symptoms to intellectual deficits in Parkinson's disease. *Neurology, 32*, 133–137.
45. PARKINSON, J. (1817). *An essay on the shaking palsy*. London: Neely and Jones.
46. PAULSON, G. W. (1961). Concept of homeostasis in the central nervous system. *Disorders of the Nervous System, 22*, 667–671.
47. PEARCE, J. (1974). The extrapyramidal disorder of Alzheimer's disease. *European Neurology, 12*, 94–103.
48. PIROZZOLO, F. J., HANSCH, E. C., MORTIMER, J. A., et al. (1982). Dementia in Parkinson disease: A neuropsychological analysis. *Brain and Cognition, 1*, 71–83.
49. POLLOCK, M., & HORNABROOK, R. W. (1966). The prevalence, natural history and dementia. *Brain, 89*, 429–448.

50. ROBBINS, A. H. (1976). Depression in patients with Parkinsonism. *British Journal of Psychiatry, 128*, 141–145.
51. SACHS, O. W., KOHL, M. S., MESSELOTT, C. R., et al. (1972). Effects of levodopa in Parkinsonism patients with dementia. *Neurology, 22*, 516–519.
52. SMITH, D. B., & CRAFT, R. B. (1984). Sudden behavioral change. In J. B. Green (Ed.), *Neurology clinics 2*. London: Saunders.
53. SULKAVA, R., HALTIA, M., PAETAN, A., et al. (1982). Clinical and neuropathological features of Alzheimer's disease. *Acta Neurologica Scandinavica, 90* (Suppl): 294–295.
54. TALLAND, G. A. (1962). Cognitive function in Parkinson's disease. *Journal of Nervous & Mental Disorders, 135*, 196–205.
55. TWEEDY, J. R., LANGER, K. G., & McDOWELL, F. M. (1982). The effect of semantic relations on the memory deficit associated with Parkinson's disease. *Journal of Clinical Neuropsychology, 4*, 235–247.
56. WARBURTON, J. W. (1967). Depressive symptoms in Parkinson patients referred for thalamotomy. *Journal of Neurology, Neurosurgery & Psychiatry, 30*, 368–370.
57. WHITEHOUSE, P. J. (1986). The concept of subcortical and cortical dementia: Another look. *Annals of Neurology, 19*, 1–6.
58. YOUNG, C., SAUNDERS, J., & PONSFORD, J. R. (1976). Mental change as an early feature of multiple sclerosis. *Journal of Neurology, Neurosurgery & Psychiatry, 39*, 1008–1013.

15

A MULTIDIMENSIONAL
APPROACH TO THE
UNDERSTANDING AND
MANAGEMENT OF BEHAVIOR
DISTURBANCE IN EPILEPSY

SHIRLEY M. FERGUSON, M.D., F.A.P.A.

Professor of Psychiatry and Neurological Surgery (Neuropsychiatry),
Medical College of Ohio, Toledo, Ohio

and

MARK RAYPORT, M.D. C.M., PH.D., F.A.C.S.

Professor and Chairman, Department of Neurological Surgery;
Director, Epilepsy Comprehensive Program,
Medical College of Ohio, Toledo, Ohio

INTRODUCTION

Epilepsy is now widely recognized as a frequent health problem. Its prevalence is estimated at 0.5 to 1 percent of the population (9,26,29). Its severity as a neurological illness ranges from minimal to fatal (9,28). When it is a mild condition, it may be readily livable; when it is an intractable disorder, it greatly burdens not only the patient but also his/her social environment.

Behavioral symptoms have been described in patients with epilepsy throughout recorded medical history (61). Currently, recognition exists among epileptologists that certain patients with epilepsy, particularly those with partial complex seizures of temporolimbic origin*, may have significant behavioral difficulties (20,23,25,37). The nature, pathogenesis, and prevalence of the behavioral problems have remained subject to uncertainty and controversy. However, it is possible, in the individual case, to gain an understanding of the mechanisms of the behavior disturbance and to evolve a therapeutic plan. This requires evaluation with careful multidimensional study and cross-disciplinary thinking. The authors will review the principal behavioral disturbances seen in patients with epilepsy. These descriptions will also exemplify the methodology of the comprehensive assessment which has been helpful to them in understanding and helping their epilepsy patients.

DIFFERENTIAL DIAGNOSIS

American and British epidemiological studies (41,68) have pointed to the difficulties in establishing prevalence rates for psychiatric disturbances in epilepsy, as well as for the proportion of people with psychiatric problems who also have seizures.

Clinical acumen is needed to avoid missing the diagnosis of cerebral seizures, or maintaining it when this diagnosis is incorrect. An apparently ictal event needs to be assessed as to whether it has or has not an organic cerebral origin. It is not rare to find a patient lying in a guarded bed who is toxic with antiepileptic drugs and still "seizing." For clarification, data from the disciplines of neurology, psychiatry, and electroencephalography are necessary. Intensive seizure monitoring with simultaneous electroencephalography (EEG) and closed-circuit television (CCTV) often settles the issue rapidly. But positive psychiatric evidence is also necessary. The

---

*Terminologic Note: The authors are adhering to the terms and definitions of the new International Classification of Seizures (10) in which a partial seizure is described as *simple* or *complex* depending on whether it is or is not associated with alteration of consciousness. Thus, an attack limited to illusion of familiarity (déjà vu) would be a *simple* partial seizure. The "dreamy state" described to Jackson (1888) (32) by his physician–patient would be classified as a *complex* partial seizure. A seizure beginning with a consciously perceived aura of déjà vu followed by automatism (unremembered behavioral episode) would be a partial seizure evolving from simple to complex. Under the new International Classification of Seizures, the term "complex partial seizure" is not synonymous with psychomotor (24) or temporal lobe, a term that denotes an unjustifiedly limited anatomical localization (21,22). A complex partial seizure can have a temporal or a nontemporal origin in the frontal, parietal, or occipital lobe. The localization of the seizure focus must therefore be conveyed with additional language.

patient should not be dismissed after a "negative EEG study" as having "nothing wrong" or be tagged with the wastebasket conclusion of "It's emotional." He/she needs to be studied psychiatrically for an understanding of the emotional factors responsible for the symptomatology. The largest subgroup among patients with pseudoepileptic seizures are those who do have an organic seizure disorder. The most prominent mechanism found among patients with pseudoepileptic seizures is conversion reaction, often with an underlying affective disorder. "Pseudoepileptic seizures" have received considerable attention in the recent literature (42,45,64). On the other hand, the manifestations of temporolimbic seizures may be mistaken for physical or psychiatric illness. Such seizures have come to be a frequent listing in the differential diagnosis of atypical, enigmatic, psychiatric conditions.

DIFFERENCES IN RESEARCH METHODOLOGY AND CLINICAL MATERIAL AS A SOURCE OF CONTROVERSY

Methodological differences may account for some of the persistent controversies and discrepancies in the behavioral literature of epilepsy.

Variations in Patient Sampling

Many reports on behavior in epilepsy are characterized by disparity in the depth and sophistication between the psychiatric and neurological investigations. In some, the diagnosis of epilepsy or of the behavior disturbance leading to inclusion in the study is established referentially: behavioral investigators rely on a nonresearched population of cases of "temporal lobe epilepsy" (2) or neurological investigations on a nonresearched population of cases of "psychosis" (51). The preponderance of published behavioral data on neurosurgically treated cases of epilepsy are neuropsychological, oriented primarily to cognitive functions. In the mental hospital or office practice setting, acquisition of neurological and electroencephalographic data is often scanty, limiting the information for seizure classification and for localization of the epileptogenic mechanism. The validity of investigations characterized by asymmetrical quality of research data must be held in question. Studies based on large numbers of cases essentially yield common factors. Longitudinal study of individual cases performed concurrently by members of a multidisciplinary group eliminates the qualitative and chronological discrepancy between the disciplinary domains of information and is uniquely effective in detecting explanatory factors in the interaction of behavioral and cerebral organic mechanisms involved in the behavioral disturbances in patients with epilepsy.

Emphasis on a Parsimonious Explanation

Among single abnormal processes that have been emphasized are atrophic brain change in the temporal lobe (52), hyperconnection (2), and laterality of the epileptogenic lesion (19). We feel that these are unlikely in themselves to account for the behavioral symptomatology in the individual case. A multifactorial explanation seems more accurate (7,14,18,38).

Emphasis on an Objective Approach

Behavior in epilepsy has been investigated also under blind research protocols with standardized psychological tests or psychiatric interviews on matched study populations of temporal lobe epilepsy (TLE), generalized epilepsy (GE), and nonepileptic control patients. The quantitative results thus obtained were statistically treated. No significant differences were found between the TLE and GE group (53,55) or these two groups and nonepileptic controls (27,53). The enumerative approach to behavioral symptoms inherent in such research designs may not be sensitive to mild or fluctuating impairment of a paroxysmal brain disorder or because the behavioral findings are necessarily acquired outside of a relational matrix. The latter would be comparable to confining the comparison of the paintings of Gainsborough and Turner to planimetric quantification of their use of selected colors. With computerized psychiatric interviews that relied on Schneiderian first-rank symptoms for diagnosis of schizophrenia, patients with epilepsy and psychosis were found to be indistinguishable from nonepileptic patients who had nuclear schizophrenia (39). Both method and results have received fundamental critique (8,38).

CLINICAL MATERIAL AND METHODS

The authors' findings are based on the longitudinal observation and treatment of over 425 patients with chronic drug-refractory seizure disorders, of whom more than 133 have received detailed multidisciplinary evaluations in the neurological, neuropsychiatric, neuroradiological, electroencephalographic, social work, and neuropsychological spheres.

Seizure histories were routinely obtained from the patient and from eyewitnesses of the seizures by at least the neurosurgeon and the neuropsychiatrist. The minimum data acquisition by the neuropsychiatrist involved a structured interview which was expanded as indicated by the opportunities of the developing information. The neuropsychiatrist's objective was to assess personality, intrapsychic dynamics, interpersonal dynamics, cognitive and other higher nervous functions, the experience of living with seizures, and the interaction between the epilepsy experience and the individual's psychological resources. The structured neuropsychiatric interview is outlined in Table 1. Electroencephalograms were obtained in the diagnostic setting with scalp leads (10–20 International System), nasopharyngeal, sphenoidal, or zygomatic electrodes, and supplementary scalp electrodes as indicated, with the patient awake, asleep, and in sleep-deprived diurnal sleep. Prior to 1975, patients being evaluated for possible neurosurgical intervention for seizure control underwent intravenous EEG activation with pentetrazol. Since 1977, spontaneous seizures have been recorded simultaneously with video and EEG, with split-screen technology, while antiepileptic drugs (AED) were being progressively withdrawn, if necessary, from all patients being evaluated presurgically. Intracarotid amobarbital injections were used preoperatively for lateralization of cerebral dominance for language and memory.

Patients with demonstrated failure of blood-level-monitored AED therapy found to have satisfactory concordance of clinical and extracranial EEG (e/cEEG) localizations were operated upon on the basis of the above data, supplemented by electrocorticography during surgery.

Patients with clinically stable unifocal drug-refractory seizure patterns and nonlocalizing e/cEEGs were offered further diagnostic studies with intracranially implanted electrodes. The biasing influence of strong monotechnical preferences in regard to level of intracranial electrode placement was obviated by a policy of using those chronically implantable electrodes that were likely to be more effective in addressing the formulation of localization of the epileptogenic focus in terms of the aggregate of the data, clinical and e/cEEG, available up to this point (43). Thus, intracerebral depth electrodes, alone or in combination with subdural electrodes, were utilized for temporolimbic cases; subdural electrodes, for partial seizures implicating the external surface of the hemisphere; and so forth. After 1969, intracerebral electrodes were implanted stereotactically (stereoelectroencephalography [SEEG]) according to the methodology of Talairach et al. (56).

Excision of the epileptogenic focus from the cerebral hemisphere dominant for language was carried out under local analgesia, and under general

Table 1
Neuropsychiatric History and Examination of
Patients with Epilepsy

I. Identification: Name, age, handedness, marital status, source of referral, list of previous psychiatric contacts and hospitalizations

II. Seizure history: Obtained separately from patient and lay eyewitness (family member if possible, or roommate, co-worker, etc.)
Age at first seizure: _____
Age at onset of chronic seizure disorder (CSD): _____

A. Spontaneous descriptions
  1. Description of first seizure
  2. Description of seizures at onset of chronic seizure disorder
  3. Subsequent seizure patterns
  4. Description of present seizure patterns (recorded in terms of pro-drome, aura, ictus, and postictal period with duration and behavioral effects of each stage)

B. Focused inquiry
  1. In regard to possible conscious seizure experiences (auras), not spontaneously mentioned
    a. Somatic motor
    b. Somatic sensory
    c. Specialized sensory: visual, auditory, gustatory, olfactory, sexual
    d. Visceral motor
    e. Visceral sensory
    f. Involving higher nervous functions:
      — illusional, e.g., auditory, visual, motility, familiarity or strangeness, etc.
      — hallucinatory, e.g., auditory, visual, emotional (fear, pleasure), etc.
      — intellectual, e.g., forced thinking, forced staring, etc.
      — complex or skilled behaviors: speech, writing
  2. Ictal behavior not remembered by the patient
    a. Alimentary pantomime
    b. Unique behavioral automatisms
    c. Laughter, smiling
    d. Other
  3. Dreams
    a. Recurrent
    b. Seizure-related

(continued)

307

Table 1
(*Continued*)

4. Precipitating factors of seizures
5. Attempts by patient at arrest of seizure
6. Frequency of seizures: Diurnal   Nocturnal
    a. At onset of CSD
    b. At present:
       average frequency
       highest frequency
       least frequency
    c. Seizure-free intervals
       none? If yes, duration? when? why?
7. Attitudes of patient toward his/her seizures
    — feelings about their cause
    — effect of having seizures
8. Antiepileptic medication
    — past
    — present
    — untoward reactions (somatic and psychiatric)
9. Contact with other persons with epilepsy
10. Attitude toward operation for seizure control

III. Personal history (exploration in each category as to interaction with and repercussions of seizure phenomena: higher-function impairments, psychodynamic conflicts, etiological factors)

A. Birth and development
B. Childhood behavioral symptomatology
C. Schooling
D. Work history
E. Interpersonal relationships
F. Sexual life
G. "Personality" (described by patient and family member)
H. Interests and activities, including writing, e.g., creative, diary, letters
I. Involvement with religion

IV. Medical and psychiatric history

A. Medical
    1. Attitude toward health in general
    2. Illnesses and operations
    3. Injuries
    4. Headaches
    5. Other complaints

(*continued*)

Table 1

(*Continued*)

B. Psychiatric
    1. Inquiry about occurrence of and relation to seizures of:
       a. Periods of depression/elation
       b. Suicidal thoughts or attempts
       c. Aggression
       d. Altered thinking
       e. Unusual experiences
    2. Professional behavioral therapy
V. Mental status examination: The mental status examination is obtained with orientation toward relating the findings to seizure phenomena and to the behavioral symptomatology
  A. Higher cortical functions
    1. Attention
    2. Concentration
    3. Orientation
    4. Memory
    5. Speech and language
    6. Calculation
    7. Gnosic functions
    8. Praxic functions
    9. Constructional ability
    10. Fund of information
    11. Ability to abstract
    12. Judgment
    13. Insight
  B. Content of thought: Inclusive of relation to seizures
    1. Spontaneous themes
    2. Illusions
       a. Simple
       b. Complex
          — ideas of unreality
          — depersonalization
          — déjà or jamais vu
    3. Hallucinations: modality?
    4. Fears, phobias
    5. Compulsions, obsessions
    6. Paranoid ideation
       — tendency
       — delusions

(*continued*)

Table 1
(*Continued*)

C. Mood state
    1. Irritability
    2. Aggressive behavior
    3. Depression or elevation of mood
VI. Psychiatric formulation
    1. Main psychiatric symptoms
    2. Mechanism(s) of these symptoms
    3. Formal nosological diagnosis
    4. Formal classification of seizures and epilepsy
VII. Summary in surgical cases
    A. Preoperative classification of seizures
        1. Clinical classification
        2. EEG classification
        3. Seizure pattern
        4. Etiology (clinically)
        5. Radiological classification
    B. Operative
        1. Electrographic localization
        2. Anatomical localization
            a. Gross abnormalities
            b. Microscopic
        3. Etiology/neuropathology
    C. Final classification:
    D. Operative procedures:
        Date

_____ 1. _____

_____ 2. _____

_____ 3. _____

anesthesia when on the nondominant side. The extent of excision was determined individually for each case.

Postoperatively, patients were followed longitudinally by the neurosurgeon or neurologist, the neuropsychiatrist, and the social worker. Of the last 30 consecutive cases of drug-refractory temporolimbic partial epilepsy with a mean duration of follow-up of 81 months (range: 20 to 198 months), 27 (90 percent) have been seizure-free for more than two years.

SOURCES OF BEHAVIORAL DIFFICULTIES ENCOUNTERED
IN TEMPOROLIMBIC PATIENTS

Although multiple interrelationships exist between the various factors impinging on the psychological state of the person with epilepsy, these factors may be considered under the headings of "extrinsic" and "intrinsic."

Extrinsic Factors

Extrinsic factors are those which derive from "living with epilepsy." They include the patient's feeling about himself as an epileptic and the interpersonal repercussions on the individual with epilepsy. The latter comprise failure of the environment to recognize seizure-engendered behavior or to provide an appropriate and humane response to knowledge of the patient's disorder.

The patient with partial complex seizures shares with other epileptics the lowering of his self-image. In the context of personality theory, a non-damaging personality outcome in epilepsy would be surprising. The person with epilepsy reacts not by feeling that he has an illness he cannot control, but may harbor primitive feelings of guilt, inferiority, and unworthiness, seeing epilepsy as a punishment for he knows not what. In the environment, knowledge that a person has epilepsy commonly produces ostracism. The patient is impeded in his life development by social or occupational prejudice and outright rejection. The child may be taunted by his peers and nicknamed "fits" or "retard." Bladder or bowel incontinence may compound his social problem. Over the years, the patient is alone, finding few who stay with him. He may be asked to leave school or work, if he was so fortunate as to have found a job. The patient's family may become desperate. Seizure-related behavior may not be recognized as such. And medications may, whether during beneficial or toxic effects, take their toll on behavior.

Such extrinsic factors are seen by many as the principal cause for the behavioral disturbances of the epileptic patient. Although extrinsic factors are unarguably operative, in some seizure patients, behavior disturbances may be causally related to the cerebral epileptogenic process.

Intrinsic Factors

Intrinsic factors leading to behavioral alteration comprise specific ictal events in a comprehensive sense, fixed or intermittent higher-function deficits, and affective changes, related to the cerebral malfunction responsible for the seizure disorder.

The experiencing of different seizure types. A significant difference exists for the patient in the experiencing of his seizure according to its type, whether generalized, partial temporolimbic, or partial nontemporolimbic.

The seizures of generalized epilepsy, major or minor, are unheralded hiatuses of consciousness and therefore of experience, with definable onset and termination. During the absence attack of generalized epilepsy ("petit mal"), consciousness is lost abruptly (for less than 20 seconds) and the typically prompt recovery is usually followed by smooth resumption of preictal activities. At the onset of a grand mal seizure, consciousness is lost abruptly; the end of the convulsive activity is readily observable. Although there may be a postictal behavioral disturbance, such as confusion, sleep, or postictal automatism, the dramatic character of the major motor attack leaves little question as to source and nature of the behavioral disturbance. During neither of the seizure types of generalized epilepsy is the patient an experiencing participant. On its part, the environment is mostly able to recognize the behavioral alteration as being seizure-related.

Partial seizures of nontemporolimbic origin are usually experienced as short episodes of physical sensations or of movement. Emotionally, their content is likely to be neutral.

In contrast, the temporolimbic partial seizure is commonly a variable and prolonged encroachment on the patient's consciousness and life. Its time boundaries are often ill defined because onset and recovery may be gradual. The minor attack of temporolimbic epilepsy may be so brief or subtle as to escape the notice of observers and of the patient, who may be amnesic for it. Or it may present as an absence of somewhat greater duration than a petit mal. The temporolimbic absence attack may be followed by affective change and/or by a prolonged period of impairment of higher nervous functions, such as receptive aphasia and dysmnesia. Because the afflicted person seemed in continuous contact, this postictal impairment may be misinterpreted by the environment as inappropriate behavior. The damage to interpersonal relationships, studies, or work from recurrent yet unexplained episodes of inability to comprehend language, or to remember, have been ruinous to some of our patients in their endeavors. Emotional experiences, shifts of affect, or paranoid sensitivity may also be prominent elements of temporolimbic seizures and are discussed below.

Conscious content of partial seizures of temporolimbic origin. Even if the specific location of the seizure focus within the temporal lobe has been found to be the same in different patients (e.g., in the anterior hippocampal formation as shown by SEEG made during spontaneous seizures), the precise pattern of their partial seizures cannot be predicted. The individual pattern and experience of the seizure vary from patient to patient. The diverse manifestations that may occur in a temporolimbic seizure reflect the different functions of the temporal lobe. The medial limbic structures are involved with affective and motivational behavior and memory. The dominant lateral temporal cortex subserves comprehension of auditory language. Interpretation and integration of sensations, sequencing, and comparing are subserved by temporal neocortex. The temporal lobe appears to be a component of the brain intimately responsible for and involved in the dynamic content of the patient's life. These observations have two sets of consequences. Temporolimbic seizure manifestations often have a very personal stamp. They may greatly disrupt ongoing experience.

The behavioral manifestations seen in partial seizures of temporolimbic origin and their repercussions are best described in relation to the successive stages in the evolution of a seizure, namely prodrome, aura, ictus, and postictal period.

The prodrome. A prodromal period, though unaccompanied by any definite EEG change, may regularly herald a seizure. The prodrome is characterized by an alteration in the patient's behavior, such as an affective shift (depression or elevation of mood), or by unprovoked irritability. This behavioral change may be stereotyped and disruptive and may last from minutes to hours or days. For example, KOT, an 18-year-old boy with complex partial seizures of frontal or temporal origin, would become aggressive and overactive several hours prior to the onset of the obvious attack. His behavior would tax the psychological resources of the family in their effort to keep him from entanglement with his siblings.

The aura. The aura is, of course, the experience of the onset of the seizure discharge. Auras involving strong affective content may be associated with psychic pain and/or disruptive behavior. In such patients, psychiatric interviewing may uncover elucidative psychodynamic material. Three cases will illustrate.

In his aura, HAX, a 15-year-old boy, had an intense feeling that anyone around him was going to kill him, a sensation so dreadful that he offered to trade an arm for its elimination. This seizure content proved to be a reflection of his emotional life, which was full of uncertainties due to realistic rejection in his personal relationships. STW, usually a meek 32-year-old man, would episodically become violent. His seizure history revealed that associated with his epigastric aura, he would have the feeling that "I am like a dummy on a string on the edge of a cliff. If anyone touches me, I think that I am going to slide off." Thus, he would fight off anyone who came into contact with him during his aura. JOD, a 35-year-old man with long-standing hostility, would have an aura of fear with hallucination of a black shadowy figure pointing a gun at him. This report and insight into his personality dynamics made it possible to help his puzzled family to understand the nature of the aggressive outbursts they had experienced.

Episodic impairment of higher cortical function may lead to disturbance of behavior. VAG, an 11-year-old girl with initially unrecognized small seizures, had been under psychiatric treatment in a child guidance center for erratic behavior with temper outbursts. Her apparent misbehavior consisted of her doing other than what had been requested of her and reacting strongly when reprimanded. Exploration of her seizure experience showed that she had auras of receptive aphasia followed by auditory hallucinations. After excision of glioma and epileptogenic focus from her left posterior temporal lobe elsewhere, seizures ceased and behavior returned to its satisfactory premorbid level.

The ictus. During the ictus, a patient's behavior may be related to the feelings belonging to life experiences prior to the onset of the seizure disorder. JAB, a 36-year-old man with a temporolimbic seizure disorder of 20 years' duration, had an aura of a strong epigastric sensation and fear that he described as "awesome terror." Becoming automatic, he would pace about with grimaces of terror and alarming screams. These episodes were disastrous for interpersonal relationships and employment. When antiepileptic medications failed to alter the seizures, they were interpreted as psychological events and he underwent psychoanalytic treatment for 10 years. Because his screaming episodes failed to respond, he was referred for epileptological evaluation. Psychiatric investigation revealed that the ictal affective behavior could be understood in terms of repeated terrorizing life experiences that had occurred at the time of onset of the seizure disorder. Excision of epileptogenic brain abscess scar tissue from the right temporal lobe elsewhere resulted in cessation of seizures and terrifying behavior.

The postictal period. Disturbance of behavior following a partial seizure of temporolimbic origin may be minimal or prolonged, from hours to days. The patient may become aggressive; he may have higher-function difficulties, with slowing of cognition and impairment of sequencing, memory, and comprehension of language; his mood may be altered.

The magnitude of the clinical seizure responsible for a postictal state may vary from an obvious ictus to a small, very brief, nearly undetectable attack. This statement is based on observations made in patients with partial seizures of temporolimbic origin proven by SEEG recording during spontaneous seizures, in some cases not visible in the simultaneous scalp EEG, and by the cessation of seizures and postictal behavior disturbances following temporal lobectomy. Such observations have been published by others (6,56) and ourselves (18).

Interictal period. In the light of what has been presented in the previous section, it should now be evident that the term "interictal" in studies of episodic behavior disturbances of patients with epilepsy may be misapplied, unless the patients are very closely observed. Episodic disturbances are likely to be ictus-related.

The pathophysiology of temporolimbic partial seizures and the experience of living with the consequences of such partial seizures have a role in the development of chronic "everyday psychopathology." In time, because of repetition of the seizure experiences and consequent occurrences, the patient's overall performance may become altered; his interpersonal relationships disrupted; and his freedom curtailed.

THE EPILEPTIC PERSONALITY

The possibility that a definite personality type occurs in the patient with temporal lobe seizures has long aroused considerable controversy, which is still ongoing. An historical review of conceptions of the epileptic personality appeared in a monograph by Guerrant et al. (27). They described the changing predominant attitudes in terms of four time periods: (1) During the "period of epileptic deterioration," which lasted until 1900, personality changes were considered to occur as a result of recurring seizures. (2) During the "period of the epileptic character," from 1900 to 1930, a constitutional defect was said to account for behavior disturbances. (3) The years after 1930 were designated as "the period of normality." This viewpoint is still held by some professionals as well as lay organizations, namely that seizure patients are like everyone else except at the moment of their seizure. This view is certainly correct for many, but cannot be generalized to all patients with epilepsy. (4) The "period of psychomotor peculiarity" began in 1948 (24) and is still ongoing. Terms used in the literature to characterize these peculiarities have been exhaustively listed by Stevens (54).

Recent attempts at defining a distinct syndrome of interictal behavior changes in temporal lobe epilepsy were initiated by Waxman and Geschwind (67) in 1975. They stated that many of these patients had alterations in sexual behavior, religiosity, and compulsive writing. Bear and Fedio (2) in 1977 produced an inventory of 18 personality traits said to be characteristic of patients with temporal lobe epilepsy. The most specific traits were humorless sobriety, dependence, and obsessionalism. They claimed distinct personality profiles for patients with left and right temporal lobe epilepsy. Subsequent investigators have not replicated their findings. Rodin and Schmaltz (49) reported on their own and other authors' unsuccessful attempts to validate the Bear-Fedio temporal lobe personality profile. They surmised that, "Inasmuch as the basic pathophysiology probably differs in individual patients in cerebral location and intensity, one could expect different personality reactions in different individuals . . . " (p. 591). We agree with this surmise but believe, on the basis of direct longitudinal observations, that the hypothesis should include the operation of multiple factors and mechanisms in the production of behavioral alterations, not limited to localization of the seizure focus, the functional organization of the seizure discharge, and the severity and frequency of seizures. We include also the presence and degree of fixed (brain-lesion-produced) and intermittent (ictus-produced) deficits of higher cerebral functions, intrapsychic dynamics, and past and ongoing life experiences (15,17,18).

In summary, a distinctive personality syndrome typical of patients with temporal lobe epilepsy has not been established.

AGGRESSIVE BEHAVIOR

Another aspect of the behavioral pathology of the patient with temporolimbic seizures is aggressive behavior. Some investigators (11,47) and lay supporters of the epileptic have denied, while others have demonstrated (1,12,13,17,36,50,58), an increased incidence of aggressiveness in these patients. We do not expect to encounter criminality in our epileptic patients. Yet, we have observed aggressive behavior, verbal or physical, in a significant number of patients with complex partial seizures.

These aggressive manifestations may vary in their form and mechanism

(17). Some of the patients may display "aggressivity," that is, a propensity to verbal or nonverbal aggression against others, self, or things. Other patients show "aggressiveness," i.e., a continuous mild pattern of verbal or nonverbal attack. Chronically irritable, they may force others to act and speak cautiously to avoid an eruption. They may have aggressive manifestations in seizures that are sometimes triggered by aggressive reference or occurrence. The response of the environment provides an operational measure of the significance and seriousness of the behavioral alteration. Thus, because of aggressive behavior, some of our temporolimbic epilepsy patients, adults and children, have been admitted to psychiatric hospitals, day-treatment centers, schools for the emotionally disturbed, and group homes, for periods of weeks to years. Other patients may show ictus-related aggression, which is discussed below.

Mechanisms responsible for aggressive manifestations may differ from patient to patient. The operational factors may be subdivided into extrinsic and intrinsic for continuity with earlier discussion. The extrinsic factors largely resemble those previously described and do not require reiteration. Intrinsic factors may, as described earlier, cause behavioral symptomatology during the stages of the epileptic seizure. We have proposed (17) that an episode of aggressive behavior related to a temporolimbic seizure may be *primary*, that is, the result of activation, by the epileptic discharge, of cerebral circuits subserving affective and motivational behavior. Although little is known about the nature of the abnormal neuronal activity underlying the prodrome, one might speculate that a continuously raised level of irritability could result from the lesser degree of epileptic discharge occurring during interictal EEG spiking. Aggressive behavior occurring during a temporolimbic seizure might be the product of the more intense ictal neuronal discharge (31). Such activation would be analogous to the paradigm of electrical brain stimulation, as illustrated by the following case. COD, a 16-year-old boy with complex partial seizures of temporolimbic origin, had a history of extended periods (hours to days) of irritable behavior during which he attacked people and things. E/cEEG showed bilateral independent temporal spiking. SEEG investigation demonstrated that spontaneous clinical seizures arose independently from either anterior hippocampus. Electrical stimulation of the right amygdala reproduced a clinical seizure: he became fearful and paranoid and threatened the staff with vigorous pawing movements (15). Aggressive behavior may also be *secondary*, being the patient's response to the mental content he experiences during the seizure (cf. case STW, p. 319). Alternatively, *secondary* aggression may be a reaction to brief ictal interruption in ongoing reality-based thinking. The subtle seizure apparently allows primary-process, uncensored, emotionally based reaction to take over. This is illustrated in the case of GEP, a 26-year-old single office worker with right temporolimbic partial seizures, who had been speaking in a rational way, during a psychiatric interview, about her good fortune with employment; after a brief interruption of such talk by a subtle seizure, she made an abrupt shift to a complaining, angry, paranoid mode of speaking about the same topic.

During an ictal or postictal automatism, the behavioral content may be consistent with the conscious experience at the beginning of the seizure or an externalization of repressed or suppressed feeling. The aggressive content may relate to the patient's psychodynamic patterns. During the postictal period there may be selective aggressivity, not aggression as a result of confusion (cf. case PAB, p. 33 ff). That is, the behavior may not be random but be directed toward individuals with whom the patient had previous negative interactions. For example, one patient said, "I never strike anyone who has been good to me," and another, "After a seizure, I don't react the way things really are."

PSYCHOSIS IN EPILEPSY

Another serious psychiatric disturbance of patients with epileptic seizures is psychosis. In 1923, Kraepelin (34) provided the last major description of epileptic psychosis prior to the introduction of the human electroencephalogram by Berger (3) in 1929. In the 1950s, Hill (30) and Pond (40) characterized epileptic psychosis as a "chronic paranoid hallucinatory state." Studies of psychosis in epilepsy became reoriented after the influential paper of Slater et al. of 1963 (52). The differences from classic schizophrenia were the maintenance of a warm affect, presence of an organic taint, and absence both of a premorbid schizoid personality and of a family history of schizophrenia. Nonetheless, subsequent authors have tended to drop the "-like," or to speak of epileptic psychosis as nuclear schizophrenia (39). Others have denied the correctness of a schizophrenia diagnosis (7,15,38).

Classifications of psychosis in epilepsy have been proposed recently (4,7,15,62). Major disturbances of thinking or of affect were viewed as interictal events, unrelated to impairment of consciousness or to ictal phenomena. Our data suggest that epileptic psychosis is not unrelated to seizure manifestations. In personally observed cases, the majority of the epileptic psychoses occurred either after a single major motor seizure, after convulsive status epilepticus, or after increase in the frequency of minor seizures. The latter can be subtle, therefore requiring very close observation for detection (see case KRS, p. 324).

Etiology and Pathogenesis of Psychosis in Epilepsy

A wide spectrum of possibilities and hypotheses has been presented in regard to the etiology and pathogenesis of epileptic psychosis. Pond (40) suggested that an experiential factor must be considered: repeated ictal experiences might eventually color the person's interpretation of reality. In our clinical material, this was illustrated by GAD, a 38-year-old woman with complex partial seizures of temporolimbic origin, chronically paranoid and grandiose. Her seizures began with a very pleasant olfactory aura. During her frequent ictal automatisms, she would continue ongoing activity or interactions. Last remembering that she was hungry, she would find her meal prepared. Last anticipating a bath, she would find it drawn; her olfactory aura made it seem delightfully fragrant. She became convinced that a guardian spirit was responsible for these activities, and she had developed delusions that the intent of the spirit was that she develop plans for interplanetary space stations.

Slater et al. (52) implicated a cerebral atrophic process. Taylor (59,60) emphasized adolescent age of onset of seizures, female sex, left-handedness, and left-sided lesions. Reynolds reported that psychosis could be due to a pharmacologically induced folate deficiency (44). In 1969, Flor-Henry (19) stated that schizophrenialike psychosis occurred in patients with left-temporal-lobe foci and affective disorders in patients with right-hemisphere foci. Others have failed to support these conclusions (25,33,35, 52,65). Sherwin et al. (51) studied the charts of 80 cases of intractable temporal lobe seizures successfully operated by Prof. J. Talairach. Seven charts had a recorded history of psychosis, which the authors did not reassess. In five of the seven cases, the focus was on the left. An association between right-sided foci and affective psychosis has not been confirmed. Bruens (7), Fenton (14), and the present authors (15,18) have emphasized the multifactorial pathogenesis of psychosis. We have also drawn attention to the role of increased frequency of seizures, whether easily recognizable or subtle, and of their often relatively prolonged cognitive deficitary and/ or affective aftermaths in the genesis of epileptic psychosis.

Psychodynamic events may also play a significant role in the precipitation of a psychosis. Thus, MIR, a 16-year-old patient with generalized tonic seizures followed by postictal automatism and subject to near-monthly bouts of status epilepticus, became psychotic only when an episode of status supervened during a period of intensified emotional pressure.

AFFECTIVE CHANGES IN SEIZURE PATIENTS

Classification of Affective Symptomatology

Affective symptomatology in seizure patients has been relatively neglected in the literature during preoccupation with the schizophrenialike psychosis. Betts (5) noted in his clinical material that depression was the most common psychiatric symptom in the epileptic patient. Robertson (46) concluded that factors responsible for depression included anticonvulsant drugs, social stigmatization, and a right-temporal-lobe lesion.

The writers classified affective symptomatology occurring in their patients as follows: (1) euphoria/elation; (2) dysphoric states, intermittent or chronic; (3) cycling disorders; (4) reactive depression (16). We found that there can be an intimate relationship between affective manifestations and the ictal process. Mechanisms included primary ictal elevation of mood with exhilaration, which colored the patient's ongoing affect, or serious depressive feelings, at times with suicidal thoughts, during a prolonged prodrome. Patients became dysphoric as postictal cognitive impairment led to misinterpretation of ongoing events and reactions. Other patients developed a chronic dysphoria as a result of environmental misinterpretations and negative reactions.

Reactive depression, seizure events, and higher-function deficits may become intertwined. One instructive case was that of FRS, a 14-year-old girl with left posterior temporal astrocytoma, who began to have daily seizures while still grieving the death from cancer of her loving and beloved mother. The child had been a steady companion during her mother's terminal illness. When the seizures began, the patient would have a vision of her mother in a shared activity, or of a television show they had watched together. Between seizures, she was continuously involved with her grief — withdrawing, talking *with* her toy animals, crying alone frequently, seeking the company of mother figures. Impairment in her verbal learning ability diminished her previous success at school. Interpersonal problems also increased as she projected the anger over her loss and difficulties to her peers, toward whom she might become aggressive. Although psychiatric treatment was recommended, the father refused, certain that these problems would resolve with time. After uneventful excision of the glioma and adjacent epileptogenic cortex, he was proved right. The seizures with their visual experiences ceased, and quite promptly the patient began to accept her mother's loss, completed the grieving process by herself, and became involved in life normally.

The behavioral repercussions of partial seizures vary with the stage of life of the patient.

During Childhood

Although adolescence is said to be the usual age of onset of temporolimbic seizures, we have repeatedly found clinical historical evidence for the presence of unrecognized ictal symptomatology at an earlier age.

During childhood, there may be misinterpretation or lack of recognition of seizures by family, teachers, and doctors. Morbid sensitivity, dysphoria, and a paranoid aggressive personality may result. School performance may suffer owing to interference by seizures, chronic higher-function deficits, or/and the stressful interpersonal setting. Medication may cause sleepiness, irritability, and cognitive slowing. The child may be expelled from school because of fear that he or others may be hurt because of seizures or behavioral reactions. The family may be accused of being overprotective. They may be told to treat the epileptic child as if he were normal. But the families see this as questionable advice. For instance, they may have to watch the child until he enters the school bus for fear he may walk into the street during an automatism.

During the Teen-age Years

During the teen-age years, seizures may become clearly manifest. Social rejection is frequent. The "empty existence" syndrome may result, as shown in the case of SHB, a 21-year-old single woman with right temporolimbic seizures, who was dismissed from school at the age of 13 without provision for a tutor. She became a recluse, reversing night and day, was unoccupied and paranoid. Those adolescents with epilepsy who do well in the structured setting of school may find transition to the outside world difficult.

In Adulthood

The adult patient often remains in a childlike role, protected by the family. Because he is prohibited from driving, his dependence greatly increases. Heterosexual experience is under the pall of feelings of unworthiness or concern because of genetic threat. Some patients are hyposexual (21,57,66). Marital problems may occur through the various misunderstandings of episodic behavior or because of affective alterations. Employment may be available only through a sympathetic employer or because the family can provide a sheltered opportunity. The patient with intractable seizures may be poorly helped by vocational counselors, who are usually more ready to work with a patient whose seizures can be controlled. The family may be immobilized by the supervision of an adult who cannot be left alone.

TREATMENT ISSUES

Diagnosis

The essential first steps in treatment are accurate diagnosis and classification of the seizures. The behavioral ramifications of the seizure disorder should be comprehensively evaluated in each case. The patient's intrapsychic and psychosocial dynamics and seizure manifestations should be reciprocally considered. The higher cortical functions must be carefully examined for their possible continuous or episodic role in behavioral alteration. Clinical neuropsychiatric examination may be supplemented by neuropsychological testing addressed to specific problem areas as determined by the clinician. After synthesis of these data, the physician can develop a therapeutic plan that addresses problems identified in these spheres.

Medications

The effect of medications on the individual patient should be evaluated: Antiepileptic drugs may cause cognitive slowing, sluggishness, impaired coordination, and sleepiness. Phenobarbitone may cause irritability and hyperactivity. Primidone (Mysoline) may be associated with a paranoid reaction. Folate deficiency occurring with phenytoin may lead to psychosis. Although clinical reports have varied, carbamazepine (Tegretol) has been reported to have a favorable effect, in some patients, on behavioral symptomatologies such as irritability, aggressive tendencies, impulsivity, dysphoria, depression, and anxiety. If epileptic psychosis develops, neuro-leptic agents may be used in conjunction with AED with full awareness that these agents may lower the convulsive threshold. If compliance is a problem, long-acting decanoate (Prolixin) may be useful. Antidepressant drugs should likewise be used as indicated. Caution should be exercised in the use of anxiolytic drugs. Chlordiazepoxide (Librium), for instance, may provoke aggressive manifestations. Detailed discussions of antiepileptic medications have been written recently by British and American authors (4,48,63).

Hospitalization

Hospitalization on a neurological/neurosurgical or psychiatric unit may be necessary, with the site chosen depending on the psychiatric indications.

Psychiatric Management

Behavioral difficulties may be understood often only after a period of observation with multiple inputs; not after one interview or test. Adequate contact with patient and family should be maintained by the clinician to assess possible relationships between seizures and behavioral events. Psy-chotherapy is utilized as necessary to evaluate and ameliorate responses of patient and/or family.

Allied Professionals

Adequate structure in the patient's life is essential. Thus, allied profes-sionals, who must be knowledgeable about epilepsy, may play important roles. The social worker, for instance, becomes a link between the patient and his family and the community. The rehabilitation counselor can be of inestimable help in the occupational preparation or employment settings.

Surgical Approach to Seizure Control

Neurosurgical intervention for seizure control may produce a lifelong improvement in the patient with intractable seizures who has an operable focus. Two surgical cases will efficiently pull together a number of the points that have been made.

The case of KRS, a 21-year-old man with partial complex seizures of left temporal origin due to gliosis of unknown cause, illustrates the diagnostic problems of chronic behavioral difficulty and acute psychotic episodes, as well as the role and interaction of subtle ictal events, higher-function deficits, and psychodynamic patterns in the genesis of the behavior disturbances.

KRS had a seizure disorder from childhood. He was viewed by his desperate family as nonfunctional and unable to adequately handle everyday situations. He was considered by the psychiatric staff of another institution as chronically psychotic. His seizure would begin with a sudden inability to understand what was being said or what he read. He would say, "A line keeps coming back, I try to figure it out. I write it down but it doesn't make any sense." After termination of his postictal behavioral automatism, difficulty with memory would continue for several hours. When he came under our observation, he was said to have suffered two periods of schizophrenic psychosis associated with status epilepticus. He had undergone an unsuccessful partial temporal lobectomy elsewhere. While he was hospitalized on the neurosurgical unit for preoperative studies, a psychotic episode developed concurrently with an increase in minor seizures. The first sign of aberrant behavior was his eating hallucinated food particles after he had refused food offered to him by a nurse. In retrospect, this behavior was interpreted as misidentification of the nurse as his mother, with whom food had become a major area in the battle for control. When his behavior became unmanageable because of overactive destructive movements, KRS was transferred to a general psychiatry ward, where he was placed in isolation. A diagnosis of schizophrenia, catatonic type, was made. In the psychiatric records, seizures were stated to be absent. However, when the epilepsy group observed the patient attentively on the psychiatry unit, it was clearly noted that he was subject to frequent, short-lasting, subtle seizures. His condition was reinterpreted as being an acute epileptic psychosis superimposed on his mild chronic brain syndrome. During gradual recovery over weeks, a resurgence of psychotic thinking was noted whenever small seizures occurred. After left anterior temporal lobectomy, he became seizure free, experienced no further psychotic episodes, and was rehabilitated, becoming an employee in a large city bank.

The second case illustrates the effects on personality development of repeated early frightening experiences and environmental punitive reactions; the enigmatic nature of interictal behavior; and the yield of longitudinal study.

PAB, a 27-year-old divorced woman, had lifelong partial complex seizures with bilateral temporal EEG spiking. Psychiatrically, she showed affective instability, paranoid ideation, and aggressive behavior, for which she was institutionalized for seven years. Her first seizure occurred at 16 months of age following closed head trauma with bleeding from one ear. At two years, she was described as placing a hand on her upper abdomen, presumably indicating an epigastric aura. At 10 years, rage outbursts appeared. The seizures and aggressivity resulted in erratic school attendance. At 18 years, she was placed in a sheltered workshop. There she met a man 20 years her senior. She married him and bore two children. At 21, she was sent to a psychiatric hospital because of aggressivity directed toward herself and others. She remained there for four years, when she was transferred to our psychiatric facility to be within the orbit of the epilepsy program for evaluation and possible surgical treatment.

Her seizures would begin with an epigastric sensation of fear associated with a paranoid feeling that she was "going to be attacked," visual illusions, and inability to speak. During the ictus, she ran, sometimes encountering dangerous situations. Postictally, she sometimes attacked other patients.

After a short time in the hospital, the patient met with considerable rejection by patients and staff. She was considered unpredictable in mood, manipulative, not trustworthy, overly complaining, paranoid, and aggressive. She was regarded by some staff members as having two concurrent diagnoses: character pathology and/or psychosis, and a seizure disorder.

Observations during her stay on the psychiatric ward led to the identification of organic mechanisms for some of the above characteristics: (1) One day the patient was found bruised, in an unexpected location on the hospital grounds. She stated that, while out walking, she had been attacked by a man and injured in the struggle as she attempted to escape. Fortunately, an objective version of these events was available from a nurse who had seen PAB walking on the grounds at some distance from a male patient. Suddenly PAB began to run at top speed, tripped, picked herself up, and ran into the nearest building. This sequence was consistent with the description of her seizures. (2) PAB got into frequent fights with other patients. Observation showed that this behavior would follow a recognized seizure and that the individuals attacked were those with whom she had previously had negative interactions. (3) The patient was seen during a prolonged period (days) of detachment when she complained of feeling afraid, pointing to her epigastrium, and giving her location as "a hotel" and calling the nurses "maids." An EEG obtained during this time showed increased temporal spike activity.

Marked fluctuations in PAB's mood state were observed on the neurosurgical unit during depth-EEG investigation with stereotactically implanted electrodes. One day she arrived in the EEG laboratory for electrical brain stimulation, morose, sullen, and irritable, exhibiting no spontaneous conversation. The next day she was spontaneous, pleasant, and talking freely. She asked, "How is it you change? Yesterday, you all looked sad; today you are happy. On some days I feel on top of the world, on other days I feel terrible, as if the world is against me." On stimulation of the right hippocampus, she said, "Voices are screaming." This was followed almost immediately by her statement that, "The tone of voice is soft and pleasant." She then described a feeling of fear and said, "I'm afraid. I don't like to talk. I would like to get away. The words are twisted." On stimulation of the right amygdala, she became dysphoric and irritable: "I feel afraid. Someone is after me. I am going to be captured." The rapid fluctuations in affect and perceptions during brain stimulation were similar to those appearing in her spontaneous behavior which had resulted in a negative reaction from her environment. A right mesial temporal localization of the epileptic mechanism was obtained by the SEEG study.

Following right anterior temporal lobectomy that included the amygdala and hippocampus, she became seizure-free. Her emotional lability and aggressivity were absent. It was possible for gradual rehabilitation to occur. She was helped to separate herself from the institutional setting, progressed to a sheltered workshop, and was briefly employed. She resided first in a group home, later at the YWCA, and currently is in her own apartment. PAB has expressed appreciation for her improvement in letters, poems, and during radio interviews which are part of her active work in support of patients with epilepsy. Her lifelong paranoid sensitivity, which had become part of her personality, has remained.

Team Approach

In the preceding sections, we have stressed a multidimensional approach that permits individualization in the design of the treatment program for patients who are significantly disabled by their chronic partial seizure disorder. That the two surgical cases made a maximal demand on the facilities of a comprehensive epilepsy program is evident. At our center, the personnel of this program comprises a neurosurgeon, who directs the program; a neurologist/electroencephalographer; a neuropsychiatrist; a nurse clinical specialist; a social worker. The reader would recognize that a similar inventory of relevant specialties can be found in most regional medical centers. Our epilepsy program, in fact, has relied at various times on resources in the community: sophisticated radiological facilities (computerized axial tomography, magnetic resonance tomography, digital video substraction angiography); neuropsychology; rehabilitation counselors; and lay social support group. Thus, as in the treatment of complex cardiological or cancer cases in their own community where the informed attending physician pulls together the necessary team, so the general psychiatrist, faced with a seizure patient with neurological and psychiatric problems, could obtain the assistance of the appropriate specialists.

CONCLUSIONS

That temporolimbic epilepsy can be associated with increased behavioral difficulty has reached a consensus in the literature. However, controversy still exists in regard to the nature of these difficulties and their mechanisms.

Attention of investigators has been directed mainly to major disturbances such as psychosis, affective symptoms, and aggressive behavior. The possibility of personality manifestations peculiar to this group of patients has also been explored, but as yet, no definite personality profile of the patient with temporolimbic seizures has been widely accepted.

The present authors have shown a more frequent association between seizure phenomena and behavioral alteration than is acknowledged by most other authors. We question the validity of the frequent reference in the literature to "interictal" behavior disturbance.

Behavioral problems range from interference with daily living by disruption in the spheres of learning, work, and interpersonal relationships to major behavioral symptomatology of aggressive, affective, or psychotic type. These problems vary from individual to individual in manifestations and mechanisms, and at different stages of life.

Overall, the authors emphasize the need for a multifactorial, crossdisciplinary, individualized approach to the understanding and treatment of behavioral difficulties in patients with temporolimbic seizures.

ACKNOWLEDGMENT

The authors thank Miss Molly Cox and W. S. Corrie, M.D., for electroencephalographic data, and Miss Carolyn A. Schell, R.N., B.S.N., for clinical observations.

REFERENCES

1. BAILEY, P., & GIBBS, F. A. (1951). The surgical treatment of psychomotor epilepsy. *Journal of the American Medical Association, 145,* 365.
2. BEAR, D. M., & FEDIO, P. (1977). Quantitative analysis of interictal behavior in temporal lobe epilepsy. *Archives of Neurology, 34,* 454.
3. BERGER, H. (1929). Ueber das Elektroenkephalogramm des Menschen. *Archiv der Psychiatrie und Nervenheilkunde, 87,* 527.
4. BETTS, T. A., MERSKEY, H., & POND, D. A. (1976). Psychiatry. In J. Laidlaw & A. Dickens (Eds.), *A textbook of epilepsy.* Edinburgh: Churchill Livingstone.
5. BETTS, T. A. (1981). Depression, anxiety and epilepsy. In E. H. Reynolds & M. R. Trimble (Eds.), *Epilepsy and psychiatry.* Edinburgh: Churchill Livingstone.
6. BONIS, A. (1979). Epilepsie et psychoses (point de vue d'un service de neurochirurgie). *Encephale, 5,* 161.
7. BRUENS, J. H. (1974). Psychoses in epilepsy. In P. J. Vinken and G. W. Bruyn (Eds.), *Clinical handbook of neurology.* New York: American Elsevier.
8. CARPENTER, W. T., JR., STRAUSS, J. S., & MULEH, S. (1973). Are there pathognomonic symptoms in schizophrenia? *Archives of General Psychiatry, 28,* 847.
9. Commission for the Control of Epilepsy and Its Consequences (1978). *Plan for nationwide action on epilepsy.* DHEW publ. no. 78-276, Vols. 1–4. Washington, DC: US Department of Health, Education and Welfare.
10. Commission on Classification and Terminology of the International League Against Epilepsy (1981). Proposal for revised clinical and electroencephalographic classification of epileptic seizures. *Epilepsia, 22,* 489.
11. CURRIE, S., HEATHFIELD, K. W. G., HENSON, R. A., & SCOTT, D. F. (1971). Clinical course and prognosis of temporal lobe epilepsy. *Brain, 94,* 173.
12. FALCONER, M. A. (1973). Reversibility by temporal lobe resection of the behavioral abnormalities of temporal lobe epilepsy. *New England Journal of Medicine, 289,* 451.
13. FALCONER, M. A., & SERAFETINIDES, E. A. (1963). A follow-up study of surgery in temporal lobe epilepsy. *Journal of Neurology, Neurosurgery & Psychiatry, 26,* 154.
14. FENTON, G. W. (1978). Epilepsy and psychosis. *Journal of the Irish Medical Association, 71,* 315.
15. FERGUSON, S. M., & RAYPORT, M. (1984). Psychosis in epilepsy. In D. Blumer (Ed.), *Psychiatric aspects of epilepsy.* Washington, DC: American Psychiatric Press.
16. FERGUSON, S. M., & RAYPORT, M. (1985). Affective symptomatology of patients with temporo-limbic seizures in a multidisciplinary neurosurgical program. Presented in Workshop on Psychosis in Epilepsy, 16th Epilepsy International Symposium, Hamburg, Federal Republic of Germany, Sept. 7.
17. FERGUSON, S. M., RAYPORT, M., & CORRIE, W. S. (1986). Brain correlates of aggressive behavior in temporal lobe epilepsy. In B. K. Doane & K. E. Livingston (Eds.), *The limbic system: Functional organization and clinical disorders.* New York: Raven Press.
18. FERGUSON, S. M., RAYPORT, M., GARDNER, R., WEINER, H., & REISER, M. (1969). Similarities in mental content of psychotic states, spontaneous seizures, dreams and responses to electrical brain stimulation in patients with temporal lobe epilepsy. *Psychosomatic Medicine, 31,* 479.
19. FLOR-HENRY, P. (1969). Psychosis and temporal lobe epilepsy. *Epilepsia, 10,* 363.
20. GASTAUT, H. (1953). So-called "psychomotor" and "temporal epilepsy." *Epilepsia, 2,* 59.
21. GASTAUT, H. (1954). Interpretation of the symptoms of psychomotor epilepsy in relation to physiological data on rhinencephalic function. *Epilepsia, 3,* 84.
22. GASTAUT, H. (1970). Clinical and electroencephalographic classification of epileptic seizures. *Epilepsia, 11,* 102.

23. GIBBS, F. A. (1951). Ictal and non-ictal psychiatric disorders in temporal lobe epilepsy. *Journal of Nervous & Mental Disorders, 113*, 522.
24. GIBBS, E. L., GIBBS, F. A., & FUSTER, B. (1948). Psychomotor epilepsy. *Archives of Neurological Psychiatry, 60*, 331.
25. GLASER, G. H. (1964). The problem of psychosis in psychomotor temporal lobe epileptics. *Epilepsia, 5*, 271.
26. GOODRIDGE, D. M., & SHORVON, S. D. (1983). Epileptic seizures in a population of 6000. I. Demography, diagnosis and classification, and role of the hospital services. *British Medical Journal, 287*, 641.
27. GUERRANT, J., ANDERSON, W. W., FISCHER, A., WEINSTEIN, M. R., JAROS, R. M., & DESKINS, A. (1962). *Personality in epilepsy*. Springfield, IL: Charles C Thomas.
28. HAUSER, W. A. (1983). Status epilepticus: Frequency, etiology and neurological sequelae. *Advances in Neurology, 34*, 3.
29. HAUSER, W. A., & KURLAND, L. T. (1975). The epidemiology of epilepsy in Rochester, Minn., 1935–1967. *Epilepsia, 16*, 1.
30. HILL, D. (1953). Psychiatric disorders of epilepsy. *Medical Press, 229*, 473.
31. JACKSON, J. H. (1873). On the anatomical, physiological and pathological investigations of the epilepsies. In J. Taylor (Ed.) (1931). *Selected writings of John Hughlings Jackson*, Vol. 1 (p. 100). London: Hodder and Stoughton.
32. JACKSON, J. H. (1888). On a particular variety of epilepsy ("intellectual aura"), one case with symptoms of organic brain disease. In J. Taylor (Ed.) (1931). *Selected writings of John Hughlings Jackson*, Vol. 1 (p. 399). London: Hodder and Stoughton.
33. JENSEN, I., & LARSEN, J. K. (1979). Mental aspects of temporal lobe epilepsy. *Journal of Neurology, Neurosurgery & Psychiatry, 42*, 256.
34. KRAEPELIN, E. (1923). *Psychiatrie*. Leipzig: Johann Ambrosius Barth.
35. KRISTENSEN, O., & SINDRUP, E. H. (1978). Psychomotor epilepsy and psychosis: II. Electroencephalographic findings. *Acta Neurologica Scandinavica, 57*, 370.
36. LINDSAY, J., OUNSTED, C., & RICHARDS, P. (1979). Long-term outcome in children with temporal lobe seizures. III: Psychiatric aspects in childhood and adult life. *Developmental Medicine & Child Neurology, 21*, 630.
37. MULDER, D. W., & DALY, D. (1952). Psychiatric symptoms associated with lesions of temporal lobe. *Journal of the American Medical Association, 150*, 173.
38. PARNAS, J., & KORSGAARD, S. (1982). Epilepsy and psychosis. *Acta Psychiatrica Scandinavica, 66*, 89.
39. PEREZ, M. M., & TRIMBLE, M. R. (1980). Epileptic psychosis: Diagnostic comparisons with process schizophrenia. *British Journal of Psychiatry, 137*, 245.
40. POND, D. A. (1957). Psychiatric aspects of epilepsy. *Journal of the Indian Med. Prof., 3*, 1421.
41. POND, D. (1981). Epidemiology of the psychiatric disorders of epilepsy. In E. H. Reynolds & M. R. Trimble (Eds.), *Epilepsy and psychiatry*. Edinburgh: Churchill Livingstone.
42. RAMANI, V., & GUMNIT, R. J. (1982). Management of hysterical seizures in epileptic patients. *Archives of Neurology, 39*, 78.
43. RAYPORT, M., FERGUSON, S. M., & CORRIE, W. S. (1986). Contributions of cerebral depth recording and electrical stimulation to the clarification of seizure patterns and behavior disturbances in patients with temporal lobe epilepsy. In B. K. Doane & K. E. Livingston (Eds.), *The limbic system: Functional organization and clinical disorders*. New York: Raven Press.
44. REYNOLDS, E. H. (1981). Biological factors in psychological disorders associated with epilepsy. In E. H. Reynolds & M. R. Trimble (Eds.), *Epilepsy and psychiatry*. Edinburgh: Churchill Livingstone.
45. RILEY, T. L., & ROY, A. (Eds.) (1982). *Pseudoseizures*. Baltimore: Williams & Wilkins.
46. ROBERTSON, M. M. (1985). Depression in patients with epilepsy: An overview and clinical

study. In M. R. Trimble (Ed.), *The psychopharmacology of epilepsy*. Chichester: John Wiley & Sons.

47. RODIN, E. (1973). Psychomotor epilepsy and aggressive behavior. *Archives of General Psychiatry, 28,* 210.

48. RODIN, E. (1984). Medical treatment of epileptic patients. In D. Blumer (Ed.), *Psychiatric aspects of epilepsy*. Washington, DC: American Psychiatric Press.

49. RODIN, E., & SCHMALTZ, S. (1984). The Bear-Fedio personality inventory and temporal lobe epilepsy. *Neurology (Minneapolis) 34,* 591.

50. SERAFETINIDES, E. A. (1965). Aggressiveness in temporal lobe epileptics and its relation to cerebral dysfunction and environmental factors. *Epilepsia, 6,* 33.

51. SHERWIN, I., PÉRON-MAGNAN, P., & BANCAUD, J. (1982). Prevalence of psychosis in epilepsy as a function of the laterality of the epileptogenic lesion. *Archives of Neurology, 39,* 621.

52. SLATER, E., BEARD, A. W., & GLITHEROE, E. (1963). The schizophrenia-like psychoses of epilepsy. *British Journal of Psychiatry, 109,* 95.

53. SMALL, J. G., MILSTEIN, V., & STEVENS, J. R. (1962). Are psychomotor epileptics different? *Archives of Neurology, 7,* 187.

54. STEVENS, J. R. (1975). Interictal manifestations of complex partial seizures. *Advances in Neurology, 11,* 85.

55. STEVENS, J. R., MILSTEIN, V., & GOLDSTEIN, S. (1972). Psychometric test performance in relation to the psychopathology of epilepsy. *Archives of General Psychiatry, 26,* 532.

56. TALAIRACH, J., BANCAUD, J., SZIKLA, G., BONIS, A., GEIER, S., & VEDRENNE, C. (1974). Approche nouvelle de la neurochirurgie de l'épilepsie. Méthodologie stéréotaxique et résultats thérapeutiques. *Neurochirurgie, 20*(Suppl. 1).

57. TAYLOR, D. C. (1969). Sexual behavior in temporal lobe epilepsy. *Archives of Neurology, 21,* 510.

58. TAYLOR, D. C. (1972). Mental state and temporal lobe epilepsy. A correlative account of 100 patients treated surgically. *Epilepsia, 13,* 727.

59. TAYLOR, D. C. (1975). Factors influencing the occurrence of schizophrenia-like psychosis in patients with temporal lobe epilepsy. *Psychological Medicine, 5,* 249.

60. TAYLOR, D. (1977). Epileptic experience, schizophrenia and the temporal lobe. *McLean Hospital Journal,* June, 22.

61. TEMKIN, O. (1971). *The falling sickness*. Baltimore: Johns Hopkins Press.

62. TOONE, B. (1981). Psychoses of epilepsy. In E. H. Reynolds and M. R. Trimble (Eds.), *Epilepsy and psychiatry*. Edinburgh: Churchill Livingstone.

63. TRIMBLE, M. (1981). Psychotropic drugs in the management of epilepsy. In E. H. Reynolds & M. R. Trimble (Eds.), *Epilepsy and psychiatry*. Edinburgh: Churchill Livingstone.

64. TRIMBLE, M. R. (1981). Hysteria and other non-epileptic convulsions. In E. H. Reynolds & M. R. Trimble (Eds.), *Epilepsy and psychiatry*. Edinburgh: Churchill Livingstone.

65. TRIMBLE, M. R., & PEREZ, M. M. (1982). The phenomenology of chronic psychoses of epilepsy. *Advances in Biological Psychiatry, 8,* 98.

66. WALKER, A. E., & BLUMER, D. (1984). Behavioral effects of temporal lobectomy for temporal lobe epilepsy. In D. Blumer (Ed.), *Psychiatric aspects of epilepsy*. Washington, DC: American Psychiatric Press.

67. WAXMAN, S. G., & GESCHWIND, N. (1975). The interictal behavior syndrome of temporal lobe epilepsy. *Archives of General Psychiatry, 32,* 1580.

68. ZIELINSKI, J. J. (1984). Epidemiologic overview of epilepsy: Morbidity, mortality, and clinical implications. In D. Blumer (Ed.), *Psychiatric aspects of epilepsy*. Washington, DC: American Psychiatric Press.

16

EMERGENCY PSYCHIATRY

GAIL M. BARTON, M.D., M.P.H.

Director of Inpatient Psychiatry, Veterans Administration
Medical and Regional Office Center, White River Junction, Vermont;
Associate Professor of Clinical Psychiatry, Dartmouth Medical School,
Hanover, New Hampshire

and

ROHN S. FRIEDMAN, M.D.

Private Practice; Instructor in Psychiatry at Harvard Medical School,
Boston, Massachusetts

INTRODUCTION: THE EMERGENCE OF EMERGENCY PSYCHIATRY

Yesterday and Today

The delivery of emergency services to the psychiatrically ill has dramatically changed over the past 30 years so that today it is high powered, substantial, and comprehensive (5). Gone are the hearses called into action as ambulances driven by the untrained drivers. Gone is an emergency room staffed by one nurse stationed in a single room with curtained-off sections. Today's emergency departments treat 200,000 people a year. Their staffs are specialists — emergency department nurses, board-certified emergency physicians, consultant psychiatrists experienced in emergency care, mental health specialists who can provide a mobile response into the community, paramedics who staff the prehospital care with quick response, care under base station medical control, and dependable transport (24). There are suites of rooms set up for orthopedic, trauma, and neonatal emergencies; there are grieving rooms, psychiatric interview rooms, and holding rooms. Computerized databases shared between facilities and across the state vie for space with elaborate laboratory equipment such as computerized tomography (CAT) scans, blood gas machines, and defibrillators.

Patients or families seeking assistance only need to dial 911 on the phone in an emergency. They can go to the hospital 24 hours a day and expect to be seen and treated there by a staff that is sensitive and skilled in emergency work. They may find themselves being given tests and medications right on the spot, their families being included in the treatment approach, and then the patient being admitted to a general hospital psychiatric unit. Admission to state hospital is rarer and for shorter periods of time.

Staff working today in emergency departments can expect flexible working hours, continuing education time, and salaries that take into consideration their special skills and the hazards of their job. They can expect to work being guided by policies and standards established by accrediting agencies, insurance companies, and governmental agencies. They can expect to work with a multidisciplinarian team and be faced with a large number of patients with a myriad of diagnostic entities both psychiatric and medical.

Changes in Therapy and Philosophy

This drastic change away from a few psychiatric patients coming into emergency rooms before the 1950s had to do with a large number of therapeutic advances and broad changes in philosophy in the mental health field (32). The wide use of the major tranquilizers in the mid-1950s allowed many "permanent" residents of state hospitals to be discharged to outpatient follow-up. They started to show up in emergency rooms whenever they got into a crisis, such as a return of symptoms, losing their housing, disagreeing with their therapist, or having medication side effects.

The Community Mental Health Act in the 1960s in the United States and socialized medicine in Great Britain allowed more patients to get a broader range of psychiatric services in the community than ever before. In 1973 the United States Emergency Medical Systems Act and the Robert Wood Johnson Foundation provided 15 million dollars to develop a mobile response system of prehospital care and acted as the impetus for regionalizing and upgrading emergency care in the United States. Specialty status and professional recognition of the staff who trained to work in the emerging emergency departments further upgraded the esteem and the care in formal facilities — the Emergency Department Nurses Association (EDNA) in 1970, the American College of Emergency Physicians (ACEP) in 1968 with a Certifying Board by 1979, and a Task Force on Psychiatric Emergency Care Issues of the American Psychiatric Association (APA) in 1978 all were part of this focus on enhancement and improvement of emergency psychiatric care.

Definition

The definition of a mental health emergency that the APA proposed states: A mental health emergency is an acute disturbance of thought, mood, behavior, or social relationship which requires an immediate intervention as defined by the patient, the family, or the community (2). Anyone may have a mental health emergency be it from illness, catastrophe, divorce, job loss, or death of a loved one (33).

Theoretical Frameworks

There are now theoretical frameworks to help conceptualize psychiatric emergencies so that the treatment can be more focused as well. These models have been discussed in detail elsewhere (32) but will be summarized here. The *biopsychosocial model* looks at the illness from a systems perspective and attempts to assign different weights to the factors that may have contributed to the state the person is in — the biological, the psychological, and the social factors. There is a *crisis intervention model*, which conceptualizes the patient as needing help at a critical time which can be a turning point in the person's life if urgent and intense help is offered. The *triage model* is more often seen in emergency departments where there is an implied constraint of limited resources so that only those are helped who can be, right then and there, with some real expectation that the help will make a drastic change for the better. Otherwise the persons are sorted out and not treated because others could benefit more.

The *developmental model* sees every crisis as having a context in a person's developmental growth. There may be a delay, a fixation, or inability to handle a crisis because of a developmental handicap.

Others draw on an *existential model* as being relevant in helping the mental health emergency: i.e., the patient may seem to be facing a question as basic as "why go on?"

Problems

Even with all this happening there are problems with the emergency psychiatry delivery of care (4). Burnout among the staff is frequent. The stresses that staff mention as contributing to the burnout include too many patients for the number of staff covering, too lengthy work hours, lack of resources, inadequate placements for the patients, lack of on-site supervision in training years, unhelpful security staff, and uncooperative team members (18). Other issues that rank high as problems include the unequal quality of care from one department to another. Without uniform standards as guides, the care is whatever the one on call decides or knows how to give. Emergency department staff often have attitudes toward patients with mental health problems which are counterproductive: "the patients tie up the rooms too long," "they are not really emergencies — they're not bleeding," "they do not need their vital signs taken — it's all in their head," "he is just drunk so why should I waste my time examining him?" (4). Mental health workers, on the other hand, may ignore signs and symptoms of medical illnesses.

Legal issues also can cause problems (17). Transporting unwilling patients, for example, may be construed as kidnapping. Child abuse laws ignore the mental health needs of the abusing parents. Holding beds are illegal in some locales. Commitment laws may be too restrictive so that persons who cannot care for themselves may be left to fend for themselves.

Economic pressures also can be problems for emergency psychiatry workers — they tend to influence care to the detriment of patient health and well-being. Some hospitals will not evaluate a person in an emergency if they have no insurance or money to pay the deposit. Insurance companies may disallow payment for the ultimate diagnosis even though the differential diagnosis for the presenting symptoms may have included an insurable cause. Lack of research funds hampers discovery of new methods of treatment and optimal care.

WHO THE PATIENTS ARE

This information has been thoroughly reviewed elsewhere (22) and is summarized below.

Young adults in their twenties and thirties are the largest single group of psychiatric emergency patients, constituting 50 percent of patients seen at present and still growing. By contrast, the elderly are underrepresented, either because they do not seek emergency psychiatric services or because they are incorrectly triaged.

Emergency patients tend to be single, separated, widowed, or divorced. Women predominate by a small margin. Lower socioeconomic classes are overrepresented in emergency populations. The ethnic, racial, and religious character of the population varies greatly from one center to another.

Why patients come to emergency services is not as simple to discover as one might hope. Diagnostic categories are fairly wide-ranging, though a rule of thirds may form a rough guide: one-third has schizophrenia and major depression, another third has personality disorders, and the other third has mixed organic-psychiatric disorders. Symptomatic behavior, rather than diagnosis, may offer a better explanation of why patients come to emergency services. Danger to self or others is the most prominent symptomatic presentation, followed by agitation and acute psychosis. Such behavior is so disruptive or life-threatening as to lead to emergency presentation.

A growing number of patients have prior outpatient, inpatient, and emergency psychiatric histories. Some have argued that the emergency department now manages predominantly nonemergency patients with complex economic and social problems along with chronic illnesses. It is the lack of social supports and available dispositions as much as psycho-pathology that leads to their presentation to the emergency service (13). The presence of such "chronic" emergency patients suggests the need to examine institutional forces (deinstitutionalization, institutional transfer-ence, and institutional expectations such as the right to immediate care) as factors in shaping the population served.

The largest group of psychiatric emergencies are self-referred. Most come unaccompanied by relatives. About half come outside of normal working hours. The nearer patients are to psychiatric emergency services, the more likely they are to present as a psychiatric emergency.

In the final analysis, patients present to a psychiatric emergency service because they or someone near to them believe that they have an urgent problem and that the emergency service is available and likely to help.

THE EMERGENCY PSYCHIATRIC STAFF

The disciplines and staffing patterns that exist for emergency psychiatric care depend on the setting, the locale, local needs, economic constraints, standards, and recruitment capability (18). Many types of disciplines serve the psychiatric emergencies. In the community it may be the visiting nurse, the paramedic, a mental health worker on a mobile response team, a police officer, a chaplain, a social worker, a local family practitioner, or a psychotherapist. In the emergency department patients may be screened at the door by a security officer, then a clerk, then a triage nurse before seeing an emergency physician, a consultant psychiatrist, and a psychiatric social worker (8).

Staffing is assigned for different purposes — patient care, education, community planning, regulations, safety, to prevent burnout, and for spe-cial needs.

For Patient Care

Staff assigned to patient care would include a physician to do a physical examination, order laboratory tests, and diagnose. A social worker would meet with the family to identify the crucial social and family factors and suggest and assist with disposition and financial considerations. Nursing would be for triage, room assignment, giving medications, observation in holding areas, restraint, continuity of care, and bodily needs. Paramedics and a mobil response team might be helping the police if staff were needed in the community.

For Education

Staffing for education would include the capability of staff to do on-site supervision, shift change supervision rounds, and formal didactics to trainees from a wide variety of disciplines.

For Community Planning

Staffing for community planning is very important so that regionalization of the care of patients can occur. This staff would function for information sharing, resource planning, formalizing transfer agreements, doing public relations, and drafting pertinent legislation.

To Prevent Burnout

Staffing to prevent burnout would mean having a diversity of disciplines to provide an interdependent, creative atmosphere to problem-solve patient issues. It would mean having enough staff to minimize overload shift by shift. It also means providing sufficient numbers so there is time for staff to meet to discuss, problem-solve, and rehash difficult cases. It means time for staff to go to continuing-education seminars and do course work to move up the job ladder.

For Regulation

Staffing for regulations is also necessary. There are records to be kept, follow-up phone calls to be made, requests for other agency records to be sent, summaries to be prepared, coding to be done, insurance and governmental forms to be completed.

For Safety

Staffing for safety is crucial. The security staff must be available 24 hours a day to protect the patients and staff. They should be educated about handling mental health emergencies and should understand who is in charge if an outburst occurs. They also can educate the mental health staff about how to prevent, decrease, and handle violence.

For Special Needs

Staffing for special patients includes having on call chaplains, rape counselors, alcohol counselors, child psychiatrists, and domestic violence counselors when special patients present (26). The patients respond initially and are more likely to continue in a follow-up relationship with these special staff if they have someone they perceive as especially understanding of their problems.

WHERE EMERGENCY PSYCHIATRY IS PRACTICED

The usual place to practice emergency psychiatry is in the emergency department. Yet, other sites include the patient's home or job, the courtroom, jail, a community mental health center, a health maintenance organization, a therapist's office, a state hospital, a disaster site, or a ward of a general hospital.

Emergency Department

In a busy urban emergency department the psychiatric service may be in a wing of its own. In such a case it has convenient access to medical screening, equipment, and laboratories of the regular emergency department. It should have some degree of privacy and screening from noise. It works best if there are interview rooms that are comfortable and large enough to include family members (16). An observation and holding area provides a place for patients to wait for transportation and transfer. There also needs to be a place for medications to be given where the patient can have time for them to take effect. There needs to be an environment where restraints may be used if necessary and ready staff to observe. A waiting room for patients and their families that has convenient access to bathrooms and food — even if the food is only from vending machines — is important (9). Telephones for both patients and staff are essential. A safe place for record storage, retrieval, and data entry needs to be near patient and staff areas. Security considerations for patients, families, and staff might include police officers at the emergency department doorway to check comings and goings and a security force who could be called on a moment's notice if violence is a possibility or has erupted or if weapons are in evidence. Conference and meeting rooms for staff are important to allow team communication, brainstorming, and supervision. These also might be the rooms where the reference books and materials are kept for the staff and students to use day to day. Some facilities also have rooms for grieving, intensive care, and seclusion.

Rural

In a rural environment psychiatric emergency care tends to be provided in the midst of the emergency department with less specialized room arrangements and more often by staff that is called to consult when a psychiatric emergency is identified.

Prehospital

Prehospital care for psychiatric emergencies occurs in the community and is handled by paramedics, the police, mental health workers, visiting nurses, clergy, and family practitioners for the most part. The main goal of working with patients in the community is to stabilize and transport them to hospital or to a community health facility.

On the Medical Ward

If the psychiatric emergency takes place on a medical or surgical ward, a consultation liaison psychiatric team is usually called in to evaluate the situation (21). Quite often, the patients are too ill to be transferred to a psychiatric unit, so they must be managed where they are. Most often the problems are related to an emotional response to the major presentation, or the staff is aware of a long-term problem that has had no easy resolution so that staff are worn out trying to deal with it piecemeal (19). The psychiatric response may be to help the staff better understand their attitudes and to educate them about the mental health problem (20). It may entail recommending use of a medication to handle a psychotic episode or depression.

Court Room

If the emergency requires commitment, the psychiatrist or mental health professional may find himself in the courtroom defending the rationale to commit the patient. Some community mental health agencies assign a court liaison person to educate the professionals who may have to testify as to the court procedure and make themselves available to the lawyers and judges to discuss alternatives to hospitalization and the types of agreements about treatment that can be worked out (35).

HOW TO APPROACH THE PATIENT

Assessment

The first step in the evaluation of a psychiatric emergency is immediate management and stabilization of the patient (28). Initial contact may be by telephone, when the patient or his family calls for help. Here the first priority is to get essential information: the patient's name, location, telephone number, and physician or therapist's name. Next the psychiatrist or screener should ask for a brief description of the situation, obtaining enough information to decide whether an on-site interview is indicated. Nonemergency situations should be handled by summarizing the clinical assessment simply and encouragingly and by referral to the patient's own therapist or an appropriate agency. If an emergency visit is in order, the clinician must ascertain whether the patient is able and willing to bring himself to the emergency service. If the patient is too disorganized or ambivalent to do so, the clinician should ask for the name of a friend or relative who can accompany him/her to the emergency service. Even when the patient is able to come by himself, it is usually advisable to have a family member provide further information and to allow the clinician to assess capability of the patient's support system.

If the patient seems in danger, the police and/or ambulance service may be called. In prehospital control and transportation it is important for workers to take a calm attitude, to speak to the patient simply and clearly, to give the patient enough physical space, to avoid precipitous action, and to try to get the patient to a quiet and unstressful environment where he/she may feel safe enough to cooperate. In most cases restraints will not be needed, but a practiced familiarity with, and protocol for, their use in such circumstances will minimize anxiety about dealing with such situations.

Once the patient arrives in the emergency service, initial management should include assessment of whether security personnel or restraints are necessary. Security personnel should be stationed in the area any time the clinician is concerned about risk, and an efficient alarm system should be included in all interview rooms. Until both staff and patient feel safe, no further evaluation is possible.

Once immediate security has been achieved, the next order of business is to obtain vital signs and to assure physiological stability. If there has been a suicidal gesture requiring medical treatment, that must take precedence. If there is evidence or suspicion of medical instability, medical consultation and clearance should be obtained.

After initial biopsychosocial stabilization has been achieved, the evaluation can proceed. The clinician must show concern without appearing either intrusive or gullible. Physical stance, tone of voice, and style of talking all help to create an initial relationship between patient and interviewer.

The next step of the evaluation is to take a succinct, but thorough psychiatric history. The emphasis in the emergency history must be on what brings the patient to the emergency service at this particular point. What has changed acutely? What is the exact sequence of events (external or internal) that led to the "emergency"? In taking the history of the current complaint, the clinician should always obtain information on alcohol use, drug use, and neurovegetative signs of depression, including change in sleep, in appetite or weight, in libido, and in bowel habits, and flattening of diurnal variation.

Past psychiatric history should take into consideration pharmacotherapy and psychotherapy, history of hospitalizations, history of suicidal gestures, and history of emergency visits. Past medical history should include any medical problems currently under treatment and any medications currently being taken. Family history includes a history of psychiatric disorders, substance abuse, suicide, hospitalizations, and use of psychotropic medications.

The personal, social, sexual, and occupational history should be covered in broad outlines. In most emergency settings there is neither the time nor the need for a detailed developmental history. However, it is essential to know whether there were major developmental arrests and to identify key traumata such as childhood parental death and physical or sexual abuse. Major past symptoms, the patient's current living and working situations, and an assessment of the highest level of functioning in relationships and social roles should also be noted.

In the emergency setting it is of the utmost importance to identify other possible sources of information: relatives, friends, co-workers or employer, landlord, minister, neighbor, physician, or therapist. They may be able to provide a coherent story when the patient is too disorganized to do so, or they may help to clarify the significance of a finding when the patient's account is suspect. This is particularly helpful when the patients may be under- or overestimating their dangerousness to themselves or others or their ability to care for themselves. The patient's permission should be sought for all such contacts, but in emergency circumstances where such outside information would affect key decisions, confidentiality may have to be waived in the interest of protecting life.

The mental status examination is a key instrument of the emergency evaluation. The patient's *appearance* and *behavior* are the first clues to the alert clinician. A neatly dressed man sitting calmly in the waiting room is quite distinct from a disheveled patient pacing rapidly up and down or from an elderly woman who averts her gaze and shows psychomotor retardation. *Cognition* includes evaluation of the patient's level of consciousness, orientation, attention span, memory, calculational ability, and constructional ability. A thorough survey of language ability or *diction* should note the amount, rate, rhythm, and articulation of spontaneous speech; the nature of the associational process (loose associations, klang associations, tangential associations); and the presence of overly abstract, concrete, illogical, metaphoric, or incoherent ways of speaking. *Emotion* is evaluated in terms of immediate affective state, subjectively and objectively reported, and in terms of the range and lability of emotional states. *Focus* or content of thought includes delusions, hallucinations, illusions, ideas of reference, overvalued ideas, obsessions, phobias, somatic concerns, helplessness or hopelessness, and suicidal or homicidal ideas as abnormal contents. The six italicized factors provide a simple alphabetical mnemonic — A,B,C,D,E,F — to ensure that all areas have been covered.

Physical and laboratory examinations must be based on the index of suspicion for an organic etiology to the psychiatric emergency. As noted above, vital signs are essential. An elevated temperature of autonomic hyperactivity may identify a patient in unsuspected alcohol withdrawal, a hypoglycemic diabetic, or the onset of neuroleptic malignant syndrome. If there is suspicion of an organic disorder on the basis of the history to this point, a physical examination and screening laboratory examination (electrolytes, electrocardiogram, chemistry profile, complete blood count, urinalysis, drug level, alcohol level, drug screen, blood gases) should be considered. Specialized tests that may be helpful include the amytal interview, the dexamethasone suppression test, and the pentobarbital challenge test. Radiological examinations and medical or neurological consultations should be available when a suspicion of medical disorder has been raised and the etiology is not clear.

The end point of the evaluation is a multiaxial DSM-III (34) diagnosis and formulation. Major diagnostic categories include major unipolar and bipolar affective disorders, schizophrenia, organic mental disorders, substance use disorders, anxiety disorders (including panic attacks and post-traumatic stress disorder), dysthymic disorder, cyclothymic disorder, adjustment disorder, disorders of impulse control, and V codes (including malingering, antisocial behavior, academic or occupational problem, marital problem, or parent-child problem) on Axis I and paranoid, schizoid, schizotypal, narcissistic, antisocial, or borderline personality disorder on Axis II.

Axis III medical disorders should be carefully specified.

Axis IV should specify the stressors and precipitants for the current emergency, including threatened and actual losses, financial stresses, interpersonal conflicts, and changes in aspects of the individual's life.

Axis V is a judgment as to where the current emergency fits relative to the patient's highest level of functioning in the past year.

Treatment

A variety of treatment modalities are available to the emergency clinician: pharmacotherapy, psychotherapy, and sociotherapy. The possible pharmacological interventions are wide- ranging. Specific treatment for unipolar and bipolar affective disorders includes tricyclic antidepressants, monoamine oxidase inhibitors, lithium carbonate, carbamazepine, and neuroleptics. Schizophrenic disorders may require neuroleptics, anti-Parkinsonian medications, and propranolol or carbamazepine for akathesia. Anxiety disorders have been responsive to treatment with benzodiazepines, antidepressants, and beta-blockers. Intermittent explosive disorders have been treated with beta-blockers, carbamazepine, and benzodiazepines. The pharmacological management of alcohol withdrawal, cholinergic syndromes, neuroleptic malignant syndrome, catatonia, and Wernicke's encephalopathy is the province of the emergency psychiatrist.

Psychotherapy in the emergency department is somewhat different from traditional long-term exploratory psychotherapy. The interventions are more active and short-term, though they may be just as definitive as longer-term therapy. Some examples include the use of breathing into a paper bag, along with instruction in relaxation techniques to deal with hyperventilation in a case of acute anxiety. Cathartic treatment following a traumatic event such as rape or a fire consists of supportive encouragement, validation of feelings, and repeated retelling of the story to "detoxify" the trauma. Clarification and interpretation may convert a terrifying onset of suicidal ideation into a more understandable response to an unrecognized loss or other life event, making the patient amenable to outpatient therapy. At times the clinician is as much arbiter and umpire as therapist in cases of marital or parent-child conflict, but skillful treatment can open channels of communication that can terminate the "emergency." Crisis theory suggests that a combination of exploratory and supportive techniques may achieve far-reaching resolution in the high- risk, high-gain context of crisis (1). Extended evaluation and crisis intervention in the emergency service can provide continuity of care and definitive resolution of a crisis, decreasing rates of hospitalization, and increasing acceptance of referrals (25).

Sociotherapy in an emergency means addressing a patient's helplessness. Financial help, temporary housing, food, and other social services are the appropriate response to many modern-day psychiatric emergencies, particularly in the population of chronic, deinstitutionalized, and homeless patients. Availability of a social worker and familiarity with community resources are valuable aspects of emergency treatment.

Disposition

Disposition decisions must be based on diagnosis and formulation of the emergency, the patient's response to the immediate treatment interventions in the emergency service, and the availability of community resources. An ideal community would have private and public psychiatric hospitals, partial-care facilities such as a day hospital, halfway houses, detoxification and rehabilitation facilities, medical-psychiatric units, drop-in centers, and home care services. Rarely are all these services available. What is essential in a psychiatric emergency service is to be familiar with the local resources, to work out mutually agreeable criteria for referral (criteria for hospitalization, for day hospitalization, and so on), and to maintain an ongoing relationship with these facilities. It is important to establish positive criteria based on which patients need and can benefit from a given service, rather than negative default criteria, which designate services "of the last resort."

Compliance with the recommendations of the emergency psychiatrist is an area of great concern. The rate of noncompliance is quite high, especially among patients without a prior connection to an institution or therapist (14). The clinician can increase the efficacy of referrals by negotiating the referral in the course of the emergency interview rather than merely presenting it to the patient at the end of the encounter; by designating a specific date, time, and place for the referral; by making direct contact with the agency rather than leaving it to the patient; and by avoiding long waits (29). If immediate referral cannot be made, the emergency clinician should be able to see the patient again or even several times. Finally, it is important to follow up with the agency and the patient to evaluate the disposition process.

WHAT MAKES EMERGENCY PSYCHIATRY WORK

A number of pragmatic considerations are important in emergency psychiatry. The backbone of successful provision of emergency care to the mentally disabled includes sound record-keeping practices, setting and following standards, establishing protocols and procedures, understanding legal issues, and maintaining a thoroughly trained staff. Research pursuit is another factor that can make a psychiatric emergency service stimulating for staff while moving the field ahead.

Records

Record keeping is best done in emergency psychiatry using a form that allows for checking off items on lists, as well as places for brief narratives cued in by heading requests for specific types of information. The usual record includes demographic information, problem list, vital signs, services provided, medications, legal constraints such as guardianship, suicide and homicide potential, staff assignment, social and developmental issues, and diagnostic impressions (10).

Standards

Standards in emergency psychiatry come from many different groups — the Joint Commission on the Accreditation of Hospitals (JCAH), the National Institute of Mental Health (NIMH), the Department of Transportation (DOT), the American College of Emergency Physicians (ACEP), the Emergency Department Nurses Association (EDNA), and the American Psychiatric Association (APA), to name major ones (7). The APA guidelines for standards, for example, describe an optimal service: 24-hour phone response, a mobile response team to evaluate patients in the community, 24-hour walk-in services, mental health personnel (not volunteers) answering the phone, designated medical direction, 24-hour nursing and social work capability, staff trained in emergency care, policy and procedure manuals to follow, triage within five minutes of presentation to the facility, vital signs taken routinely, initial signs and symptoms reported to a medical professional, medical screening, logbook, written treatment plan, evaluation and disposition, sharing of information to transfer agency, written transfer agreements, 24-hour access to dispositions, 24-hour availability of a physician, immediate recording of information, immediate retrievability of records information (11). Locales differ in their degrees of compliance and completeness relative to these standards (3).

Protocols

Protocols are particularly helpful in emergency care since there is usually a multitude of staff servicing the emergency department, each with its own set of attitudes, upbringing, and training background. Protocols provide consistency and continuity of care. Typical topics for emergency psychiatric facilities include violence, safety, child abuse, triage, rape, domestic violence, restraints, and seclusion (12). The format of protocols may be a simple outline or algorithm or a combination of both. They should pictorially and verbally show, in quick, easy-to-read style, step-by-step directions to follow for each case presentation.

Procedures

Procedure manuals should include protocols, administrative agreements, staffing roles, commitment procedures, admission procedures, copies of forms, and phone numbers and addresses of potential dispositions (15).

Legal Issues

The legal issues that are important for emergency psychiatric staff to be aware of include (1) *implied consent* — when someone comes to the emergency department, he is consenting by implication to treatment or laboratory tests; (2) *assault and battery* (threat of touching) — staff should have firmly documented justification to touch or restrain a patient; (3) *false imprisonment* — staff must justify holding someone more than 24 hours against his will; (4) *negligence* — this can be active or passive breech of duty with a patient suffering damages; (5) *confidentiality* — patients' statements to a physician and other mental health professionals are protected, as are laboratory findings and records — but not in every state or county and not if an illegal act or dangerous weapons were involved; (6) *right to refuse treatment* — an incompetent patient may not have this right in some states; (7) *informed consent* — a person has a right to know whether there are possible adverse effects to a medication; (8) *involuntary hospitalization* — the state is the caretaker of the weak and helpless, so that patients who are mentally ill and are a danger to themselves or others may be involuntarily committed (17). Some states allow for commitment if there is inability to care for self also.

Training

Training in emergency psychiatry is crucial to good care. The curriculum should include ennunciation of the goals, communication skills, therapy approaches, differential diagnosis, medication management, resource identification, team approach, burnout and stress reduction, protocols, record keeping, different patient presentations, and staff response (27). The methods a trainer might utilize in teaching emergency psychiatry are vast and include use of tapes, films, video, patient simulations, role playing, graded experiences, skill testing, on-site supervision, small group discussions, lectures, home study, and workshops (23). There are different opportunities to reach the trainees as well — in undergraduate and graduate training years, at board examination and recertification times, or as a continuing education opportunity.

Research

The research potential in emergency psychiatry is still very much unrealized. Funding has been poor; staff has felt pressured for time. Yet there is a need to pool demographic and outcome data (31). It is known that staff attitudes influence diagnostics and disposition, but these need study to see whether attitudes can be altered to enhance patient care (23). Cost benefit issues are not clearly identified, let alone studied. Accessibility due to geography, ethnicity, transportation, and economic barriers may be worthwhile studying, if even on the local level. Whether there is a level of care consistent with standards is not known — a far-reaching survey would soon identify where we are (3).

THE FUTURE OF EMERGENCY PSYCHIATRY

The future will be in more refined diagnostics and referral capability. Economic restraints will restrict the number of casual visits to emergency departments and may encroach on existing dispositional options. Research could be increased, but only if money is available for it. Hopefully all psychiatric residents will get emergency psychiatry training and all staff who supervise emergency psychiatry trainees will have had emergency psychiatric training themselves. Better and more efficient coordination of resources, as well as specialized services to children, the multiple drug abuser, and those who are both mentally ill and drug abusing, is needed (6). It will be important to get regional planning and clearinghouse activities started. The emergency department has evolved as a hub of a wheel of resource coordination. Therefore, it will be important for emergency psychiatry to remain an integral part of the emergency department so that patients will have their medical as well as their psychiatric needs met, so that alternatives to state hospital care are thought through, so that access to involuntary treatment remains available, so that training remains an integrative, sharing experience for all disciplines (30).

ACKNOWLEDGMENT

Portions of this chapter have been adapted from the text, *Handbook of Emergency Psychiatry for Clinical Administrators*, edited by Gail M. Barton, M.D., M.P.H., and Rohn S. Friedman, M.D., published by the Haworth Press, Inc., 1986, with permission of the publisher.

REFERENCES

1. BARTOLUCCI, G., & DRAYER, C. S. (1973). An overview of crisis intervention in the emergency rooms of general hospitals. *American Journal of Psychiatry, 130,* 953.
2. BARTON, G. M. (1978). Mental health emergency. In *Task force on psychiatric emergency care issues draft.* Washington, DC: American Psychiatric Association.
3. BARTON, G. M. (1981). Psychiatric emergency care standards: A survey of hospitals in Michigan. Lecture in the postgraduate course in emergency psychiatry at Towsley Center. Ann Arbor, MI: University of Michigan.

4. BARTON, G. M. (1981). The psychiatrist in the emergency department: Problems and resistances as determined by a national opinion survey. Lecture in the postgraduate course in emergency psychiatry. Ann Arbor, MI: University of Michigan.
5. BARTON, G. M. (1981). The emergence of emergency psychiatry. *Hospital & Community Psychiatry, 32*, 667.
6. BARTON, G. M. (1982). Emergency psychiatry: The outlook for the future. *Psychiatric Annals, 12*, 807.
7. BARTON, G. M. (1982). Standards of care. In J. G. Gorton & R. Partridge (Eds.), *Practice and management of psychiatric emergency care.* St. Louis: Mosby.
8. BARTON, G. M. (1983). Psychiatric staff and the emergency department: Roles, responsibilities, and reciprocation. *Psychiatric Clinics of North America: Emergency Psychiatry, 6*, 317.
9. BARTON, G. M. (1985/1986). Architectural model considerations in planning a psychiatric emergency service. *Emergency Health Services Review, 3*(2/3), 55–62.
10. BARTON, G. M. (1985/1986). Emergency psychiatric records. *Emergency Health Services Review, 3*(2/3), 217–236.
11. BARTON, G. M. (1985–1986). Standards for emergency psychiatry. *Emergency Health Services Review, 3*(2/3), 237–260.
12. BARTON, G. M., & COMSTOCK, B. S. (1985/1986). Protocols, algorithms, and procedures in emergency psychiatry. *Emergency Health Services Review, 3*(2/3), 185–216.
13. BASSUK, E. L., & GERSON, S. (1979). Into the breach: Emergency psychiatry in the general hospital. *General Hospital Psychiatry, 1*, 31.
14. BLOUIN, A., PERES, E., & MINOLETTI, A. (1985). Compliance to referrals from the psychiatric emergency room. *Canadian Journal of Psychiatry, 30*, 103.
15. COMSTOCK, B. S. (1980). *Program manual in emergency psychiatry.* Houston: Ben Taub General Hospital.
16. COMSTOCK, B. S. (1985/1986). The structure of one emergency psychiatry service. *Emergency Health Services Review, 3*(2/3), 159–168.
17. FAUMAN, B. J. (1985/1986). Legal issues in emergency psychiatry. *Emergency Health Services Review, 3*(2/3), 75–86.
18. FAUMAN, B. J. (1985/1986). Personnel: The psychiatric emergency care team. *Emergency Health Services Review, 3*(2/3), 37–48.
19. FAUMAN, M. A. (1981). Psychiatric components of medical and surgical practice: I: A survey of general hospital physicians. *American Journal of Psychiatry, 138*, 1298.
20. FAUMAN, M. A. (1983). Psychiatric components of medical and surgical practice, II: Referral and treatment of psychiatric disorders. *American Journal of Psychiatry, 140*, 760.
21. FAUMAN, M. A. (1985/1986). Emergency psychiatric services for medical and surgical inpatients. *Emergency Health Services Review, 3*(2/3), 123–132.
22. FRIEDMAN, R. S. (1985/1986). The profile of psychiatric emergency patients. *Emergency Health Services Review, 3*(2/3), 25–36.
23. FRIEDMAN, R. S., BARTON, G. M., COMSTOCK, B. S., & WALKER, E. (1985/1986). Training and research in emergency psychiatry. *Emergency Health Services Review, 3*(2/3), 87–104.
24. FRIEDMAN, R., SOREFF, S., & BARTON, G. M. (1986). The development of emergency psychiatry. In G. Barton & R. Friedman (Eds.), *The handbook of emergency psychiatry for clinical administrators.* New York: Haworth Press.
25. GERSON, S., & BASSUK, E. (1980). Psychiatric emergencies: An overview. *American Journal of Psychiatry, 137*, 1.
26. GOMEZ, R., & BARTON, G. M. (1985/1986). Staff attitudes towards psychiatric emergency patients with special needs. *Emergency Health Services Review, 3*(2/3), 49–54.
27. HAZEL, J. P., & ESTRADA, E. G. (1980). Nursing process in crisis intervention. In J. P.

Hazel & E. G. Estrada (Eds.), *Core curriculum* (pp. 333–356). Chicago: Emergency Department Nurses Association.

28. HYMAN, S. E. (Ed.) (1984). *Manual of psychiatric emergencies.* Boston: Little, Brown.

29. JELLINEK, M. (1978). Referrals from a psychiatric emergency room: Relationship of compliance to demographic and interview variables. *American Journal of Psychiatry, 135,* 209.

30. SLABY, A. E. (1981). Emergency psychiatry: An update. *Hospital & Community Psychiatry, 32,* 687.

31. SLABY, A. E. (1983). Research strategies in emergency psychiatry. *Psychiatric Clinics of North America: Emergency Psychiatry, 6,* 347.

32. SLABY, A. E. (1985/1986). Definitions and conceptual framework of psychiatric emergencies. *Emergency Health Services Review, 3*(2/3), 9–24.

33. SLABY, A. E., LIEB, J., & TANCREDI, L. R. (1986). *Handbook of psychiatric emergencies* (3rd ed.). Garden City, NY: Medical Examination Publishing Co.

34. SPITZER, R. L., & TASK FORCE ON NOMENCLATURE AND STATISTICS (1980). *Diagnostic and statistical manual of mental disorders* (3rd ed.). Washington, DC: American Psychiatric Association.

35. STROTKAMP, J., & BARTON, G. M. (1985/1986). Liaison with the courts and corrections. *Emergency Health Services Review, 3*(2/3), 261–276.

17

RECENT ADVANCES IN THE CLINICAL USE OF LITHIUM

PETER WEIDEN, M.D.

Instructor in Psychiatry,
The New York Hospital, Payne Whitney Clinic,
New York City, New York

and

JAMES KOCSIS, M.D.

Associate Professor of Psychiatry,
The New York Hospital, Payne Whitney Clinic,
New York City, New York

INTRODUCTION

A review of lithium treatment 10 years ago might have focused on its efficacy in acute mania and in prophylaxis of bipolar illness. While the role of lithium salts in the treatment of these conditions is now unquestioned, new issues are emerging. Current areas of critical clinical importance include new potential indicators for lithium, increased awareness of the problems involved in long-term lithium management, and alternative or adjunctive treatments when lithium fails. The goal of this chapter is to review advances in the clinical uses of lithium that have occurred over the past decade, including: (1) identification of other illnesses that might be lithium responsive; (2) development of alternative treatment possibilities for lithium-unresponsive, relapsing bipolar patients; (3) methods of better recognition and management of lithium side effects; and (4) more effective management of the multiple factors involved in lithium noncompliance.

350

Acute Mania

Although lithium has been shown to be effective in placebo-controlled trials in acute mania (26), clinicians still face major problems and choices while treating acutely manic patients. For example, there are options involving rapid lithium dosing. In order to achieve a clinical response, plasma lithium levels need to be raised as high as tolerated during an acute manic episode (26,27,56). Because of increasing pressure for short hospitalizations in the United States, fairly aggressive dosing is required to achieve to a target level of 1.2–1.4 mEq/liter (recommended for young, physically healthy patients) within 1 week. One empirical method is to begin with lithium carbonate, 300 mg capsules three times a day, and following dosage requirements with daily lithium levels. Alternatively, another approach is to estimate lithium requirements via a single dose of 600 mg of lithium followed by a serum lithium determination 24 hours later (7). The frequent resistance to treatment found in acute mania further complicates dosage adjustments. Approaches that facilitate compliance despite the typical symptoms of grandiosity, paranoia, and denial include careful training of hospital staff in use of lithium, early family and patient education about the benefits of lithium, and use of adjuvant agents such as neuroleptics for faster symptom relief. Liquid lithium citrate preparation (instead of carbonate capsules) may be used to ensure the patient is not "cheeking" the capsules (27). Because lithium can take up to six weeks to control acute symptoms, treatment with lithium alone requires hospital staff patience and tolerance for manic behavior. If the patient's past history or extent of manic symptoms (paranoia, denial, or assaultiveness) prohibit the use of lithium alone, concomitant neuroleptics or sedatives are indicated (26).

However, combined treatment with lithium and neuroleptic introduces other potential complications. Lithium/neuroleptic toxicity is of concern because of reports of neurological syndromes as a result of high doses of combined haloperidol/lithium administration (29). These syndromes probably represent variants of neuroleptic malignant syndrome (NMS). The risk of NMS has been found to depend primarily on neuroleptic dosage rather than lithium levels or class of neuroleptic (13,35). A clear understanding of the etiology of NMS in patients receiving lithium and neuroleptic is complicated by the fact that severe toxicity can arise from either one. However, since parkinsonian signs including rigidity almost always predate NMS (13), NMS may be prevented by lowering or discontinuing neuroleptic treatment when significant or progressive parkinsonian signs (rigidity, tremor, and akinesia) develop. Progressive extrapyramidal symptoms (EPS) in acute mania should be closely followed and vigorously treated (i.e., neuroleptic dosage reduction or concomitant use of anticholinergic agents). A cautious approach to neuroleptic dosing should be taken with elderly and medically ill patients (35). Because lithium can augment EPS effects (50), neuroleptics may have to be lowered if lithium is added later.

Another potential complication introduced by neuroleptic use is tardive dyskinesia (TD). Unfortunately, bipolar affective illness seems to be a risk factor for TD. The intermittent nature of neuroleptic administration often prescribed for recurrent mania may actually increase the patient's risk of TD. It is not surprising, therefore, that a recent survey found a high incidence of TD in a chronically ill bipolar outpatient sample (37). Therefore, neuroleptics probably should not be used in manic patients who have signs of TD or a history of frequent relapses that require multiple exposures to neuroleptics. In these situations, alternate adjunctive medications other than neuroleptics, such as benzodiazepines, might be considered (36). Physical examination for signs of TD should be done and documented at least yearly between acute episodes.

The problems of neuroleptic toxicity in bipolar patients have led to a search for alternative treatments. Recently benzodiazepines (lorazepam) have been reported to be effective as adjuvant treatment in acute (even psychotic) mania (36). Although these findings need replication in controlled studies, benzodiazepines (especially lorazepam, which is easily administered intramuscularly) may represent an alternate adjunctive treatment for manic patients who either refuse or cannot tolerate neuroleptics, or for those who have signs of TD. Nevertheless, combined neuroleptic/lithium treatment usually is a safe, effective treatment for acute mania.

Lithium-unresponsive acute manics may also benefit from treatment with carbamazepine (41, 42) or clonazepam (5), alone or in combination with lithium. Rapid-cycling or mixed bipolar patients may be bipolar subtypes who are more likely to respond from these alternate treatments (49,51), especially in the setting of documented previous lithium failure. However, before treatment is changed, one should evaluate whether the patient's plasma lithium had been at adequately high therapeutic levels for a long enough period of time. Inadequate lithium trials are an indication for more vigorous lithium treatment rather than its abandonment (25,26).

Prophylaxis in Bipolar Disorder

Lithium has been repeatedly shown to prevent or diminish manic and depressive episodes in bipolar patients. Nevertheless, attenuated affective episodes frequently occur despite lithium maintenance. Such episodes are generally milder than those expected in the same individual without lithium (25). In many patients there is tendency for a positive response to lithium maintenance to develop only with time. Thus, early management of maintenance bipolar patients often means encouraging patients to persist with lithium despite relapses that occur. The frequency of relapse for lithium patients is directly proportional to their serum levels (25), so raising the maintenance dosage should be tried for those who have repeated full relapses. When patients are educated about lithium, emphasis on the important benefits of maintenance therapy needs to be offset with avoiding conveying *excessively* high expectations of lithium's efficacy (52). This is most true at the beginning of treatment (usually just as the patient is recovering from a devastating first episode) before the patient's individual lithium response is known. Lithium is not always the "miracle" it is thought to be by the lay public.

Recommendations for duration of lithium prophylaxis need to be individualized. Illness severity, abruptness of onset, potential consequences of relapse, and the severity and discomfort of adverse effects should go into a risk/benefit analysis that is made by both patient and doctor (9). Severely ill patients often require lifelong treatment, whereas indications for long-term treatment in the less severely ill bipolar patients are less clear-cut. Most studies of lithium prophylaxis have tended to use a severely ill, frequently relapsing cohort of patients (9,43). Therefore, few research studies are available for clinical guidance in terms of duration of treatment for bipolar patients who have less severe or infrequent episodes. Most authors recommend plasma levels of lithium from 0.6 to 1.2 mEq/liter for maintenance therapy (19,21); however, dosages and plasma levels should be individualized according to the clinical situation. When possible, such dosage decisions should be based on the patient's past history of minimal effective dosages and/or knowledge at what serum level the side effects become intolerable.

Another important clinical issue is the usefulness of combined maintenance lithium and tricyclic antidepressants (TCA). One recent large study of long-term outcome in bipolar patients demonstrated that maintenance imipramine in combination with lithium did not offer additional benefits compared to lithium alone (23,43). Indeed, such a regimen may increase the risk of manic episodes during lithium maintenance (although the question of whether antidepressants precipitate mania continues to be controversial) (30). TCAs or monoamine oxidase inhibitors (MAOI) should usually not be used on a *long-term* basis during maintenance therapy for bipolar patients. They are best reserved for *short-term* use during acute depressions. TCAs and MAOIs should be discontinued shortly after the acute depression resolves. Although TCAs are the usual first-line agent in bipolar depression, some recent evidence suggests that the MAOI tranylcypramine may be the most effective antidepressant for bipolar depressions with predominant symptoms of hypersomnia and psychomotor retardation (14).

Recurrent Major Depression

An exciting new development has been the repeated finding that lithium can be helpful when combined with either TCAs or MAOIs for unipolar-depressed patients who are refractory to treatment with antidepressant agents alone (10). When effective, the antidepressant response to adjuvant lithium will usually be observed within one week. A goal of future research will be to attempt to identify clinical characteristics of those refractory individuals who will specifically benefit from lithium augmentation or TCA or MAOI treatment.

Lithium use for prophylaxis of unipolar depression is controversial. A review by Davis in 1976 of a small number of early studies concluded that lithium was just as effective as a TCA for this purpose (9). A relative advantage of lithium in unipolar patients is that lithium, unlike the usual antidepressants, does not increase the patient's risk of first-episode mania. Despite these considerations most investigators conclude that lithium is less effective than TCAs for the *unipolar*-depressed population. The lithium response rate has been lower than that seen with TCAs and recovery has tended to take longer (19,21). A recent multicenter collaborative study found that severely ill unipolar depressives fared relatively better on TCA maintenance compared to lithium (43). Despite conflicting reports, it seems reasonable to utilize lithium as a second-line rather than a primary agent in prophylaxis of unipolar depression. Therefore, lithium as a sole agent for treatment of unipolar depression cannot generally be recommended. Lithium as the primary prophylactic medication should be considered for TCA-unresponsive patients, patients with family histories of bipolar disorder, women with histories of postpartum depression, depressed patients with bipolar II or cyclothymic disorders, and patients intolerant to side effects of other antidepressant medications (21).

Atypical Affective Disorders

Bipolar variants include (1) mixed affective states with persistent coexisting manic and depressive symptoms, (2) rapid cycling (usually defined as four or more affective episodes per year), (3) cyclothymic disorders and the so-called "emotionally-unstable personality disorder" described by Rifkin et al. (47), (4) organic mania and mania coexisting with brain disease (6,28). Not surprisingly, lithium has been used to treat all of these presumed bipolar variants.

Mixed or rapid-cycling types of bipolar illness have tended to be poorly responsive to lithium. As reviewed by Roy-Byrne et al. (49), rapid-cycling patients were more likely to have underlying medical problems (e.g., multiple sclerosis or thyroid disease) and were perhaps more sensitive to mood-dysregulating effects of time zone changes, concomitant medications (e.g., thyroid supplement), and antidepressant therapies. While the sensitivity of rapid-cycling patients to exogenous or endogenous stressors may attentuate the therapeutic gain possible from lithium, it is our recommendation that lithium remain the first-line treatment. Careful attention should be given to any coexisting stressors and/or underlying medical problems exacerbating the affective episodes. If rapid-cycling patients do not improve after a substantial trial of lithium treatment (i.e., one year at serum levels greater than 1.0 mEq/liter), one might consider alternate or adjunctive therapies, such as carbamazepine, clonazepam, valproic acid, or levo-thyroxine.

The clinical aspects of the cyclothymic–bipolar II spectrum have been well reviewed by Akiskal and associates (1), who underscored methodological problems in evaluation of lithium treatment for patients with these bipolar spectrum disorders. They present with symptoms of insomnia, promiscuity, "dilettantism," repeated marital failures, and drug and alcohol abuse. These kinds of problems are frequently viewed as personality disorders, and the affective syndrome is missed. Such patients also often derive considerable social benefit from their hypomania and do not comply with psychological or medical therapies. Nonetheless, lithium can be very helpful for patients who do comply. Dramatic and sustained clinical improvements may occur, including decreased illicit drug use, improved insomnia, or a subjective sense of an improved quality of life. Lithium should be considered for so-called "personality disorder," affectively unstable, predominantly hypomanic patients (1,47). Therefore, a careful clinical evaluation for possible hypomanic symptoms should be done in patients who present with apparent personality disorders or substance abuse diagnoses.

Lithium has also been found to be efficacious for treatment of mania secondary to certain types of organic brain disease (DSM-III diagnosis of organic affective syndrome) (6,28). Lithium may be used for symptomatic control, especially in cases where the underlying cerebral pathology cannot be corrected (i.e., stroke) (38). In mentally retarded individuals who suffer from coexisting bipolar illness, lithium treatment has improved cognitive performance as well as decreasing bizarre, violent and uncontrollable behavior (6). It is important to note that the co-occurrence of mental retardation and bipolar illness often results in atypical clinical presentations without classical bipolar signs. Such patients are at high risk for TD and other complications of chronic neuroleptic therapy. For this population, lithium has the advantage of efficacy and safety compared to the more commonly used neuroleptics.

Alcoholism

Lithium has been used as a preventive agent in the treatment of alcoholism. At least two controlled studies demonstrate that alcoholics on lithium maintenance had a lower relapse rate than those taking placebo (34). However, these results were limited by the confounding factor that compliance to any medication by alcoholic patients is a good prognostic sign. The lithium-compliant alcoholic group (which is clearly established via lithium levels) may have represented a better prognosis population than its placebo control (where compliance is uncertain). Therefore, despite some encouraging data, the effectiveness of lithium treatment to promote alcohol abstinence has not been established. Furthermore, alcoholics are at great danger of iatrogenic lithium toxicity. Until further research is done that accounts for compliance, lithium should not be recommended as a primary treatment modality for alcoholism. The important and common clinical exception are patients whose alcohol abuse is secondary to an underlying primary bipolar disorder. For these patients, lithium is a primary and essential treatment.

Schizophrenic and Schizoaffective Disorders

Before considering lithium in schizophrenic disorders, the following questions need to be addressed. (1) Is lithium helpful for secondary manic-like symptoms in schizophrenia, or is it efficacious (without neuroleptic) for "core" schizophrenic symptoms (i.e., thought disorder, unrelatedness)? (2) Is schizoaffective disorder (where lithium is commonly used) a "true" disease or actually a latent form of either bipolar disorder or schizophrenia only to be clarified later in the course of the illness? (3) If schizoaffective disorder is a separate illness, does its natural history more closely resemble schizophrenia or bipolar disorder? (4) Do changes in diagnostic criteria for schizoaffective disorder change the likelihood of a lithium response?

Although none of these major issues have been definitively resolved, how these problems are viewed impacts on clinical decisions for lithium use.

Bipolar disorder versus schizophrenia. Long-term studies have shown that many "schizoaffective" patients eventually develop clear schizophrenia or bipolar disorders (24). Presumably at the time of presentation when schizoaffective disorder is diagnosed, the "true" illness has not yet assumed a typical clinical form. Lithium might be expected to be efficacious in patients who will later develop typical bipolar patterns, but clinical predictors to specifically identify those patients are not established. In addition, it is well known that there is significant overlap between "schizophrenic" and "manic" symptoms during an acute manic psychosis. Acutely ill manic patients may display a full range of schizophrenic (i.e., Schniederian first rank) symptoms, thus obscuring the bipolar diagnosis. Making a correct diagnosis is further complicated by the frequent occurrence of marked affective features in young first-episode schizophrenics. In light of these observations, we recommend a cautious diagnostic approach in distinguishing bipolar disorder from schizophrenia in unclear first-episode cases. Assessments should emphasize longitudinal course and family history in addition to the acute symptom complex. It goes without saying that one should avoid (as best possible) misdiagnosing psychotic bipolar patients as schizophrenics, and vice versa. Clinicians treating schizoaffective patients early in the course of illness should be prepared to shift diagnosis and treatment if the clinical picture changes over time. Lithium is, of course, the primary treatment for patients who eventually develop unequivocal bipolar illness.

Treatment of secondary manic symptoms versus core schizophrenic symptoms. Because one would intuitively expect lithium to be most helpful in cases of schizophrenia with secondary manic symptoms, it is not surprising that most reports of use of lithium in schizophrenia have involved "schizoaffective" samples. The definitions of this disorder, however, have varied among authors. Procci (44), in an excellent review, combined data from a number of studies and found that lithium alone was helpful in 74 percent of schizoaffective patients (here defined as having both manic and schizophrenic symptoms), but that improvement on lithium was usually limited to affective symptoms.

However, Donaldson and colleagues (11) have reviewed three studies that attempted to separate schizoaffective disorder from chronic schizophrenia. They did not find any difference in lithium responsiveness between these groups. They concluded that "affective symptoms are neither necessary nor sufficient to predict a beneficial response to lithium treatment" (p. 508). An example is a study by Hirschowitz and colleagues that found DSM-III *schizophreniform* (*not* schizoaffective) psychosis responded better to lithium than did schizophrenia. In addition, Mattes and Nayak (32) did not find lithium helpful for schizophreniclike schizoaffective patients. These findings, taken together, suggest that *good-prognosis* acute schizophrenics might respond relatively well to lithium. The presence or absence of affective symptoms may be less important than was once believed. In contrast, chronic schizophrenia with or without affective symptoms has generally been found to be lithium unresponsive.

Changing diagnostic criteria. When evaluating the question of lithium in schizophrenia and schizoaffective disorder, it is important to consider that key studies represent patient samples selected according to definitions of schizoaffective disorder (39,44) that substantially differ from American DSM-III-R criteria. DSM-III-R criteria for schizoaffective disorder specifically exclude as bipolar patients with a manic syndrome and bizarre mood-incongruent delusions. Thus, many schizoaffective patients, as defined earlier by Procci, would be currently diagnosed as having either bipolar or schizophreniform disorders. DSM-III-R schizoaffective patients usually represent more chronically psychotic patients who display intermittent affective syndromes. Because of the studies described above (10,15,30), lithium treatment for those DSM-III-R schizoaffective disorders may thus be less effective than for schizoaffective patients diagnosed by Research Diagnostic Criteria, a system more clinically similar to Procci's definition.

Conclusion. Therapeutic indications for a lithium trial as an adjunct to neuroleptics might be broadened to include acutely ill, good-prognosis schizophrenic or schizophreniform patients with or without affective symptoms (39), particularly when neuroleptics alone have been shown to be ineffective. On the other hand, lithium alone may be relatively ineffective for schizoaffective patients as diagnosed by DSM-III-R criteria.

COMPLICATIONS AND SIDE EFFECTS OF LITHIUM THERAPY

Lithium-induced side effects range from toxic syndromes to subtle and often unreported problems. Toxicity usually occurs at high (>1.5 mEq/liter) while expected side effects occur at therapeutic (<1.5 mEq/liter) serum lithium levels. However, overlap exists and the patient's complaints and symptoms are more clinically meaningful than the serum level. Because the signs, symptoms, and management of severe lithium toxicity have been well described in standard textbooks, we shall consider only the subtle problems often encountered at therapeutic serum levels.

The frequency of occurrence of side effects will depend on the vigor with which a clinician sets out to find them. "Minor" (to the physician) side effects are a major contributor to an extremely high lithium noncompliance rate (58% the first year of treatment in one major study) (33). Active inquiry about specific lithium side effects will provide more valid information than waiting for spontaneous complaints. Furthermore, some "side effects" (as reported by a patient) may actually represent misinterpreted therapeutic effects (i.e., loss of the manic euphoria). Patients experience significant distress from these psychological losses and often require psychological and pharmacological management, just as one would for more straightforward side effects.

Neuropsychological Effects

Recent research has yielded information about adverse effects of lithium on cognition, memory, and creativity. These findings may be helpful in understanding patient complaints and noncompliance to lithium. Although clinicians have long suspected such cognitive effects (54), lack of methodologies for distinguishing between affective symptoms and lithium-induced cognitive impairment has limited investigations. Earlier studies of lithium side effects did not include systemized objective or subjective ratings of cognitive or memory problems, thus limiting the recognition and reporting of these side effects (58). Only recently have sensitive neuropsychological measures been applied that demonstrate lithium-induced cognitive syndromes (52). Nonetheless, patients on lithium frequently do report subjective memory loss and cognitive impairment. Such subjective complaints have been objectively confirmed by Shaw and colleagues (52). Their study used euthymic as well as affectively ill subjects. Euthymic patients had a reversible, lithium-induced neuropsychological syndrome, marked by memory impairment and decreased thinking and motor speed. These deficits were found in patients who had remained on lithium for long periods of time and presumably were maximally accommodated to these effects. It seems reasonable to assume that patients recently started on lithium could experience even more acute effects and notice greater memory impairment. These effects may contribute to the high noncompliance rates observed during the first year of lithium treatment. Despite the difficulties inherent in interpreting reports of cognitive dysfunction in patients just recovering from affective episodes, such symptoms warrant serious consideration as being valid. Judd (22) found that subtle lithium-induced cognitive impairments in normal subjects are better observed by family and friends compared to trained investigators rating adverse effects. This observation demonstrates the usefulness of interviewing family members in the evaluation of potential lithium side effects.

As suggested by Vestergaard and colleagues, many patients are reluctant to complain about memory and cognitive effects and such information needs to be actively drawn out in the interview. Although concern may be raised about "putting ideas into the patient's head," probably the net effect of questioning for cognitive problems would be increased compliance. Patients expressed *relief* at the knowledge that their memory problems were from lithium rather than their illness (52). No patient in the sample studied refused lithium after being told of lithium-induced memory effects. A clinical approach to a euthymic, recently lithium-stabilized bipolar patient might include (1) active inquiry (including asking family members) about the presence of subtle cognitive problems, (2) ruling out a prodromal affective relapse or lithium-induced hypothyroidism as the cause of memory complaints, (3) acknowledging as valid the patient's complaints of memory and creativity difficulties, (4) discussion of the benefits of lithium, (5) willingness to work to minimize these side effects, such as lowering maintenance dosages whenever possible (52,53).

Another related area that can be considered a side effect (from the patient's point of view) is the lithium-induced loss of productivity and creativity experienced during hypomanic phases of bipolar disorders. Jamison and associates (18) questioned their bipolar outpatients about various psychosocial aspects of their illness, including interpersonal sensitivity, sexuality, productivity, social ease, and creativity. Over 80 percent of the sample reported experiencing benefits from their bipolar illness along one of these dimensions. Presumably, effective lithium treatment produces a loss of these perceived benefits and could be considered (at least to the patient) as an "adverse effect." We recommend that clinicians discuss such issues with their patients and consider them as possible "adverse effects" of lithium therapy (17). Psychotherapy around these issues can be helpful; clinicians have tended to underestimate its importance for lithium compliance.

Thyroid

Lithium can cause a range of thyroid abnormalities from euthyroid goiter to frank hypothyroidism. Although the mechanism of lithium's effect on the thyroid is not fully understood, lithium does block the cAMP second messenger system when thyroid-stimulating hormone (TSH) stimulates thyroid release at the gland site, which could account for this effect. A sensitive laboratory test for lithium effects on thyroid is serum TSH.

The relationship between thyroid disease, bipolar psychopathology, and lithium is not fully understood (3). Bipolar patients, without lithium exposure, seem more likely to have underlying thyroid illness than the general population. Patients with preexisting laboratory values consistent with Hashimoto's thryroiditis (high antithyroid titers) are more likely to develop lithium-induced hypothyroidism. It also seems that "rapid cyclers" in particular are more likely to having preexisting thyroid disorders and developing lithium-induced hypothyroidism (3,8).

We recommend the following for the evaluation and management of thyroid function in lithium patients: (1) routine measurement of serum TSH (at least yearly); (2) evaluation of autoimmune function (i.e., antithyroid antibody titers) in all cases of lithium-induced hypothyroidism (4); (3) thorough investigation of thyroid status in rapid-cycling patients (8,49); (4) thyroid evaluation (TSH and physical examination) in any lithium patient developing depression or paranoia (even when the symptoms resemble primary psychopathology) to rule out organic affective syndromes secondary to thyroid dysfunction (28); (5) evaluation of thyroid status (TSH) when patients complain of cognitive or memory problems (50); (6) levothyroxine as a possible adjunctive treatment for lithium-unresponsive rapid-cycling patients, whether or not thyroid indices are abnormal (12,55).

Parathyroid

Lithium has recently been reported to cause hypercalcemia secondary to increased parathyroid hormone activity (48). This rare complication should be considered in cases of unexplained hypercalcemia in lithium patients.

Renal

Lithium is primarily eliminated from the body through excretion by the kidneys. Renal handling of lithium parallels sodium; conditions leading to physiological renal resorption of sodium (i.e., low salt intake or dehydration) may cause lithium retention. Toxicity may arise from clinical states involving sodium depletion (i.e., low salt intake) or a prerenal decrease in glomerular filtration rate (i.e., dehydration). It is important to educate patients to maintain salt and fluid intake. Patients should be instructed not to take (without consultation) diuretics prescribed by other physicians.

Lithium is known to decrease the action of ADH on the distal tubule, the site of much water and salt resorption. This can lead to nephrogenic diabetes insipidus (DI), which can arise at any point in long-term lithium therapy. Clinical symptoms include polyuria, nocturia, and polydipsia. Laboratory abnormalities include decreased renal concentrating capacity and mild hypernatremia (57). Patients with nephrogenic DI may require larger lithium dosages than usual to achieve therapeutic serum concentrations because of the increased renal loss of lithium. Nephrogenic DI can be distinguished from the psychogenic polydipsia often seen in psychiatric patients by measurement of serum sodium. Sodium is slightly lower than normal (<140 mEq/liter) in psychogenic polydipsia and elevated (>140 mEq/liter) in DI. Fluid deprivation followed by a measurement of renal concentrating ability is a more definitive test differentiating psychogenic from lithium-induced polyuria, but requires considerable patient cooperation.

Several treatments are possible for lithium-induced DI. Because the symptoms are sometimes dose-dependent, lowering maintenance lithium dose and serum levels may suffice. Various diuretics may paradoxically be helpful in refractory patients by increasing lithium and sodium resorption in the proximal tubules. Thiazide diuretics have traditionally been used for this purpose, and recently the potassium-sparing diuretic amiloride (2) has been reported effective. It is necessary to monitor serum lithium levels closely (daily) when treating nephrogenic DI with diuretics because of the possibility of inducing rapidly increasing lithium levels with subsequent toxicity.

Some controversy persists about whether lithium causes long-term renal damage. Early reports of interstitial nephritis in chronic lithium treatment patients have not been confirmed in later studies. Vestergaard and Amdisen (57) followed 147 long-term lithium patients for an average of 1.7 years and found no difference in serum creatinine or 24-hour creatinine clearance between lithium patients and bipolar unmedicated controls. We agree with most authorities that while baseline renal function tests should be obtained before initiation of lithium therapy and that serum creatinine should be measured yearly during lithium treatment, renal toxicity should not be considered a likely risk of treatment (45). Finally, lithium use is safe in patients with end-stage renal disease, when the appropriate dosage is given immediately after dialysis (31).

Gastrointestinal

Lithium at therapeutic dosages may cause nausea, vomiting, and diarrhea. These symptoms correlate with the rate of rise of the serum levels as well as the absolute level and hence are more likely to occur as doses are being increased. Taking lithium with food slows down rapid gastrointestinal absorption and may decrease nausea related to direct gastric irritation (21). Slow-release lithium preparations can cause diarrhea from the osmotic load of undigested tablets reaching the colon.

Respiratory

Lithium has recently been found to exacerbate respiratory failure in patients with preexisting lung disease (60). Presumably the mechanism of action involves lithium-induced neuromuscular blockade. Obviously this is of concern in chronic pulmonary patients with already impaired ventilatory capacity who also require lithium. In those circumstances clinical judgment weighing the relative risks and benefits of lithium is necessary. Also of note is that concomitant theophylline lowers serum lithium levels (40).

Hemopoietic

Lithium causes a benign leukocytosis (and also thrombocytosis) (20) not associated with any increased risk of leukemia or other blood dyscrasias. The leukocytosis, if not familiar to the physician, can lead to unnecessary workups for infection. Lithium leukocytosis, unlike infection, does not cause a relative increase of immature neutrophils ("a shift to the left").

Pregnancy, Postpartum, and Lactation

Lithium administration during pregnancy and the postpartum period requires special management (59). Lithium has been found to be teratogenic in the first trimester. Exposure during that period substantially increases the risk of Ebstein's anomaly (atresia of the tricuspid value) relative to other reported fetal abnormalities. Therefore, Ebstein's anomaly represents a real lithium risk rather than an artifact of case reporting. Since Ebstein's anomaly can be a fatal malformation, minimizing fetal exposure to lithium during the first trimester is important. The following steps may be helpful in management of women with childbearing potential who require lithium. (1) Serum beta human choriogonadotrophin (BHCG) should be determined prior to lithium treatment in any woman of childbearing potential. (2) The patient and her sexual partner should be educated about the risks of pregnancy while taking lithium. If precautions are not adequate, there should be appropriate birth control counseling with basic review of contraceptive methods. (3) Whenever clinically possible, lithium should be discontinued before attempting conception. Neuroleptics may substitute temporarily since they are less likely to be associated with first-trimester teratogenicity. If by history the patient requires continuous lithium and desires pregnancy, the psychiatrist should develop a coordinated treatment program with an obstetrician knowledgeable about lithium-related risks to the fetus.

If indicated, after the first trimester, lithium may be reintroduced since it no longer is teratogenic. This is often necessary as pregnancy and the postpartum period, both for psychological and physiological reasons, represent a high-risk time for affective relapse. Because of increased plasma volume in pregnancy, higher-than-usual lithium dosages are often required to maintain serum levels until the immediate postpartum period, when plasma volume falls to normal. Most authorities recommend reduction of dose before delivery to avoid acute postpartum lithium toxicity (59). Since lithium readily passes the placenta, newborns should be evaluated promptly and carefully for signs of acute lithium toxicity and/or lithium-induced hypothyroidism (lethargy or "floppy baby" syndrome) (61). Since lithium is secreted in breast milk, breast feeding while on lithium is contraindicated.

CONCLUSION

Lithium was once regarded as a mysterious and dangerous treatment. Now it has become a part of standard psychiatric practice and has achieved widespread acceptance by the lay public. These gains are real, but much work still needs to be done to explore the expanding indications of lithium's use, effective management of lithium noncompliance, and alternate treatments when lithium fails. In the meantime, a thorough understanding of lithium's indications, time course of action, side effects, and the differential diagnosis of lithium noncompliance is essential for maximizing its effectiveness.

REFERENCES

1. AKISKAL, H. S., KHANI, M. K., & SCOTT-STRAUSS, A. (1983). Cyclothymic temperamental disorders. *Psychiatric Clinics of North America, 2,* 527–554.
2. BATTLE, D. C., VON RIOTT, A. B., GAVIRIA M., et al. (1985). Amelioration of polyuria by amiloride in patients receiving longterm lithium therapy. *New England Journal of Medicine, 312,* 408–414.
3. BAUER, M. S., & WHYBROW, P. C. (1986). The effect of changing thyroid function on cyclic affective illness in a human subject. *American Journal of Psychiatry, 143,* 633–636.
4. CALABRESE, J. R., GULLEDGE, A. D., HALIN, H., et al. (1985). Autoimmune thyroiditis in manic-depressive patients treated with lithium. *American Journal of Psychiatry, 142,* 1318–1321.
5. CHOUINARD, G., YOUNG, S. N., & ANNABLE, L. (1983). Antimanic effect of clonazepam. *Biologic Psychiatry, 18,* 451–466.
6. CARLSON, G. (1979). Affective psychoses in mental retardates. *Psychiatric Clinics of North America, 2,* 499–510.
7. COOPER, T. B., & SIMPSON, G. M. (1976). The 24-hour lithium level as a prognosticator of dosage requirements: A two year follow-up study. *American Journal of Psychiatry, 133,* 440–443.
8. COWDRY, R., WEHR, T., ZIS, A., et al. (1983). Thyroid abnormalities associated with rapid-cycling bipolar illness. *Archives of General Psychiatry, 40,* 414–420.
9. DAVIS, J. M. (1976). Overview: Maintenance therapy in psychiatry: II Affective disorders. *American Journal of Psychiatry, 133,* 1–13.
10. DeMONTIGNEY, C., GREENBERG, F., & MAYER, H. (1981). Lithium induces rapid relief of depression in tricyclic nonresponders. *British Journal of Psychiatry, 138,* 324–327.
11. DONALDSON, S. R., GELENBERG, A. J., & BALDESSARINI, R. J. (1983). The pharmacologic treatment of schizophrenia: A progress report. *Schizophrenia Bulletin, 9,* 504–527.
12. EXTEIN, I., POTTASH, A., & GOLD, M. (1982). Does subclinical hypothyroidism predispose to tricyclic-induced rapid mood swings? *Journal of Clinical Psychiatry, 43,* 290–291.
13. FOGEL, B. S., & GOLDBERG, R. J. (1985). Neuroleptic malignant syndrome (letter). *New England Journal of Medicine, 313,* 1292.
14. HIMMELHOCH, J. M., THASE, M. E., MALLINGER, A. G., & FUCHS, C. Z. (1986). Tranylcypromine versus imipramine in manic depression. Presented at the American Psychiatric Association Annual Meeting, Washington, DC, New Research.

15. HIRSCHOWITZ, J., CASPER, R., GARVER, D. L., & CHANG, S. (1986). Lithium response in good prognosis schizophrenia. *American Journal of Psychiatry, 137*, 916–920.
16. JAMISON, K. P., & AKISKAL, H. S. (1983). Medication compliance in patients with bipolar disorder. *Psychiatric Clinics of North America, 6*, 175–192.
17. JAMISON, K. R., GERNER, R. H., & GOODWIN, F. K. (1979). Patient and physician attitudes toward lithium. *Archives of General Psychiatry, 36*, 866–869.
18. JAMISON, K. R., GERNER, R. H., HAMMER, C., & PADESKY, C. (1980). Clouds and silver linings: Positive experiences associated with primary affective disorders. *American Journal of Psychiatry, 137*, 198–202.
19. JEFFERSON, J. W., & GREIST, J. H. (1977). *Primer of lithium therapy.* Baltimore: Wilkins & Wilkins.
20. JOFFE, R. T., KELLNER, C. H., POST, R. M., & UHDE, T. W. (1984). Lithium increases platelet count (letter). *New England Journal of Medicine, 3*, 674–675.
21. JOHNSON, F. N. (Ed.) (1980). *Handbook of lithium therapy.* Lancaster, UK: MPT Press.
22. JUDD, L. L. (1979). Effect of lithium on mood, cognition, and personality function in normal subjects. *Archives of General Psychiatry, 36*, 860–865.
23. KANE, J. M., QUITKIN, F. M., RIFKIN, A., et al. (1981). Prophylactic lithium with and without imipramine for bipolar I patients: A double blind study. *Psychopharmacology Bulletin, 17*, 144–145.
24. KENDLER, K. S., GRUENBERG, A. M., & TSUANG, M. T. (1986). A DSM III family study of the nonschizophrenic psychotic disorders. *American Journal of Psychiatry, 143*, 1098–1105.
25. KOCSIS, J. H., & STOKES, P. E. (1979). Lithium maintenance: Factors affecting outcome. *American Journal of Psychiatry, 136*, 563–566.
26. KOCSIS, J. H. (1981): Treatment of mania. *Comprehensive Psychiatry, 22*, 596–602.
27. KOCSIS, J. H. (1980). Lithium in the acute treatment of mania. In F. N. Johnson (Ed.), *A handbook of lithium therapy.* Lancaster, UK: MPT Press.
28. KRAUTHAMMER, C., & KLERMAN, G. L. (1978). Secondary mania: Manic syndromes associated with antecedent physical illness or drugs. *Archives of General Psychiatry, 35*, 1333–1339.
29. LEVENSON, J. L. (1985). Neuroleptic malignant syndrome. *American Journal of Psychiatry, 142*, 1137–1145.
30. LEWIS, J. L., & WINOKUR, G. (1982). The induction of mania. *Archives of General Psychiatry, 39*, 303–306.
31. LIPPMAN, S. B., MANSHADI, M. S., & GULTEKIN, A. (1984). Lithium in a patient with renal failure on hemodialysis (letter). *Journal of Clinical Psychiatry, 45*, 449.
32. MATTES, J. A., & NAYAK, D. (1984). Lithium versus fluphenazine for prophylaxis in mainly schizophrenic schizo-affectives. *Biological Psychiatry, 19*, 445–449.
33. McCREADIE, R. G., & MORRISON, D. P. (1985). The impact of lithium in South-West Scotland. III. The discontinuation of lithium. *British Journal of Psychiatry, 146*, 77–80.
34. McMILLAN, T. M. (1981). Lithium and the treatment of alcoholism: A critical review. *British Journal of Addiction, 76*, 245–258.
35. MILLER, F., MENNINGER, J., & WHITCUP, S. (1986). Lithium-neuroleptic neurotoxicity in the elderly bipolar patients. *Journal of Clinical Psychopharmacology, 6*, 176–178.
36. MODELL, J. G., LENOX, R. H., & WEINER, S. (1985). Inpatient clinical trial of lorazepam for the management of manic agitation. *Journal of Clinical Psychopharmacology, 5*, 109–113.
37. MUKHERJEE, S., ROSEN, A. M., CARACCI, G., & SHUKLA, S. (1986). Persistent tardive dyskinesia in bipolar patients. *Archives of General Psychiatry, 43*, 335–342.
38. OYEWUM, L. K., & LAPIERRE, Y. O. (1981). Efficacy of lithium in treating mood disorder occurring after brainstem injury. *American Journal of Psychiatry, 137*, 847–848.
39. PERRIS, C. (1978). Morbidity suppressive effect of lithium carbonate in cycloid psychosis. *Archives of General Psychiatry, 35*, 328–331.
40. PERRY, P. J., CALLOWAY, R. A., COOK, B. L., & SMITH, R. E. (1984). Theophylline-

precipitated alterations of lithium clearance. *Acta Psychiatrica Scandinavica, 69*, 528–537.

41. Post, R. M. (1982). Use of the anticonvulsant carbamazepine in primary and secondary affective illness: Clinical and theoretical implications. *Psychological Medicine, 12*, 701–704.

42. Post, R. M., Uhde, T. W., Ballenger, J. C., & Squillace, K. M. (1983). Prophylactic efficacy of carbamazepine in manic-depressive illness. *American Journal of Psychiatry, 140*, 1602–1604.

43. Prien, R. F., Kupfer, D. J., Mansky, P. A., et al. (1984). Drug therapy in the prevention of recurrences in unipolar and bipolar affective disorders. *Archives of General Psychiatry, 41*, 1096–1104.

44. Procci, W. R. (1976). Schizo-affective psychosis: Fact or fiction? *Archives of General Psychiatry, 33*, 1167–1178.

45. Ramsey, T. A., & Cox, M. (1982). Lithium and the kidney: A review. *American Journal of Psychiatry, 139*, 443–449.

46. Reisbert, B., & Gershon, S. (1979). Side effects associated with lithium therapy. *Archives of General Psychiatry, 36*, 879–887.

47. Rifkin, A., Quitkin, F., Carillo, C. et al. (1972). Lithium carbonate in emotionally unstable character disorders. *Archives of General Psychiatry, 27*, 519–523.

48. Rothman, M. (1982). Acute hyperparathyroidism in a patient after initiation of lithium therapy. *American Journal of Psychiatry, 139*, 362–363.

49. Roy-Byrne, P. P., Joffee, R. T., Unde, T. W., & Post, R. M. (1984). Approaches to the evaluation and treatment of rapid-cycling affective illness. *British Journal of Psychiatry, 145*, 543–550.

50. Sachdev P. S. (1986). Lithium potentiation of neuroleptic-related extrapyramidal side effects (letter). *American Journal of Psychiatry, 143*, 942.

51. Secunda, S. K., Katz, M., & Croughan, J. (1985). Mixed mania: Diagnosis and treatment. Presented at the American Psychiatric Association Annual Meeting, Dallas, May 22, 1985.

52. Shaw, E. D., Mann, J. J., Stokes, P. E., & Manevitz, Z. A. (1986). Effects of lithium carbonate on associative productivity and idiosyncracy in bipolar outpatients. *American Journal of Psychiatry, 143*, 1166–1169.

53. Shaw, E. D. (1986). Lithium noncompliance. *Psychiatric Annals, 16*, 583–587.

54. Schou, M. (1979). Artistic productivity and lithium prophylaxis in manic depressive illness. *British Journal of Psychiatry, 135*, 97–103.

55. Stancer, H. C. & Persad, E. (1982). Treatment of intractable rapid-cycling manicdepressive disorder with levothyroxine. *Archives of General Psychiatry, 39*, 311–312.

56. Stokes, P. E., Kocsis, J. H., & Orestes, J. A. (1976). Relationship of lithium chloride dose to treatment response in acute mania. *Archives of General Psychiatry, 33*, 1080–1084.

57. Vestergaard, P., & Amdisen, A. (1981). Lithium treatment and kidney function: A follow-up study of 237 patients in long-term treatment. *Acta Psychiatric Scandinavia, 63*, 333–345.

58. Vestergaard, P., Amdisen, A., & Schou, M. (1980). Clinically significant side effects of lithium treatment. A survey of 237 patients in long-term treatment. *Acta Psychiatrica Scandinavica, 62*, 193–200.

59. Weinstein, M. R. (1980). Lithium treatment of women during pregnancy and in the post delivery period. In F. N. Johnson (Ed.), *Handbook of lithium therapy.* Lancaster, England: MPT Press.

60. Wolpert, E., Chausow, A., & Szidon, J. P. (1985). Respiratory failure and lithium (letter). *Psychiatric Research, 15*, 249–252.

61. Woody, J. N., London, W. L., & Wilbanks, G. D. (1971). Lithium toxicity in a newborn. *Pediatrics, 47*, 94–96.

NAME INDEX

369

SUBJECT INDEX